Psycholinguistics

Hans Hörmann

Psycholinguistics

An Introduction to Research and Theory

Second Edition, Revised

Translated by H. H. Stern and Peter Leppmann

With 60 illustrations

 Springer-Verlag New York Heidelberg Berlin

Dr. Hans Hörmann, o. Professor der Psychologie an der Ruhr-Universität, Bochum, Psychologisches Institut der Ruhr-Universität, Universitätstrasse 150, 463 Bochum, Federal Republic of Germany

Dr. H. H. Stern, Director of the Modern Language Center, Ontario Institute for Studies in Education, 252 Bloor Street West, Toronto, Ontario, Canada

Dr. Peter Leppmann, Department of Psychology, College of Social Sciences, University of Guelph, Guelph, Ontario, Canada

This English edition is a revised version of the second revised German edition, *Psychologie der Sprache*.

Library of Congress Cataloging in Publication Data

Hörmann, Hans, 1924–
   Psycholinguistics: an introduction to research and theory.

   Bibliography: p.
   Includes indexes.
   1. Psycholinguistics.   I.   Title.
P37.H6313   1979   401'.9   79-18600

Printed in the United States of America

9 8 7 6 5 4 3 2 1

ISBN 0-387-90417-4   Springer-Verlag   New York   Heidelberg   Berlin
ISBN 3-540-90417-4   Springer-Verlag   Berlin   Heidelberg   New York

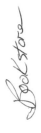

Preface to the Second English Edition

The first edition of this book received wide circulation: It was translated from German into English, French, Spanish, Italian and Japanese. In the decade since publication of the original edition, the field of psycholinguistics has grown enormously, both in scope and in theoretical and experimental sophistication. The main trend reflected in this growth has no doubt been away from the domain of linguistics and toward a psychology of language.

To accommodate these developments in the second edition, some topics were deleted, while others have been treated in a summary fashion; otherwise the book would have lost its convenient textbook character. Some readers will be interested in a more extensive treatment of the many-faceted problems related to some of the concepts discussed here; I invite them to consult my recently published book *Meinen und Verstehen,* which is presently being translated into English.

This second edition maintains an eclectic attitude so that the reader may become aware of the various approaches to these issues. There is still no single "school of psychology" which offers adequate treatment of all questions in psycholinguistics.

Some of the critical reviews of the first edition have been most helpful in the preparation of the second edition. I am particularly grateful to the members of our section "Psychology of Language and Information Processing" at the Ruhr-Universität, Bochum, for their suggestions and support.

Hans Hörmann

Bochum, September 1979

75059

Contents

Chapter 1   Introduction: Organism, Language, and World   1

Characterization of the field in which language becomes possible and necessary—Organism and environment—Language as stimulus—Language as response—Speaker and listener—Language as a system of signs—Development from a historical to a structural orientation in linguistics—Saussure's distinction between *langue* and *parole*—Carroll's definition of language—Linguistics and psycholinguistics.

Chapter 2   Sign, Expression, and Symbol   21

Bühler's *organon* model—Different conceptions of the nature of signs—Problems concerning the language of animals—The language of bees—The performance of Washoe, the chimpanzee—The origin of language in symbolic behavior—Communicative intentions.

Chapter 3   Linguistic Units and the Rules for Their Connection   33

Schema of the speech event—Articulation—Processes of categorization in perception—Phoneme and morpheme—Distinctive features—Definition of the word—The sentence as the playing field of grammar—Principles of generative transformational grammar—Competence and performance—Surface and deep structures—The theory of semantics of Katz and Fodor—Dimensions of the lexicon.

Chapter 4   Language, Information, and Communication   57

The concept of information—Code—Information value and uncertainty—The bit—Utilization of the communication channel—Classification and identification—The motor theory of speech perception—Analysis by synthesis—Interference in the speech channel—The concept of channel capacity.

Chapter 5   Frequency and Probability   85

The role of hypotheses in perception—Frequency and expectation—Diversification of the vocabulary—Formulas of readability—Possibility and probability—The concept of redundancy—Joint and transitional probabilities—Approximations to genuine speech—Lexical units and logogens.

Chapter 6   Verbal Association and the Problem of Meaning   111

From a sequential to an associationist viewpoint—The concept of association—
Galton and Marbe—Association experiments and everyday verbal behavior—
Norms of association and their range of application—Group and personality
factors in the differentiation of verbal habits—Jung's investigations and Laffal's
critique—Elements of meaning—Clark—The concept of semantic field—Deese's
studies of association.

Chapter 7   The Philosophical Background to Modern
              Psychology of Language   137

Meaning as natural bipolar connection—The designating function of language—
Adaequatio rei et intellectus—Language and meta-language—Empiricist criteria
of truth—Pragmatism and operationalism—Between-world of meaning—Meaning
as context—Role of language user—Morris—Meaning as behavior—Wittgenstein's language game—Searle's speech acts.

Chapter 8   Sign and Object Signified: Classical Theories of
              the Development of Meaning   153

Association through conditioning—Skinner's *Verbal Behavior*—Chomsky's
critique of it—Meaning as a response—Meaning as disposition—MacKay's and
Deese's contribution to it—Bloomfield's model—Mediational theories of
meaning—Osgood and the semantic differential—Bilingualism and semantic
satiation—A cognitive model of meaning.

Chapter 9   Imitation of Sound, Sound Symbolism,
              Expression   185

Imitation of sounds as the germ of human speech—Humboldt's dichotomy—
Evolution of onomatopoeia—Traces of sound symbolish in linguistic behavior—
"Maluma" and "takete"—Matching experiments in the mother tongue and an
unknown second language—Concept of physiognomy—Werner's theory of symbol formation—Ertel's psychophonetics.

Chapter 10   The Psychological Reality of Grammar   201

Limitations of Markov's model—The concept of grammaticality—Effects of syntactical structure on learning and retention—Temporal features of speech perception and speech production—The concept of the plan—Surface and deep structure
viewed psychologically—Johnson's model of sentence-generating—Semantic factors of sentence structure—The semantic organization of memory—Paivio's dual
coding hypothesis—Predicate/argument structure and their influence on sentence
processing.

Chapter 11   The Developmental Psychology of Language
              Acquisition   233

The role of imitation—The language acquisition device (LAD)—Pivot-
grammars—R. Brown's studies of Adam and Eve—The sensory-motor stage of

intelligence—McNamara's theory—The role of intention in language learning—Global behavior as the basis for language acquisition—The problem of the one-word sentence—The grammar of action—Strategies in language acquisition.

Chapter 12   Language Comprehension and Man's View of the
               World   265

Olson's cognitive theory of semantics—Situational determinants of meaning—Comprehension as constructive process—Levels of comprehension—Influence of language on the speaker's view of the world—Categories as guides to attention—Linguistic determinism and linguistic relativity—Whorf—Studies of color coding—Language universals—*General Semantics*.

Bibliography   301

Author Index   329

Subject Index   334

CHAPTER 1

Introduction: Organism, Language, and World

Characterization of the field in which language becomes possible and necessary—Organism and environment—Language as stimulus—Language as response—Speaker and listener—Language as a system of signs—Development from a historical to a structural orientation in linguistics—Saussure's distinction between *langue* and *parole*—Carroll's definition of language—Linguistics and psycholinguistics.

The possession of language distinguishes man from animal. Our whole capacity of being truly human is implicit in language. Truth is only possible in language or, at least, by means of language. Even a lie presupposes language.

Language, it has been said, is "man's greatest invention" (Thorndike, 1943, p. 60). As we think about this statement, a number of questions arise which serve as our first landmarks at the beginning of our inquiry. Was the inventor of language already human before his invention? What kind of situation made such an invention possible and necessary? Can it be studied phylogenetically by comparing man and animal in relation to language? Or ontogenetically by tracing the development of language from prelinguistic infancy to early childhood?

The feature of language is so specifically human that it would be hopeless to think that we might be able to trace and observe the gradual evolution of this feature itself. Phylogenetic comparisons can, at best, give us hints from what points of view to study the complex speech act of man. Needless to say, this limitation is not a comment upon the relevance of a biologic perspective. Lenneberg (1964b) has established the notion that a definite constellation of biologic peculiarities accounts for the presence of language in man and only in man: linguistic behavior correlates highly with a large number of special morphological and functional developments; the onset and the course of linguistic development in the child are an extraordinarily regular process; even in case of serious handicaps, such as blindness or deafness, language is still possible; no nonhuman species can acquire language, in the sense in which it is here understood; there are linguistic universals (see pp. 228 f.), i.e., universal principles found in natural languages, which cannot be explained in terms of historical causation. According to Lenneberg, the capacity to acquire and employ a human language does not depend upon the intelligence of the organism or the size of its brain, but upon the fact that it is a human organism.

Moreover, a biologic or genetic viewpoint will be useful to us in a different sense. We will attempt to explain the function of language by observing the genesis and process of the individual speech act. "Speech, in its true essence, is constantly and at any moment ephemeral. It is itself not a product (*ergon*) but an activity (*energeia*). Its true definition must therefore be a genetic one. Language is the ever recurring activity of the mind endeavoring to make the articulated sound express thought. Taking it quite literally and strictly, this is the definition of each act of speech; but in a more real and fundamental sense, only the totality of these speech acts can, as it were, be understood as language" (Humboldt, translated from the 1949 edition, p. 44).

It is at this point that Humboldt, the linguistic scholar and philosopher, has raised the question of the fundamental nature of language. For a psycholinguistic study, this orientation is hardly appropriate because psychology does not ask questions about the *nature* of the object it studies, e.g., the nature of the psyche; but, presupposing its existence, it asks how the psychic event happens. The question of the nature of language is beyond the domain of an empirical psychology. That does not mean, however, that the psycholinguist can totally ignore this question, he must be aware of the philosophical foundation and the scientific bases of the concepts which direct his analysis of the phenomena. If language, which interests him from a psychological point of view, is seen as a static system, then the psycholinguist must proceed differently in explaining the use of this system, and perhaps encounter greater difficulties, than if he conceives of language as an activity. Yet, if the philosopher recognizes the nature of language as an *energeia,* an activity or a process, this approach offers a basis which is entirely acceptable to the psychologist because in other branches of psychology as well, e.g., in the psychology of learning or of motivation, psychological insight is increased if we treat the object of scientific inquiry as a process. Such a dynamic viewpoint gives a clear and broad perspective, especially for a study of language, but in principle also for psychology as a whole. It is our intention to adopt this point of view, although with some caution, so as to be able to analyze the factors which determine speech events and language. We will discover what the nature of these factors is if, before examining language itself, we begin our inquiry at an earlier stage, so to speak, or at a more fundamental level.

The event which we call "organism" can be described in terms of two groups of factors: broadly speaking, and without being unduly inhibited by theological or philosophical considerations, there is what, on the one hand, might be called *spontaneity* or the life force which, from inside the organism, strives towards fulfilment, Bergson's *élan vital*. On the other hand, this spontaneity is surrounded by the *life space* within which the vital process takes place. Determinants of the "life space" shape the spontaneous strivings of the organism's capacities and potentialities into its unique, precise, and recognizable biography. The spirituality of the highest form of life, man, manifesting itself through the will, adds a further dimension of freedom to this interplay of spontaneity and life space.

In psychology, v. Allesch adheres most clearly to such a dynamic-biologic basic viewpoint, which is characterized by the assumption that spontaneity and life space are in harmony with each other. For a particular kind of spontaneity, a characteristic life space is, as it were, "pre-determined"; e.g., the bird's instinctive nesting behavior is designed for an environment which provides twigs.

The relationship between spontaneity and life space can be more or less intimate, more or less variable. Varying degrees of closeness of fit characterize different organisms. Some organisms fit so precisely and neatly into their vital space that even a slight variation in the environment is sufficient to exceed the tolerance level of the organism which then succumbs. Interesting instances of this interplay are certain cases of symbiosis and similar forms of interaction: thus, future generations of the yucca plant are endangered by anyone who disturbs the yucca moth.

The relationship between life force and life space can attain greater degrees of freedom in other species. Here a variation in one group of factors is not always nor inevitably accompanied by definite variations in the other. In these organisms the framework within which the events of life take place is much less fixed, and the life of the organism is no longer dependent upon a definite realization within a narrowly defined life space.

We come to a similar point of view if we compare, as Uexküll (1928) has, environment in lower organisms and in man. In the animal, spontaneity and milieu are almost like a closed world that is nearly perfectly divided into the two hemispheres of action (*Wirkwelt*) and perception (*Merkwelt*). Uexküll says about the animal, "The stimuli of the environment surround the animal like the walls of a self-made dwelling cutting off the entire world outside it" (translated from Cassirer, 1932).

Life in such an enclosed space is unlike human life because it can never transcend its own field of action and look at it from outside (Cassirer, 1932). To make this possible the close fit must be relaxed; this tight world must somehow come apart so that finally consciousness, representation, language, and knowledge can develop. Such a loosening has already begun at the lower levels of phylogenesis, and we must be able to recognize such early beginnings if we want to come to grips with the psychological dynamics of speech events. This is not to say that language has gradually evolved from nonlinguistic preformations.[1] What it does mean is that the concepts with which we operate in explaining the linguistic event have something in common with those factors which, at a prelinguistic stage, determine the relationship between spontaneity and environment.

At this point it may be appropriate to interrupt the argument briefly in order to consider an obvious objection. It may be argued that such biologic and teleological interpretations are inappropriate in general psychology, hence equally so in psycholinguistics. Concepts such as Bergson's *élan vital* are in bad odor in an empirical science—and psychology is an empirical science.

Of course such an objection would be valid only if one were to try to develop a psychology of language based exclusively on such teleological methods of observation, to the exclusion of an empirical basis. Through the mathematical and physical analysis of goal-oriented servomechanisms and cybernetic relay systems, however, we have learned that causal and teleological explanations cannot be excluded as categorically as was thought earlier. Thus the question, What for? cannot be avoided, for it serves to direct the basic conceptions and the collection of empirical data. This is especially true in the case of the psychology of language, because speaking, the use of speech, as we will see, is always a means toward an end. It follows then that the intentional aspect is always an integral part of the object which we wish to examine psychologically.

In general, this book represents the view that it is helpful in psycholinguistics to be able to vary procedures and approaches. To uphold a method which has proved fruitful at one point, knowing that few new insights can be gained, would be less desirable than a certain flexibility in method. Such flexibility must, however, fulfil one condition, namely, that we are always aware of the change of method and its implications. Only such a procedure would offer the prospect of steering us safely between the simplification of a pure stimulus-response model and the premature systematization of linguistic philosophy. We want to avoid the "mystification of age-old anthropomorphisms" and study psycholinguistics in a way which does full justice to the epistemological criteria of psychology as well as to the object of enquiry itself, viz, language, ranging from "the physics of air vibrations to the philosophy of the objective mind."

After this digression let us return to our principal argument. The loosening of the tight interlocking fit between spontaneity and life space creates the precondition for the emergence of speech. The disturbance in the adjustment gives rise to a new group of devices whose function is to compensate for the discrepancies and the imbalances. Such devices which control the adapta-

---

[1] This problem is the starting point of Toulmin's (1971) criticism of Chomsky. It will not be discussed here, but see Hörmann (1976).

tion to the environment are unnecessary as long as the organism—assuming a borderline case—fits so perfectly into its environment that, for example, periodic changes in the environment are taken care of by simultaneous changes in the plan and structure of the organism. In this case the organism would not require, for instance, sense receptors to be informed about the momentary state of the environment.

However, if spontaneity and life space are no longer perfectly attuned, and if they no longer obey the same rules and rhythms, and if, in consequence, discrepancies and tensions occur, a controlling device is needed to bridge the two worlds which have moved apart. This bridging operation makes behavior possible and indeed necessary.

Perception, for example, may be looked upon as such a controlling device; for perception is not primarily the cause or initiator of behavior. Behavior, after all, occurs continuously from the moment the organism begins to live. Perception steers behavior and is one of its codeterminants. A school of psychology that views behavior and especially perception as a sequence of stimuli (S) and responses (R) can, indeed, explain a great deal but it remains incomplete. We shall later examine more closely the potentialities of an S-R analysis in the field of psycholinguistics.

Behavior, then, is viewed here as the process in which the interaction of life space and spontaneity becomes manifest. Perception is, in a peculiar way, both a part and a determinant of this process. If we adopt this point of view, language may be considered to be similar. It originates, too, in the indeterminate sphere between the spontaneous impulses of the individual and his life space. In the last resort, language is, as Aristotle already said, an *organon* or tool which comes into use between the self and its surrounding world as a means of coming to terms with its environment. But whereas perception links the self and objective reality, speech links man with other kinds of realities: he is surrounded by the social world of his speech community. Verbal thinking relates him to the world of the mind; and in the "intercourse of mind with itself" (Plato) man creates the world of his own self. If, in this preliminary and sweeping way, we ascribe to language a function which, in principle, is analogous to perception, it is tempting to test this analogy a little further and to examine the applicability to language of the notions of stimulus and response.

Speech as stimulus: verbal signals can guide and determine behavior. But speech can also be perceived. The nature and conditions of such speech perception will therefore have to be investigated.

Speech as response: we note that many chains of events end in a verbal utterance, just as other chains of events end in motor behavior. The question is what are the antecedents to the verbal response.

Within the framework of an S-R analysis, we must not simply look upon language as stimulus and response but also as an intervening variable, using this term in its widest sense. In other words, language intervenes in the bond between stimulus and response. If a particular R and no other follows a specific S, this may well be the result of the kind of linguistic categories which are at our disposal in dealing with a particular S. Or looking at it differently, an empirically discovered relationship between a given R and an S can sometimes only be explained if we assume linguistic links as mediating elements. The mechanism of an action can often only make sense if it is assumed that a verbal component, without necessarily appearing overtly, modifies the S-R sequence in a qualitative way. For instance, purposeful human acts which extend over a period of time, almost inevitably involve intermediate purposes expressed in verbal forms that are like bridge supports carrying the event from the original stimulus to the final response. The concept of *mediation* which should be mentioned here is one that must engage our attention to a considerable extent at a later stage.

These initial reflections on an S-R analysis of language already indicate that the explanation of language demands, under certain conditions, that we have to operate with variables that have no equivalent in externally observable behavior. The question of how necessary and yet how risky it is to go beyond observable behavior has been an important aspect in the discussion on behaviorism in general and has affected the psychology of language.

One important distinguishing feature of *speech as stimulus* is that it is, at least in principle, a stimulus directed towards us with intent by other members of our species. With this observation, we touch a problem which we will take up again later. In the psychology of perception, once we are beyond the purely physical description, we face this question, Is the "real" stimulus the light waves, or is it a discharge in the receptor? Is it the glass of water before us, or is it the object of our thirst? Similarly, in psycholinguistics, the air vibrations which we can regard as stimuli do not so much exercise their effect because of the energy they hold (a bang could have as much) but they act as stimuli because they convey meaning. It is as if the physical stimulus, at the same time, was a stimulus carrier of a totally different order.

It is tempting to try to account for this fact by asserting that the physical stimulus is the conveyor of *meaning* (or that it is a sign), but this formulation could open the door to new difficulties. Is meaning something that is conveyed by the physical stimulus? To what extent does meaning "stimulate"? Particularly in the area of speech perception we encounter the problem of this peculiar overlapping of physical and semiotic aspects of stimulation. What does a listener actually perceive? Is it the speaker-generated sound waves, the articulated sounds, the expressed words, or possibly the intended meaning that is perceived?

Similar distinguishing characteristics can be noted in looking upon *language as response*. The speech event produced by an individual A is hardly ever the last link in a stimulus-response chain; it is generally a directed response transmitted from A to B. The linguistic response is produced by A with the intention of making B react. In other words, a verbal response can only be regarded as the last link in a chain of events if the unit of observation is the individual. But the social nature of language demands the embedding of the speech event into a social field which comprises a speaker and a hearer. The dynamic structure of this field arises from the fact "that the essentials of language reside in purpose. Looked at teleologically, language is particularly powerful as a means of communication" (Révész, 1946, p. 109). Freytag-Loeringhoff has described communication as the ontological locus of language. If we want to understand language, he argues, we must inquire into the nature of interpersonal communication (1962, p. 240).

The conceptualization of language as stimulus-response events, therefore, must always remain as just one among several approaches. This approach may be useful for the analysis of the manipulatory aspects of language, which is one of its several functions, but one encounters difficulties if one tries to apply a rigorous S-R schema to the "manipulation of consciousness" through language. This approach becomes totally inadequate at the point where one's concern is directed toward what we call the transparency of language, i.e., the fact that we recognize the intended meaning of the speaker "beyond" just his vocal expression. But let us now return to the social field which was mentioned above. The social field in which speaker and hearer represent the two poles is characterized by certain lines of force. Speech as an event occurring in this field manifests the influence of these lines of force in various ways. While we initially discussed in very general terms the dynamics of the processes occurring between organism and environment, we shall now, in a parallel manner, but closer to language, discuss the social field as a language-forming structure. In doing so, we will not treat language as a unitary substance (see Cassirer, 1944, pp. 129f.) but will attempt to analyze it from ever-changing perspectives in such a way that the totality of the various components will reveal the functional unity of language.

One line of force which marks this field is relatively simple: it is the social contact between the "I" and "thou" in its quite primitive form. Speech as *contact-sound* is, according to Révész, the first and lowest stage of linguistic evolution. The contact-sound repeats, as it were, the most reassuring of messages, which says, "Here too is someone," and thus maintains a social bond.

> We operate with Révész' concepts, not because we believe language has developed according to the sequences which Révész proposed, but because these notions—outside their evolutionary context—are convenient in making apparent the forces at work to which a language, even at its most advanced level, is subjected.

This first and most simple line of force in the social field appears in many different manifestations. It occurs, in the animal kingdom, well below the mammals, e.g., in the cry of wild geese on the wing. It ranges from the phatic communion—as Malinowski (see Ogden and Richards, 1923) has called the vocal utterances which serve to establish social relations—to the highly stylized forms of social conversation, where talk occurs because it would be rude to be silent. Hayakawa calls the prevention of silence an important function of speech (1949, p. 72).

Close to the line of force represented by the undirected primitive contact-call, the social field in which speech events occur carries another similar line of force. To make it evident, we adopt Hayakawa's presentation. According to Hayakawa, a community or a social group is a network of "mutual agreements." Being in vocal contact with one another is not insignificant; it has affective meaning. The *emotional charge* of the sound turns a mere sound into a call which moves the listener to establish or demonstrate the "mutual agreements" which, according to Hayakawa, are the framework of society.

Now two things which are of importance for our later discussions become clear: Language does not develop within a vacuum, it does not develop from or function as a *tabula rasa*. It arises from a broad basis of nonverbal communication that supports it and with which it is totally integrated. Communication, information exchange, and mutual manipulation by individuals are "older" than verbal communication, verbal information exchange, and manipulation by means of language.

Furthermore, speech is more than an exchange of information; for example, a question can be more than, or different from, a request for factual knowledge. It may well be an attempt to seek confirmation, to be assured of the mutual agreement and thus to orient oneself with regard to one's own place in a social situation. Like Hayakawa, Glinz writes in an essay devoted to this function of language, "The effect on talk among two or more persons is that it interposes between them values which are already held in common or have yet to be accepted. In this way, it is not only that objects or phenomena find their place and are related to people but lines of thought are drawn between persons like streamers stretched from one to another" (1959, p. 104).

The manifestations of this line of force range from the *hailing-call* (*Zuruf*), which Révész considers to be the second stage of language above the contact-sound, to the postsymbolic use of words which are no longer intended to transmit information but "merely" serve the ritualized communion of social contact. Between these extremes is the area of social manipulation through language.

It was stated earlier that the field of force in which speech events occur has two poles, speaker and listener, transmitter and receiver. The "existential situation" of the speech event lies in the imbalance between the two poles. This discrepancy or gradient produces the tensions that we are investigating.

There is either an imbalance of information or an imbalance of intention and awareness. The imbalance of information—or, to put it more precisely, of informed-ness—causes the person who has less information to be on the look-out for information-bearing signals or to question the other person who has "more" and who makes this "more" available in some form of presentation. The imbalance of intention impels the one to send out signals or commands and the other to act or cogitate upon these signals or commands.

It is because of this dynamic imbalance that language functions as a tool—in this case in the social field, in other cases, to be explained later, in the area of thought or philosophic orientation.

Language is a tool for the speaker, because with its help he can obtain from someone else what he himself lacks, or he can get someone else to do what he himself is unable or unwilling to do. But language is also a means to give help *to* the other fellow. Information or signals which are useful to the receiver may be transmitted to him. In the *demand-call* (*Anruf*)—the third stage of the evolutionary scale of Révész—the imperatives in both directions are combined; the demand-call "come here" is meant to get the listener moving: it may be for *my* benefit, because *I* want something from him, or for *his* benefit, because I want to guide him round a treacherous stretch of the road.

Höpp (1970) in a similar but more differentiated manner, views the imperative "hailing-call" (*Zuruf*) as the origin of language that arose from the mutual sharing of tasks of two individuals. A hundred years earlier Steinthal had already emphasized that one must "conceptualize the origin of language in such a way that it is not created in the mind of the individual as such, but arises from a common context" (1871, p. 386).

The imbalance between speaker and listener is of course not the only factor in the force-field of language. The dynamic which is produced by this imbalance becomes standardized and coded in order to serve effectively as a means for communicating differentiated intentions.

With this observation we reach a point which has bearing on the social function of language but which at the same time transcends it: language is essentially a system of signs. Signs, meaning, signification are concepts which in every treatment of psycholinguistics play a decisive role. But, fundamentally, they are not so much psychological as philosophical concepts.

> It follows that it will not be possible to allocate them a definite place in a system, to treat them, and then to move on, relieved of this somewhat awkward baggage. Instead we will find that these notions crop up again and again, and only after numerous encounters can we hope to get the psychological aspects of these concepts into some perspective.

Language, we said, is essentially a system of signs, but signs are possible even before any language. A Pavlovian dog, conditioned to the sound of a bell, accepts this sound as a sign or signal that food is on its way, and he reacts to this sign. The rat, which in a Lashley "jump" box faces one card with stripes and another with squares, treats the sight of the striped card as a sign for food behind it and acts accordingly. The animal in a Tolman maze learns to react to signs, to expect signs, and to be guided by signs. The sign directs to something that is not the sign itself. The sign is generally a biologically irrelevant object (e.g., striped cards are totally irrelevant to rats not trained in a Lashley "jump" box) which gains biologic value only through learning and experience and thus becomes relevant for the behavior of the animal.

We discussed earlier in detail the phylogenetically increasing separation of organism and environment necessitating simultaneously the creation of control mechanisms by means of which mutual adjustment becomes possible. The most important part in this control mechanism is played by the sign. Nowhere is this so clearly expressed as in the work of Russian psychologists. Leontiev writes, for example: "The fundamental fact is that initially the direct, unmediated connection of organisms with the external medium at a certain stage in evolution formed the basis for the development of connections which were indirect and mediated. Animals acquired the capacity to react in the same way to agents which *of themselves* had no biological significance for them . . . This type of agent . . . became a signal stimulus" (1961, p. 228). This *first signal-system,* which already exists in the animal world, leads, in man, to a second one, based on language (Pavlov, 1960, 1963). In this *second signal-system* the immediate sense impressions are transformed. "The second signal-system must not be treated as a kind of abstraction. It is rather the neurodynamic system of conditioned associations, which, in turn, are indirect and generalized signals of reality. Human concepts result from the generalization of conditioned associations in the first signal-system. This process of generalization occurs on the basis of the verbal repertoire" (Albrecht, 1959, p. 129).

The possibility of generalization is one of the most important functions of language. But it must be remembered that even below language, within the first signal-system, a form of generalization is already possible, i.e., *stimulus generalization.* A dog conditioned to a tone of 1000 cps. reacts also to a similar tone of 800 cps. But the generalizations in the first signal-system run along physically or biologically given dimensions (in our example, the dimension of pitch measured in cps.) In the linguistic medium generalization is not predetermined in extent or direction and, as a result, is open to ideational or sociological influences.

Signs, then, occur wherever purposive behavior occurs. The act of substitution, distinct from direct action, or the sign which stands for something else originates at a prelinguistic stage; but the sign comes truly into its own only in language, for only in language does it become a sign which can be used at will. "Between the clearest animal call of love or warning or anger, and a man's least trivial *word* there lies a whole day of *Creation*—or in modern phrase, a whole chapter of evolution" (Langer, 1963, p. 103). For the whole further mode of procedure in psycholinguistics it is important to recognize these two sides: the parallels and analogies between animal and human behavior, and the distinctively new in human language. Language opens up the dimension of the intellect and, at the same time, is an expression of this dimension, a duality already thoroughly explored by Humboldt. By making available the not-here and the not-now, language enables us to step out of the firm stimulus-response chain. An event may be "wished," an action "planned," an experience "remembered" and "told." Whereas the speechless animal remains almost completely in the prison of action and reaction and only makes, as it were, preliminary moves towards breaking out with the help of its primitive use of signals, language makes possible explicit representation, and thus the possibility is given of drawing on knowledge at will.

The making of generalizations creates order which transcends the sequence of concrete events, gives each single event a place in a hierarchy and treats it as "a case of . . ." or "an instance of . . . ," an instance of bread, kindness, schizophrenia, etc. This higher-order something is no longer concretely accessible; it is a fact of language, which we create, or of which we can take possession because it is already available to us through culture and society. Language enables us to extract from the fleeting mass of phenomena the common elements or qualities essential for our experience, and to give them permanence. The Greek word *logos* expresses this function of language. Stenzel (1934) speaks of the primal phenomenon of the "crystallization, from the buzzing confusion, of an object by means of the word. The word is so powerful that without it the object would not exist for the mind, but once the mind has a word it seems to be able to do what it likes with it. Mental activity, which reaches awareness only through language, helps to define more clearly the essential qualities of an object in all its manifestations and makes it possible to ask questions about the essence of the object, and thus the mind itself shapes it in the way it will appear to consciousness. . . . As a result (the word) now becomes an inherent part of the object and expresses it, and must henceforth be used to refer to it" (p. 38). "The transformation of experience into concepts . . . is the motive of language" (Langer, 1963, p. 126). The close connection between language and thought is the consequence of all this. Certainly language and thought cannot be treated as identical, but language is "thought made directly real" (K. Marx).

The abstraction of essentials, conveyed by language, makes it possible to accumulate experience in form of knowledge and thus, in the long run, to establish a culture. Human cunning and human rationality are based on the capacity to operate with signs.

In language biologic, psychological, and sociohistorical determinants converge. Language is a product of the social field; consciousness in the individual is largely verbal in character: the consequence of these two facts is that man is basically a *zoon politikon*.

Thus language presents itself to us as the characteristically human instrument. With a minimum of energy this instrument reaches beyond the arm's length of the language user; it surrounds the speaker and in its applications is not confined to straight-line communication, nor is it—like vision—restricted to use in daylight. Community and consciousness, rationality and knowledge are in their human form only possible with the aid of language. Its influence, as Humboldt says, extends over everything man thinks or feels, decides and achieves. "It transforms the world into a possession of the mind" (Humboldt, 1905b edition, p. 420).

This transformation of the world into a possession of the mind—in Humboldt's view, the primary achievement of language—is of interest to many sciences. Hardly anywhere else can one see so clearly as here that the sciences differ from each other not so much in the object of inquiry, as in their approach, the unit of analysis and the methodology they employ. Linguistic events engage the attention of such diverse disciplines as phonology and historical linguistics, acoustics and psycholinguistics. We shall understand better the procedures, viewpoints, possibilities and limitations of the psychology of language or psycholinguistics if we give some thought to the relationship of the other disciplines to language, the common object of study.

The science of language or linguistics was, right into the nineteenth century, a discipline with a historical orientation. Its development shows a history of speculation about the origin of language, the genesis of a single word or of a grammatical category (Lohmann, 1962). In the early 19th century, the discipline gradually gained methodologically more stringent characteristics, particularly through the works of Bopp (1833 and later),[2] who developed the comparative and reconstructive science of language, using Sanskrit as an example. The model which formed the basis of the development of language soon came under the influence of Darwin. Here language was seen as an "organism with physical and mechanical laws" which were to be identified. The diversification of today's languages can be traced back to a common primary language. The Neogrammarians (Junggrammatiker), who also had a strong historical bent, were in agreement with the psychologist Wundt, believing that historically caused changes in a language ought to be explained psychologically. Paul called psychology "the most eminent foundation for the humanities, where these are concerned with higher mental processes (1909, p. 6).

But this psychologizing in historical linguistics confined itself to the construction of motives for particular historical processes after the event, based on psychological insight. For Wundt, language belonged to the psychology of nations (*Völkerpsychologie*) which he conceived in ideographic terms; it was not—as in the modern conception—part of general psychology which

---

[2] Short sketches of the history of the science of language can be found in Figge (1974) and in Jakobson (1973).

has a nomothetic orientation and is fundamentally ahistorical (cf. Sommer-felt, 1962a).

This kind of linguistic science was therefore close to comparative gram-mar and to philology with its texts and consequently also to classical educa-tion, as Martinet (1962) has rightly pointed out. Language, for 19th-century linguistics, was a product of the human mind which was final and static, but had a history, just as a landscape was the static product of a geological evolution which could be laboriously reconstructed.

A second characteristic of the conception of language which was current at the time was the view represented, for example, by Becker (1841), that the whole of grammar could be derived from formal logic. The logical order of the world is "explicitly used as the theoretically demonstrable measuring rod for linguistic order" (Apel, 1962, p. 205), a conception which goes back to Ockham: language as a system of signs, fitted as an afterthought upon a "given" primary, prelinguistic world, and presenting an undistorted picture of this world. This fundamental conception—as we shall see later—is of decisive importance for all sciences which study the problem of *meaning*.

The rejection of these two features of 19th-century linguistics (i.e., his-toricism and the identification of laws of language with laws of nature) and the consequent emancipation of modern linguistics go back to Humboldt. After Humboldt language was viewed not as an invention of the human mind, or *ergon,* but as *energeia.* As a result, its psychological interest became something quite different from that in Paul's work: an activity can only be understood psychologically if agent and objective are included in the analysis.

In contrast to Kant, Humboldt has also recognized the determining role of language in the way humans construct a world-view: language does not so much reflect a world which exists apart from it; language moulds a world. "Language is the thought-shaping organ. The subjective activity of thinking gives form to an object" (1949 edition, pp. 53 and 55). This aspect will be treated in greater detail at a later stage. We now turn to a line of thought in the development of modern linguistics which has quite recently become important for the psychology of language.

The proposal to view language as *energeia,* i.e., as an activity, provided the impetus for a far-reaching change in many of the disciplines interested in the totality of language. This change, without which psycholinguistics in the contemporary sense would have been impossible, was furthered through the influence of Durkheim on the one hand and Husserl on the other, and was finally carried out by De Saussure. Durkheim intimated that language should be regarded as a social phenomenon; he was interested in how social facts, scattered throughout a society, have an existence of their own, independent of individual manifestations, and, because of this nonindividualized exis-tence, exercise *une contrainte extérieure,* i.e., external constraints, upon the individual. The further development of Humboldtian thought in the work of

Sapir and Whorf will later show that language imposes not only external but also internal constraints. To consider speech as a social event, as a process comprising speaker and listener in a social field, is axiomatic for any modern form of linguistics which has not a purely historical orientation.

By emphasizing a general and a priori grammar (which stands in contrast to the "exclusively empirical grammars") Husserl[3] prepared the way for the position primarily taken by the members of the circle of linguists in Prague and Copenhagen, namely that the *structure* of language is an independent object in science and therefore also subject to autonomic theorization. This structure can neither be deduced from nor reduced to its elements. It must be added here that the concept of intentionality, which for Husserl played an important role, has found little support in structural linguistics.

The confrontation, already indicated in Durkheim's work, of supra-individual facts on the one hand and of individual manifestations on the other was given a precise form—probably independently of Durkheim—by the Swiss linguist Saussure (1916, posthumously): *language* is divided into *langue,* the system of language existing in the abstract, and *parole,* the individual speech acts. The form in which *langue* exists is, according to Saussure, that of a totality of impressions, deposited in the brain of each member of a speech community, rather like a dictionary of which many identical copies have been distributed. In other words, *langue* is present in every individual, but it has no individuality.

Parole is, at every moment, in a process of creation under the determining and prescribing influence of *langue.* For psycholinguistics the genesis of *parole* is the central issue; Saussure had practically no interest in it.

> An even greater problem is the fact that the relationship of *langue* and *parole* to each other remains as unclear as the relationship of each of these concepts to the everyday reality of spoken language. Is *la langue* an immediate given, can it be studied scientifically, or can it be inferred only via *parole*? If the latter is the case, is *la parole* a "segment" of *la langue,* is *la parole* solely subject to the laws of *la langue,* or is it subject to others as well? We find the same lack of clarity in the contemporary "school" of linguistics (influenced by Saussure) with respect to the relationship between the concepts of competence and performance. But let us now return to the exposition of Saussure's deliberations.
>
> The distinction between *langue* and *parole* recurs in similar forms repeatedly. In the analysis offered by information theory "code" equals *langue,* whereas "message" corresponds to *parole.* Herdan (1956) who understands *langue* as the engrams of language plus the statistical probability of the appearance of these engrams, views *langue* as statistical population, while *parole* assumes the character of a sample of this population. Malmberg (1953), however, raises the objection to this viewpoint that it does not adequately describe

[3] Jakobson (1973) places particular emphasis on Husserl's contribution; cf. also Holenstein (1976).

the relationship between *langue* and *parole: langue* provides rules for what is possible or impossible in *parole;* and this regulating function, as we shall see, cannot be fully grasped in terms of probability. Also worth mentioning is Jakobson's conception of *langue* as a totality of prearranged and available possibilities. The totality of possibilities—it will be shown—plays an important part in information theory. Buber (1951) distinguishes three modes of language: available repertoire (*präsenter Bestand*), potential repertoire (*potentialer Bestand*) and actual event (*aktuelles Begebnis*). But he points out emphatically that the repertoire (*Bestand*) cannot be regarded as something that can be found outside the human being.

Both *langue* and *parole* are characterized by form rather than substance. The linguistic reality lies in their function and in the dynamic relationships among the units into which language can be divided.

Saussure traces these dynamic relations in two different directions, diachronically and synchronically. The diachronic approach is approximately in line with that which is customary in a historically oriented science of language, whereas synchrony represents a "transverse cut through diachrony" (Merleau-Ponty, 1952, p. 95). As for the time dimensions with which Saussure tacitly operates, diachrony predominates in the scientific exploration of *langue,* synchrony in the treatment of *parole.* We shall later become acquainted with sequential psycholinguistics which lies between diachrony and synchrony.

Synchronic linguistics describes *états de langue,* snapshots of temporal cross-sections, or whatever lies "along the axis of simultaneity."

Next, we have to ask ourselves *what* it is that can be arranged diachronically in a sequence, or side by side synchronically. Here we face the problem of the search for units of linguistic analysis. "Language then has the strange, striking characteristic of not having entities that are perceptible at the outset and yet of not permitting us to doubt that they exist and that their functioning constitutes it" (Saussure, 1959 edition, p. 107). This unit is the *sign.*

The history of modern linguistics (and psycholinguistics which evolved from it) was extensively moulded by Saussure's point of view. The sign is the elementary unit of which language is composed and which constitutes the structure of language. This explains why the modern science of language has focused almost exclusively on the problems of syntax. After all, syntax is concerned with the rules for the combining of signs.

Before we continue in this direction, it should be noted that there might have been another way of conceptualizing language, one which does not start with sign-characteristic elements and the rules for combining them, but which begins with the dynamic of people living and working together in the real world. In that case, the conveyance of intentions would become the primary characteristic, which would later become more and more formalized, standardized, and codified in the course of phylogeny and ontogeny. In this view, signs would not be something of which language is composed, but signifying would be one aspect characterizing certain processes and accomplishments.

According to the commonly accepted view in linguistics, the sign was there first, so to speak, it could (then) be used (also) by the speaker for purposes of communication. But according to the second view, understanding would be the primary fact. In order to arrive at such functional understanding, the common behavioral mode of two individuals must be transferred to a representative plane, i.e., a linguistic medium. This approach to the problem of meaning, however, still lacks clarity with respect to its philosophical foundation and its conceptualization of a theoretical framework acceptable to contemporary theories of science.

Saussure defines the term *sign* in two different ways. In the first case it denotes a combining of content (*signifié*) with the vocal form (*signifiant*). The term "content" is used here to identify the concept itself, e.g., the concept of a tree which is also associated with the sound sequence t-r-e-e. In this way Saussure recognized one of the important tasks of linguistics, namely to draw a clear demarcation line between these two components. For example, in French, I must know the demarcation of one *signifié* from another in order to articulate properly the vocal sequence "*sichlapra*" as either *si je la prends* or *si je l'apprends* (in English, "if I take her" or "when I learn it"). In other words, Saussure puts emphasis on the fact that the vocal unit can be delineated only on the basis of knowledge about the conceptual unit.

This was an important insight for the development of linguistics, but the majority of investigators chose to ignore it. Their search, for the most part, focused on elementary vocal units and rarely included a search for elementary meanings.[4]

The second definition given by Saussure still largely determines the contemporary views of linguistics and psycholinguistics. A sign is something which can be differentiated from other signs. The proposition that *dans la langue il n'y a que des différences, sans termes positifs,* signifies that the linguistic form as such is meaningless and without content (cf. Lohmann, 1962). The entire mechanism of language rests upon differences and similarities. "In language, as in any other semiological system, whatever differentiates one sign from the other constitutes it" (Saussure, 1959, p. 121). Therefore, in reference to *la langue,* synchronic linguistics is concerned with a system of linguistic signs, which has validity for all members of a particular speech community. In such a system, every sign is delineated by its neighboring signs, each segment of the system supports the other. In this way, linguistics becomes structuralistic; each element becomes determined in a unique way by means of the encompassing structure, i.e., the lawfulness that characterizes the entire system. Speech is in and of itself a structure

---

[4] Cf. Chafe (1971).

(Hjelmslev); its function as a tool for communication, etc., becomes secondary. We find this to be the case even in the most influential contemporary school of structuralistic linguistics, the so-called generative grammar of Chomsky. There is no longer the search for methods with which to discover the constituent components of an utterance. Instead, the sentence is the starting point and the question is, What does a native speaker need to know about the structure of his language in order to generate all of the grammatically correct sentences of his language and avoid the incorrect ones?

This brief historical sketch of developments in linguistics in more recent times, incomplete though it is, is adequate for the purpose of further discussion here.

We now take up the fact which Saussure had emphasized, viz, that language can be looked upon as a system transcending the individual or as a structure characterized by formal relations. This system or structure has a direct effect on individual acts of speech inasmuch as it commands how things may be said.

This approach, which is formal rather than substantial, goes well with nomothetic procedures which are as customary in modern linguistics as they are in modern psychology. Carroll has significantly called linguistics the *science* of language.

If we take the two key concepts which we evolved earlier—*language as a tool* and *language as a social phenomenon* and add to that *language as structure* we are now ready for a first definition of language which originates from Carroll (1955, p. 10) and reads as follows: "A language is a structured system of arbitrary vocal sounds and sequences of sounds which is used, or can be used, in interpersonal communication by an aggregation of human beings, and which rather exhaustively catalogs the things, events, and processes in the human environment."

The determination of purpose contained in this statement makes Carroll's definition particularly good as a point of departure for a *psychological* study of language, because—as we have repeatedly emphasized—in psychology purposive activity in social beings plays a decisive role.

With the help of a diagram (Fig. 1) we shall now describe that event which psycholinguistics attempts to elucidate. We start from the fact that language occurs in a social field, determined by the two poles, speaker and listener (or source and receiver). The information links the two. The information or message is that part of the speaker's *output* which, simultaneously, forms the listener's *input*. Under output we understand here what the speaker

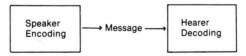

Fig. 1 (Adapted from Osgood and Sebeok, 1954)

produces and under input what the listener receives. The activity of the speaker which constructs and edits the message and sends it on its way is called *encoding;* the activity of the listener which, in turn, makes sense out of sound waves is called *decoding.*

The concepts "encoding" and "decoding" suggest translating into and from a code. *Code* represents the systematic aspect which has proved so important in the analysis of the linguistic event. Linguistic communication is always communication by means of a system; this is what distinguishes it from primitive communication, e.g., by means of contact-sound. It must be emphasized again that the above schema not only differentiates between psycholinguistics and linguistics, but also implies a particular assignment of roles to each of the two disciplines.

With the help of Fig. 1 we can now demarcate psycholinguistics from linguistics proper. Linguistics deals with the structure of messages. The linguist describes the message—*en route,* so to speak—as an objective configuration, whose rules of organization have to be discovered. Linguistics "confines itself to the analysis of the characteristics of signal systems or 'codes', as it may be derived from the structure of messages" (Lounsbury, 1956, p. 158). Naturally the analysis of the language system of a speech community is only possible through the study of particular instances, i.e., concrete speech events; but the object of the linguistic effort is the presentation of the system which underlies all the particular manifestations. In the terminology of Bühler or Kainz we might say: the linguist studies *Sprachgebilde* (linguistic forms).

The object of psycholinguistics is not to describe language scientifically, but to describe the processes of language use. Psycholinguistics is concerned with the relation between messages and the individual transmitting or receiving these messages.

Going back to the model in Fig. 1 we might say, following Osgood, "Psycholinguistics deals . . . with the processes of encoding and decoding as they relate states of messages to states of communicators" (Osgood and Sebeok, 1954, p. 4).

Encoding and decoding are transitions from one behavior modality to another. In encoding, the perceptions, thoughts and feelings of the speaker are translated into a behavior modality, i.e., verbal behavior. This sequence can be made explicit in Fig. 2 (following Carroll and others).

| Intentive behavior of speaker | → | Encoding behavior of speaker | → | Message | → | Decoding behavior of hearer | → | Interpretive behavior of hearer |

Fig. 2

The markedly behavioristic flavor of this conception is evident. What the speaker has to encode, and what happens when the listener decodes is, of course, behavior and certainly nothing so "mentalistic" as imaging or knowing.

Speech behavior is not only anchored in the stimuli on the one side and the responses on the other, but is also subject to the determining influences on the part of the superordinate system which is the structured *langue* of Saussure.

Furthermore, linguistic events are more than just behavior, they must also embrace states, linguistic knowledge at the various levels of consciousness.

Even if we cannot accept completely the implications arising from the terminology employed by the above schema, it can serve as a point of departure in three directions:

First, encoding and decoding can be treated as series of decisions. Decisions occur between discrete choices. This leads us to the problem of what to consider as the unit of linguistic analysis and further to interpretations of information theory.

Second, the model shows that the linguistic process involves a kind of translation in two places. The sound cluster is produced by the speaker in lieu of something else and is understood by the listener as standing for something else; in other words, the sound complex functions as a sign; it has meaning.

Third, if *linguistics* is concerned with the structural aspects of messages, it seems reasonable that *psycholinguistics* should make use of the structures identified by this linguistics in the former's attempt to find a relationship between the states of messages and the states of transmitter and receiver. Psycholinguistics assumes, therefore, that the structures of messages described by linguistics are those which are also psychologically relevant. That view characterized the historical development of psycholinguistics beginning in the mid-1950s (the publication of the above schema) and continuing to the end of the 1960s. Much effort was expended in identifying the "psychological reality" of those concepts which were introduced by linguistics for its own purposes (cf. Hörmann, 1974). Only recently has psycholinguistics raised the question of the appropriateness of the linguistic description of messages for purposes of psychological consideration and investigations.[5]

In the following pages we shall take up again (and indeed not the only time in this book) the character and function of signs, while the ideas which lead from this model to information theory will be discussed in a later chapter.

---

[5] Along with Bierwisch one could draw a distinction between psycholinguistics and psychology of language. Psycholinguistics investigates language behavior and acquisition based on specific findings of linguistics, whereas the psychology of language is not committed to linguistic hypotheses.

CHAPTER 2

Sign, Expression, and Symbol

Bühler's *organon* model—Different conceptions of the nature of signs—
Problems concerning the language of animals—The language of bees—
The performance of Washoe, the chimpanzee—The origin of language in
symbolic behavior—Communicative intentions.

Bühler in his work *Sprachtheorie* (1934), a monumental investigation on
the concept of the sign, set out from the *stat aliquid pro aliquo* of Scholasticism. This "standing for something else" can occur in different modes,
which are not distinguished so much by substance as by function. Bühler
conceives these modes of sign-quality in terms of an "organon model" of
language (or more precisely of the sign), in keeping with the Platonic statement that language is a tool or *organum* so that "one person can talk to
another about things." One person (A)—to another (B)—about things: these
are the three elements which are related to each other in Fig. 3.

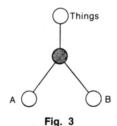

Fig. 3

Bühler gives the following example: A hears the patter of rain and says to
B, "It's raining." B on hearing these words looks towards the window. To
represent these events with greater accuracy the first drawing can be developed in Fig. 4.

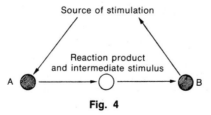

Fig. 4

Let us note, however, that even in the interpretations of a scholar such as Bühler, who can hardly be suspected of behavioristic inclinations, the analysis of sign function leads to a presentation in terms of stimulus and response. "Reaction product and intermediate stimulus" are central to what modern mediating-response theories are about (see chap. 10).

At the next stage Bühler makes use of a more powerful magnification which permits him to identify differences in the various relations. In the center we find again the concrete event or phenomenon (Ph) (Fig. 5).

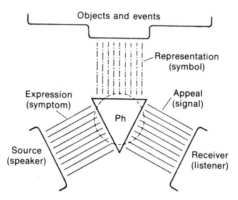

Fig. 5. Bühler's *organon* model. (Adapted from Bühler, 1934, p. 28)

Three features of this phenomenon turn it in a threefold way into a sign. Bühler represents these three features as a triangle. Corresponding to its three sides are the three modes of sign-quality. The phenomenon is a *symbol* in relation to objects and events; it is a *symptom* because of its dependence on the speaker whose inner state it expresses, and it is a *signal* because of its appeal to the receiver whose behavior it guides.

Representation, expression, and appeal—these are, according to Bühler, the three characteristic functions of language (or of signs, as we would more cautiously be inclined to say).

Suppose we want to understand two people talking to each other in a foreign language, we can undertake the analysis under the three aspects; the phenomena, i.e., the sound patterns, may be related to: (1) the events in the real world ("Whenever it rains, he utters this sound"); (2) the state of the speaker ("Whenever he is afraid, he utters this sound"); (3) the effect on the hearer ("Whenever he hears this sound, he comes").

In the first case the sound pattern is viewed for its representational function, i.e., it functions as a symbol; in the second case it is taken as an expression or symptom, and in the third case as a signal that directs an appeal to the receiver.

By treating a sign as an expression or symptom, we infer something: because we know of, or assume, a connection, we conclude that the appearance of the phenomenon implies the occurrence of what is connected with it, although it cannot be directly observed. Thus, if we observe marked variations in voice intensity we conclude that the speaker is excited. This is, according to Bühler, the inference *quoad existentiam*. It is quite different in the case of the representational function of the sign. Here the perceived phenomenon does not act as an indicator by its appearance, *quoad existentiam* with which it is linked through *connexio rerum;* it stands *quoad essentiam* for something outside itself (Bühler, 1932, p. 102 f.). Although a high color on the cheeks is connected with a fever (*connexio rerum*), the fever does not draw the curve on the temperature chart; the chart represents certain abstract moments of the course of the fever. In this form of representational relatedness, there is no *connexio rerum,* but an *ordo rerum,* produced by the ordering activity of the mind.

If we consider the cogency of the relationship between the sign and the object signified we find, in Bühler's model, only two possibilities: either the relationship is natural (derived from a *connexio rerum*) and thus compelling and universal, or it is conventional (i.e., arbitrarily established).

A more detailed scale of necessity in the relation between sign and what it designates has been established by Peirce (1932): he distinguishes *icon* (the sign has similarity to what is signified), *index* (the sign is causally connected with the thing signified), and *symbol* (the sign is connected with what it designates according to a conventional rule). The varying degrees of necessity in the connection between sign and denotatum will be discussed once more in greater detail in connection with the claim of an "inner relationship" between sign and the thing signified: in onomatopoeia, in Werner's theory of linguistic physiognomy and in sound symbolism, also in connection with the reverse of this theory, the *General Semantics* of Korzybski and Hayakawa.

Saussure stresses the arbitrariness of the connection between the sign and what it signifies. *Signe* is the unit which is produced by the association of *signifié* and *signifiant*. *Signifié* is not the object itself but the concept, *signifiant* not the sound, but the psychological trace of the sound. *Signifié* and *signifiant* are, therefore, abstractions which in the system are placed into the area of *langue* (cf. Malmberg, 1963). A consequence of this shift of *signe* into the "objective" sphere of *langue* is that it unwittingly confirms the Saussurian view of the meaning of a word as something definite. The inevitable relativity of meaning produced by the situation is a feature still to be discussed in greater detail. The point here is that we now meet for the first time the difference of opinion as to what the object really is in the dual relationship between sign and signified object.

In Bühler's model (see Fig. 5), the three modes of sign quality are represented by a triangle. This triangle is somewhat smaller in places than the circle which represents the concrete phenomenon. If a concrete object or process (e.g., a sound pattern) functions as a sign, the sign function is exercised by certain features—and only those (1932, p. 110). In traffic signals only the color functions as a sign, not their size or degree of brightness. This is what Bühler calls "abstractive relevance" (*abstraktive Relevanz*). This principle, according to which only part of a sound cluster has sign function, whereas all the rest is irrelevant, is important for the discussion of linguistic units (see chap. 3).

The triangle which represents the three modes of sign quality (Fig. 5) in certain places extends beyond the circle of concrete phenomena. According to Bühler this is meant to indicate that the acoustic data are supplemented by others which cannot be immediately perceived by the senses, but derive, for example, from memory, motivation and so on. This filling-out process by the organism occurs according to principles which in modern psychology are studied under the headings of social perception or under analysis-by-synthesis. At the basis of this approach is a fact which is all too often overlooked; namely that man is subjectively always oriented toward meaning. This spontaneous supplementation of perception was emphasized as early as 1909 by v. Allesch, who stated that "this comprehension and supplementation is nothing else than the apprehending of an appearance in terms of specific prior knowledge. This supplementation proceeds step by step and is guided by the subjective need which shapes our perception" (1909, p. 498).

This relates to another question which Bühler, although he recognized it in another context, does not take into consideration in his model. Can one say that the specific function of a sign is inherent in that sign, or is that function constituted only through the intentions of its user who gives it a particular direction? (For a discussion of significative intention, see Husserl, 1929; Merleau-Ponty, 1952; Wittgenstein, 1960; and Höpp, 1970.)

Another deficiency in Bühler's model, which results from the philosophical climate of his time, is that the world of objects and events is treated as completely detached from language. This is the Aristotelian notion that language depicts the world. There is no place in this model for the object-creating function of language which was stressed by Humboldt, and later by Cassirer, Sapir, Whorf, and others.

The sign is undoubtedly the nucleus of language, but language is more than mere sign. The blurring of these distinctions has caused an old controversy: to what extent can expression—mime, facial expression, gesture, and certain phenomena of the autonomic nervous system—be considered to be a language or to belong to language? One can speak of "the language of the human face" or of a "telling" blush.

Such views can be accommodated in the model under discussion; in Bühler's conception the sign is a symptom whenever it can be understood as an expression of the inner state of the speaker. The symptom relationship between sign and what is signified is in this case, as we have seen, a natural one because of the *connexio rerum*. But Malmberg rightly notes in this connection that a symptom does not have to be natural. Even such apparently "primitive" utterances as cries of pain have a different form in different languages; i.e., they are, to a certain extent at least, codetermined by conventions. Where the sign functions as a symbol (i.e., for reference), the arbitrary conventional association is dominant, but even in these cases, as we shall see in the discussion on sound symbolism, there are, so to speak, "natural" preferences. In the signal and the symbol functions, then, the border-line between conventional and natural causation is either vague or nonexistent. If the poet says that the heart is worn like a posy of violets—is this using language for representation or as expression?

And again, Is the presence of the expressive function alone sufficient to speak of "language"? This question may seem to lead to a purely terminological dispute about the definition of language; but it is this kind of questioning which has for centuries given the impetus to thought about the origin and evolution of speech.

The expressive movements and sounds in animals manifest themselves for emotional reasons or in connection with instinctive actions. Can animals speak? Herder (1772) has answered this question succinctly by saying that the sounds of emotion can only become language if an intellect is added which can cause the sound to be uttered intentionally.

Consequently, the similarity of animal and human language is external; it refers purely to the appearance of sound, but not "to the specifically linguistic sound which emanates from the urge to speak and which is determined by an inner faculty of language" (Révész, 1946, p. 37). The total character and intention of the uttered sounds indicate that animal language is not language in the real sense. In these observations, Révész shows that he is still entirely in the tradition of the psychology of consciousness. "If the tendency or intention of entering into contact with others is added to the expressive movement, the latter ceases to be purely expressive movement and becomes either a signalling sign or a linguistic symbol" (1946, p. 39). Révész, therefore, assumes that expression and what is expressed are coexistent poles in a psychic unity. It follows that expression, produced with intent or employed for whatever purpose, e.g., to make contact, is no longer simply expression. If, on the other hand, expression—or, more precisely, expressive behavior—is in principle regarded as separable from an inner state, as was discussed above, there is no clear distinction between expression on the one hand and symbol and sign on the other. According to our present state of knowledge on the role of tradition in expression, of the directive function of expressive movements and the role of learning in understanding of expression (cf. Kirchhoff, 1965, on this point), it is certain that expression can, to a certain extent, be used purposefully. We must therefore assume a broad field of transition between symptom, signal, and symbol; one might place in this area, for example, threatening gestures of animals or the display behavior of geese. These result in communication and, yet, we do not have to presuppose communicative intent in the source.

Révész would be prepared to ascribe a language to certain animal species, if they disposed of a well-ordered system of signs, or, to use the terms of our earlier discussions, of a structured *langue* or *code*. In this case animals would have to have "e.g., not one warning call but several, one for the approach of a human, another for a member of his family coming into view (*sic*), another again for a hostile animal" (1946, p. 47). Révész no doubt believed that it would not be possible to find animal utterances which satisfied these criteria. He was mistaken. It is known, thanks to observations by Heinroth and Lorenz, that various species of birds make just these distinctions in their warning sounds. For instance, one may find in one and the same species different warning sounds for flying enemies and for enemies on the ground.

The point of view, which has thus been introduced into the discussion, of a systematic differentiation of messages has never been more clearly demonstrated than in the fascinating researches of Frisch on the language of bees. One can hardly think about the psychology of language without taking note of the results of these investigations. They are therefore briefly described here.

In 1919 Frisch observed a bee which, having just returned from a feeding place to the hive, danced around and caused excitement among the worker-bees. After a three-year period of intensive research he believed he had come to understand the language of bees. Forty years later, Frisch himself remarked that he had overlooked the most important factor and that the language of bees was exceedingly complex (1962a).

When a honey bee returns from a forage and performs a dance, the other worker-bees experience the characteristic smell of the feeding place because of the scent which adheres to the returning scout. Frisch held at first that it would be impossible for the bee to provide, in addition, an exact description of the location. But when the foragers fly off they search at the right distance as well as in the right direction. Has the language of bees a word for distance? A bee coming from a nearby feeding place performs a round-dance; if it returns from a more distant place it executes a tail-wagging-dance. But the indication of distance is even more differentiated. The message transmitted through the wagging-dance contains more information than merely "more than 50 meters." If the goal is at a distance of 100 meters the bee repeats the straight run of the dance pattern approximately 9 or 10 times in 15 seconds. At greater distances the speed of the dance declines in a regular manner; a definite tempo corresponds to each distance (Fig. 6).

This is the internationally accepted form of communication among bees; various strains of the species *apis mellifera* can communicate with one another; but there are "dialects." Austrian and Italian bees can cooperate

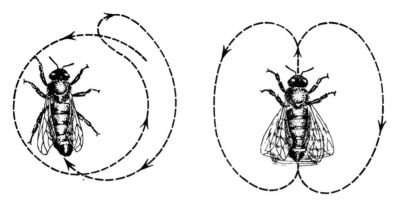

Fig. 6. Dance patterns of the bee: round dance (left) and wagging dance (right). (From Frisch, 1962a, p. 126)

harmoniously: the Austrian dance stimulates the Italian bee; but the indication of a distance of 100 meters is misinterpreted as 80 meters, whereas 100 meters danced in the Italian dialect is interpreted by the Austrian bee as 120 meters (Frisch, 1962b).

The direction of the target is indicated by the direction of the straight line in the wagging-dance pattern, with the position of the sun as a point of reference. In the darkened beehive this angle on the sun is represented by a corresponding angle on the direction of gravity. The differences in the dialects described above stand in contrast to a phylogenitically earlier and simpler form of communication: Indian dwarf bees, a more primitive ancestor of the *apis mellifera*, are not capable of this transposition from light to gravity. A less developed language corresponds to a more primitive social organization. Even lower in the phylogenetic scale are the stingless *meliponini*; in this strain the information about the target is not transmitted to the foragers in the hive, but traces of scent and pilot bees act as guides (Lindauer, 1961).

It had been thought for a long time that the capacity of the communicative system in the honey bee is restricted to transmission of information on quality and position of feeding places. Lindauer (1955 and later) was able to demonstrate that swarming bees can signal the position of a good place for a dwelling with a similar code.

The communicative system of the honey bee is also important for linguistics from another point of view. A number of different sense modalities are brought into use to transmit information: the kind of food found by the scout is indicated by a minute particle of the substance itself or by the scent of the substance, and the distance of the feeding place is communicated by the dance. Investigations by Esch (1961) suggest that sound utterances of bees equally contain information on quality and distance.

Different strands of development lead from the communicative achievements of honey bees to phylogenetically higher species. These strands seem to disappear in one place, reappear in a changed form elsewhere and finally lead to strange and puzzling forms of "linguistic" behavior, such as those which are found in dolphins and chimpanzees in the wild (Goodall, 1963). It will be seen that the various strands or components are sometimes cumulative, sometimes disappear and reappear in a new place and develop afresh. The study of communication in the animal world can present informative analogies for the study of human speech, as, for instance, Carmichael (1964) has brilliantly demonstrated.

Bühler has regarded the signals used in a colony of bees as steering devices which represent a prehuman analogue to language. Greenberg (1961), who "as a human" insisted on giving the bees not just "a technical knockout," has claimed that genuine (i.e., human) language must be capable of being used metalinguistically: one must be able to speak in language about language, e.g., to exchange opinions on the meaning of an utterance. But it is not certain whether even this criterion enables us to keep apart animal and human language; rhesus monkeys exchange metalinguistic information in order to distinguish between play and reality (Sebeok, 1963).

The question, Can animals speak? turns out to be a terminological one; it can in fact only be answered by a definition of what one is prepared to recognize as language. But the lengthy discussion on this question has not been useless; it has taught linguistic science and psycholinguistics to take note of certain aspects and to make distinctions which, in quite a general way,—also outside this particular problem area—have proved to be important and fruitful.

The studies by Gardner and Gardner (1969) and Premack (1966), added a new dimension to the discussion about animal language. Instead of studying the species-specific communication system of chimpanzees, these investigators attempted to teach the animals the rudimentary elements of a man-made language system. What was shown here to be possible and impossible is by its very nature more closely related to conventional linguistics and psycholinguistics.

On the basis of a series of earlier, unsuccessful attempts to teach chimpanzees to articulate English words, the Gardners decided to bypass the monkey larynx which apparently was unsuitable for generating human speech sounds. They taught a female chimpanzee named Washoe part of American Sign Language (ASL). Washoe lived in the Gardners' home and they communicated with her daily as if she was a deaf-mute child. The success of this procedure exceeded all expectations. After three years Washoe knew and was able to use nearly 100 different ASL signs, even chaining three or four signs in a row.

Even more revealing to the psychologist interested in human speech are the findings beyond those concerning this "absolute" performance. For example, if Washoe learns with respect to a particular door, that a specific sign denotes "open" and she is then able to apply this sign immediately, without further training, to a closed briefcase, a water faucet, and a capped cola bottle, we can assume that even in the case of animals there is a nonverbal, general schema to which a linguistic designation will be "attached." This is a point of view that we should keep in mind for our discussion of speech learning in children.[1]

Neither Washoe's performance nor the surprising cognitive skills performed by Premack's Sarah, who was able to arrive at logical conclusions by means of a "language" of plastic signs on a magnetic board, permit us to give a genuine answer to the question whether animals can speak. What we can conclude based on this lengthy discussion is that apparently speech is not something uniform, functioning only according to *one* particular principle. If one views speech and speaking psychologically, one must differentiate between the various components and partial elements that are acquired through the total phenomenon of speech.

In our inquiries on the behavior of bees the communicative aspect of language was prominent. But it is by no means certain whether from an evolutionary point of view communication is the earliest strand in the tissue of language.

In more recent times, Suzanne Langer (1963) has approached this problem in a way which is particularly interesting for a *psychology* of language and we shall therefore briefly describe it. She starts out from a view expressed by Sapir, who has declared that the attempts to unravel the origin of language are hardly more than exercises in speculative imagination. As for the reason for this failure, Sapir argues as follows: "The primary function of language is generally said to be communication . . . The autistic speech of children seems to show that the purely communicative aspect of language has been exaggerated. It is best to admit that language is primarily a vocal actualization of the tendency to see reality symbolically, that it is precisely this quality which renders it a fit instrument for communication and that it is in the actual give and take of social intercourse that it has been complicated and refined into the form in which it is known today" (Sapir, 1933, p. 159). This "tendency to see reality symbolically" is for Langer the nucleus from which language has originated. It follows that the search for the roots of language should not be directed so much towards preformations of communication as towards earlier forms of symbolic behavior.

What should we imagine these early forms of *symbols* to have been like? To begin with, there was probably no more than a vague feeling that an object, a certain pattern or a sound is not insignificant, but that it has some meaning. Langer documents with a series of examples that in certain anthropoid apes there are indications of an aesthetic sense or of superstitious fear directed towards objects which in themselves were trivial. Often such an

---

[1] The importance of this study is discussed in detail in Ploog (1972) and in Brown (1973).

object is treated literally as a fetish. Such behavior is evidence for the tendency to see more in an object than what is immediately and objectively given: the emotional tendency is a rudimentary form of symbolic behavior.

A genuine symbol evolves from these earlier forms through a process of dissociation and objectivization. The process originates most clearly "where some object, sound, or act is provided which has no *practical* meaning, yet tends to elicit an emotional response and thus hold one's undivided attention" (Langer 1965, p. 121).

The proposition that the symbol evolves through the attachment of affective components to previously neutral behavioral elements is contrary to the one which was mentioned earlier and will be discussed in more detail later. This opposing view states that the basis for the genesis of communication by means of verbal symbols is the practice of communal acts and behaviors which relates to the division of labor.

If the earliest symbolic value of words originates in a vague emotional arrest at the use of words, then only a later stage can free the symbol "from its original instinctive utterance and marks its deliberate *use, outside of the total situation that gave it birth*" (Langer, 1963, p. 133). Thus, connotation becomes denotation, the factual relationship of the sign to the object signified is established, and this, as Langer says, is the essense of language.

Langer traces here the same line of development as Cassirer[2] who sees it as a transition from emotional to propositional language or, in other words, to the power of conceptual use of language. The symbolic transformation makes possible the great discovery that in principle everything has a name.

Basically, then, these considerations lead us to a final criterion: whether something is or is not a symbol depends on the subjective manner of possessing it, or, in other words, on the awareness of having full control over it and of being able to use it at will. If, thus, we accord a decisive role to the subjective factor in symbol formation we touch upon problems and difficulties that reach beyond the question of the origin of speech.

Is it actually possible to speak of communication if the sender (who in this case would be better called symptom carrier) does not have any intentions to communicate? Is it proper to go so far as to expand the concept of communication to include every reception of information by a receiver? It has become fashionable today to label as communication everything which permits the receiver to draw inferences. It is not possible for us to enter into a detailed discussion of this question which properly belongs to the field of semiotics. Those who are interested in this issue will find an excellent discussion in Wiener et al. (1972). We are going to accept in principle the definition of MacKay (1972), that we can speak of *information* if an event causes us to know or believe something that we did not know or believe before. "Information-about-X determines the form of our readiness-to-reckon-

---

[2] See particularly the fourth edition of *Philosophie der Symbolischen Formen* (1964).

with-X in appropriate circumstances'' (1972, p. 8). MacKay defines communication this way: In order for individual A to recognize individual B as communicating, A must recognize B as acting with a goal orientation. Without recognition of this goal-oriented action, B may in fact convey information to A but he does not communicate. From this vantage point we can look back once more to Bühler. The sign and what it signifies, symptom and inner state, symbol and object, are for him, and not just for him, concepts that always imply a relation between two poles. The goal-oriented behavior which gives impetus and meaning to this polarization is not always considered in the organon model of language. But other authors on the subject of sign and speech usually ignore it completely.

CHAPTER 3

Linguistic Units and the Rules for Their Connection

Schema of the speech event—Articulation—Process of categorization in perception—Phoneme and morpheme—Distinctive features—Definition of the word—The sentence as the playing field of grammar—Principles of generative transformational grammar—Competence and performance— Surface and deep structures—The theory of semantics of Katz and Fodor—Dimensions of the lexicon.

In the preceding chapters the attempt was made to fit together biological, philosophical, and epistemological ideas in order to lay a general foundation for psycholinguistics. This attempt cannot be said to have been successful; we have not discovered a readily available philosophical basis for empirical inquiries in psycholinguistics. However, these chapters can give us points of view, hints and warnings which we would be well advised to bear in mind in our forthcoming discussions. We will find that, from time to time, the empirical inquiries will yield new glimpses of the epistemological questions which we have already considered.

Let us start once more from the model of the speech event we had outlined in Chapter 1 (Fig. 7).

Encoding and decoding are processes of translation—from and into language. The translator must choose among the possibilities which the lexicon and the grammar put at his disposal. Language, understood in this way, demands a series of decisions or choices; it is not an undivided total stream, but a sequence of different, separable events.

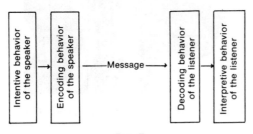

Fig. 7

With that we return to the thought expressed earlier: Speech events consist of single, more or less elementary units. In order to investigate the psychological processes it becomes necessary to identify the nature of these units, the possibilities for chaining them, i.e., the possibilities for structuring them, which form the basis for the use of speech.

We shall examine various attempts to discover and/or define such units of speech events. These attempts can be differentiated first and foremost in terms of their point of origin. To begin with, the description of a speech event can be undertaken from two points of view: (a) *articulation,* i.e., the production of sound sequences; and (b) *acoustics,* i.e., the physical characteristics of the sound sequences, thus produced. It is not uncommon to find a good deal of switching from articulatory to acoustic description, as the need arises.

A corresponding description of the listening event can equally be undertaken from two points of view: (a) the physical characteristics of the sound sequence which acts as a stimulus, in other words, from an *acoustic* point of view, and (b) what is heard by the receiver, the *auditory description.*

The total event comprising speaker and hearer can therefore be divided into three different phases and be described in three different terminologies: *articulatory, acoustic,* and *auditory.*

Speech sounds are made by modifications of the air-stream which is produced by exhalation. (We are not, at this point, taking note of exceptions.) The two cavities which participate in the modification of the air-stream, the chest, and the pharyngeal-oral cavity are separated by the larynx which contains mobile folds of tissue, ligaments, and muscles, the *vocal cords* (Fig. 8).

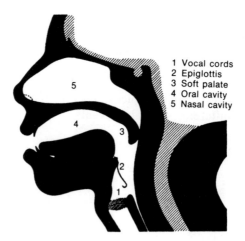

1 Vocal cords
2 Epiglottis
3 Soft palate
4 Oral cavity
5 Nasal cavity

Fig. 8. Schematic diagram of the organs of speech. (From Steinbuch, 1965, p. 90)

Partly with the help of primitive resonators, attempts to understand the physical nature of speech sounds and the physical consequences of the processes of articulation have a long history. The acoustic analysis of speech sounds undertaken in the framework of phonetics recognizes three dimensions: intensity, frequency, and duration. Through sound spectrography acoustic patterns can be converted into visual ones and thus be made more amenable to investigation (Fig. 9). Thanks to the spectrograph the energy of continuous speech is distributed, by means of filters, over 10 to 20 frequency-bands. The moving, light-sensitive paper is blackened according to the relative intensity of the energy at different bands.

An even more ingenious instrument, called a pattern playback, can reconvert graphic patterns into sound. It is possible, first, to darken the paper in order to indicate certain intensities and distributions, and in this way emphasize some frequencies and omit others, and then to hear what the sound, constructed by this procedure, is like. The analysis of a sound pattern can thus be tested by a subsequent synthesis for accuracy and exhaustiveness.

The following outlines certain phonetic outcomes which have important implications for psycholinguistics.

The cavities through which the air-stream passes act as filters, filtering out some frequencies, and as resonators, reinforcing others. The principle involved is well-known: if we blow over the opening of a bottle, the size and shape of the cavity determine the frequency of the sound produced in this way. This principle is at the basis of vowel sounds. If we examine a spectrogram for the frequencies which are produced, for example, by the vowel sound [i], the pattern will normally reveal two peaks. In other words, two frequencies have more energy than others. These are the so-called *formants*. A formant is a concentration of energy in a relatively narrow frequency-band.

That vowels are characterized by such formants has been made known

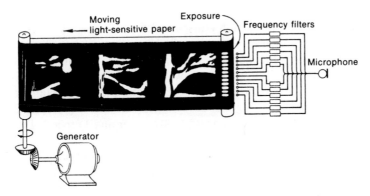

Fig. 9. Principle of "visible speech" record. (From Steinbuch, 1965, p. 97)

above all through the research of Carl Stumpf (1926) whose work—without any electronic devices—has led to astonishingly exact results even by present-day standards.

Position and number of formants, however, are not the only constituents of a given vowel. The formants of the vowel [a] spoken by a man are different from those spoken by a woman; and yet both can be clearly recognized as [a]. Nor is the relative position of the formants the only decisive factor; it may well be that learning and experience play a part.

The mark of a consonant is a sudden change in the even pattern of the formants. While in vowels the time dimension plays no important part, it is decisive for consonants. The change in the structure of the formants can be caused by a sudden complete stoppage or by transition to an irregular nonperiodic noise spectrum. The open vocal tract is closed once or several times and thus variation and repetition, having the effect of a disturbance, are brought into the even course of sound production. We do not have to go into detail here on further differences caused by stops, fricatives, and so on.

So far we have described the sounds of speech in acoustic or physical terms. If such a description is greatly refined, it will be found that no speaker can twice produce the same sound, nor can different speakers produce two sounds which are the same. Since, strictly speaking, there are no events which can be repeated, this account of a physical event could not be lawfully related to other processes, e.g., the comprehension of spoken utterances. In order to establish regularities, the separate events must be classified, as we have already done by speaking of "vowels" and "consonants."

The same conclusion is reached, i.e., a categorizing process must be assumed, if we leave the articulatory-acoustic interpretation of speech production and move on to the acoustic-auditive description of speech perception.

An experiment of the Haskins Laboratories is perhaps a suitable link between the production phase and studies on speech perception (cf. Liberman, 1957, and Liberman et al., 1963).

Seven different vowels, each consisting of two formants, were recorded on magnetic tape. Each of these vowels was preceded by a burst of noise lasting 1.5 cs. The frequency span of this explosion remained 600 cps; but the absolute height of the explosion was varied. Different [a] sounds and different [i] sounds were produced, etc.; among them, for example, an [a] preceded by a noise lasting 1.5 cs between 400 and 1000 cps, or an [a] preceded by a noise between 600 and 1200 cps, or an [i] preceded by a noise between 400 and 1000 cps.

What does a subject hear who listens to these sound sequences? If the noise explosion lies at a level above 3000 cps it is generally heard as [t]; if it is below 3000 cps it is heard as [k], as long as it occurs above the second formant of the vowel; otherwise it is heard as [p]. This means different explosions are heard as identical consonants, provided they occur above

3000 cps; on the other hand, identical explosions are perceived as different consonants depending on the relationship to the subsequent vowel.

This experiment has three interesting implications for us:

1. What we perceive as vowels and consonants are not invariant sounds or noises, but classes or categories of different noises. The differences between classes determine our perceptions; differences between noises within the same class are overheard or disregarded. The processing of a speech event—and, as we shall see later, both in its articulatory and its perceptive phase—has a built-in device which takes note of certain distinctions and orients itself in accordance with them, but it ignores other distinctions and declares them as nonexistent. We are reminded of Saussure's "differences and identities" which are decisive for language. By introducing the concept of classification, i.e., both noting and ignoring differences, we have of necessity come to include a psychological point of view.

2. In physical terms a sound is always fully defined by the characteristics of the sound wave. But what sort of consonant this sound is perceived as, is psychologically determined by the subsequent vowel, or by the sequence within which the sound is embedded. We shall return to this sequential feature.

3. The three aspects which we have so far distinguished in a speech event—the articulatory, acoustic, and auditory aspect—are not completely compatible. This means that, for instance, not all articulatory movements of the speech organs have an acoustic effect, and it further implies that a particular acoustic process does not always result in the same auditory experience. To put it differently: the articulatory space has different dimensions from the acoustic one, and the acoustic space, in turn, has different dimensions from the auditory space. There is a higher degree of agreement between the articulatory and the auditory dimensions than between the acoustic and the auditory ones: this peculiar state of affairs will occupy us again at a later stage when we discuss Liberman's theory (see p. 72).

We now return to the question we discussed before our digression on the Haskins experiment. The search for linguistically and psycholinguistically relevant units, which we began in the field of phonetics with the help of the Saussurian "clues" of likenesses and differences, has yielded the following results: differences that the speaker produces are not necessarily perceived as differences; identical utterances do not always exercise identical effects. The attempt of phonetics to determine the sounds of speech as events in their own right has shown that psychological factors must inevitably be taken into account. But this is not surprising; the speech sounds produced by the human voice are not random vocalizations, they are *linguistic* sounds. That is important in two respects. First, a particular, acoustically defined event can be perceived differentially by the hearer, depending on whether he knows that it is a speech event or not. The tuning-in to verbal communication initiates in the listener a kind of special perceptual program. Here we find again the projective nature of perception, which we encounter repeatedly, and which also forms the basis of the analysis-by-synthesis theories of contemporary perceptual research.

The second aspect is that speech sounds produced by the human voice have sign characteristics, they carry meaning. A sign, as we learned in our discussion of Saussure, is constituted in terms of that which differentiates it from other signs. In searching for linguistically relevant units, we have seen that the route via absolute *physical* characteristics does not lead very far. Recognizing that, one will then use the difference or identity of *meaning* as an instrument for the discovery of relevant units. (The question here, however, is *not* what meaning two units have, but only whether their meaning is identical or different.)

A similar position is reached from the point of view of communication theory: "To be a practicable medium for the transmission of information, a language must be susceptible of description by a finite number of distinguishable, mutually exclusive sounds. That is, the language must be representable in terms of basic linguistic units which have the property that if one replaces another in an utterance, the meaning is changed" (Flanagan, 1965, p. 14).

In order to discover linguistic units, or to recognize distinct boundaries between them an analysis of the choice processes which occur during the speech act must be made. The speaker and the hearer must make a series of decisions. For each unit a choice has to be made or, conversely, what is selected at each single choice point constitutes a unit.

In the sentence, "The beer is good," a choice has been made before "good." During speaking (encoding) or listening (decoding) the decision might have been "bitter," or "stale," or "pale." Another decision has to be made before "is": "tastes" or "was" might well have been chosen. And instead of "beer" the decision might have been to say "house" or "child."

The units which thus occur are, following Martinet (1960), called "units of the first articulation" or *monemes;* another common designation is also *morpheme.* It should be added that these units are not identical with words: the sentence, "He feels unwell," has five morphemes: "he," "feel," "s," "un," "well."

Each of the units of the first level of articulation displays meaning and phonic shape. Some thousands of such units in every new combination serve to communicate whatever we want to say. "What characterizes linguistic communication and opposes it to prelinguistic groans is precisely this analysis into a number of units which, because of their vocal nature, are to be presented successively in a linear fashion. These are the units which many contemporary linguists call 'morphemes' " (Martinet, 1962, p. 22).[1]

---

[1] Cf. Bierwisch (1966) concerning the problem of this approach to isolating or defining morphemes.

If a morpheme is analyzed further, its meaning is lost. The meaning of "toe" is not a combination of the meanings of /t/ and /o/. The only analysis that is still possible is that of the phonic shape. It follows that the morpheme is the smallest meaningful unit. It is a segment of an utterance which recurs in different utterances with more or less the same meaning. The word "older" consists of two morphemes, because the suffix "-er" has independent meaning. It is the comparative. The same sound "-er" in the word "hunter" represents a different morpheme; it is an operator appended to a verb (from Berko and Brown, 1960).

> While here the same sound (or as we shall call it below: the same "phoneme") is recognized as two morphemes according to the environment in which it occurs, the morpheme can be said to form a class or category. In English, for example, we find the morpheme /s/ with the meaning of plural. This constitutes a class, composed of various *allomorphs,* with the same meaning: "cats" with voiceless /s/, "boys" with voiced /z/, "roses" with /iz/. Which of these allomorphs is selected, is determined by what precedes and is not open to the free choice of the speaker; hence these three forms are not three different units, but only one. Sometimes the allomorphs of a morpheme are totally different in sound. "Am, is, are" are allomorphs of the morpheme "be"; which of these is used in a given utterance is not determined by the speaker but by the context; for example, the allomorph "am" occurs only together with "I."

The morpheme as the "smallest semantic vehicle" (Jakobson and Halle, 1956, p. 3) is not the lowest level of decision making. The morpheme "toe," phonemically /to/, can be further analyzed into units, which—although they no longer *contain* meaning—still *convey* meaning. If instead of /o:/ we choose /i:/, we signal a different meaning: "tea."

This "articulation at the second level" (Martinet) into units of sound, the *phonemes,* again makes it possible to use decision making as a criterion: for each unit a particular choice must be made; what is selected through one such act of decision, constitutes a unit.

The first articulation may be found in nearly all symbol systems, whereas the possibility of the lower-level articulation is the mark only of human language (Malmberg, 1963). It is therefore possible to construct signs and messages of infinite length from a small number of units which themselves are not signs.

This dual articulation is so fundamental to language that Martinet has placed it in the center of his definition of language. "A language is a medium of communication according to which human experience is analyzed, differently in each community, into units (monemes) with a semantic content and a phonic shape. This phonic shape, in its turn, is articulated in distinctive and successive units (phonemes) whose number in a given language is fixed and whose nature and mutual relations also vary from language to language" (1962, p. 26). In the same way Schnelle (1970) views this double articulation, i.e., "the fusing of meaning conveying units from purely meaning differentiating units, the phonemes and graphemes,'' as an essential characteristic of *the* language.

The great merit of this dual articulation is the economy that is thus attained. With the help of some 12 to 65 phonemes on the second level and some thousands of morphemes on the first it is possible to say everything that ever has been or ever will be spoken. The number of phonemes and the length of morphemes stand in a relationship to each other which can easily be established on the grounds of information theory. If a language had only a small number of phonemes, the morphemes must correspondingly be longer (i.e., consist of more phonemes) in order to be mutually exclusive. If it had a large number of phonemes, the phonemes would be less easy to differentiate (Carroll, 1964a).

In *phonetics* we have become acquainted with a discipline which investigates the physical characteristics of human speech sounds in their own right (Bühler).

Phonology is concerned with those aspects of speech-sounds that are relevant for the purpose of sign-functioning. The development of phonology has been decisively influenced by the Russian prince Trubetzkoy (1929) and the so-called Prague Circle, a group with which, incidentally, Karl Bühler was closely associated. Phonology classifies the sounds of a language according to the smallest units which account for differences between various utterances in this language.

With the concept of the phoneme we have moved once more into the neighborhood of Bühler's arguments on the nature and function of the sign. The example with which Bühler in his *Sprachtheorie* introduces the phoneme makes this clear:

> Suppose two persons agree to communicate by means of flag signals. In the code they arrange, the size and shape of the flags are irrelevant, only the shade of the color matters. Three grades of color saturation are agreed upon as relevant for meaning. Firstly, the shades of the black-white range with the least degree of saturation have meaning A; secondly, an intermediate degree of saturation is said to always have meaning B, but whether the color is sky-blue, pink or brown does not matter. Thirdly, the most saturated colors always have meaning C. Whether in a particular case a rich red, blue, green, or yellow appears makes no difference.

> Supposing one of the partners wishes to send message C, the weather, his mood or his supply of flags may dictate whether he chooses dark-red, dark-yellow, dark-green, or dark-blue. Thus, weather, mood, or supply influence the particular choice, and yet are irrelevant for the sign function of the flags.

Let us now move from this hypothetical example to a concrete illustration. A West-Caucasian language has vowel sounds not unlike those of German. Among them, for example, are the sounds /u/, /y/ and /i/. But whereas in German it is possible to distinguish two words through the contrast of /u/ and /i/, e.g., "Tusche" (India ink) vs. "Tische" (tables), this is not possible in the West-Caucasian language, because in this language /u/, /y/ and /i/ have no distinguishing or diacritical significance. In German /u/ and /i/ function as two different phonemes; in the West-Caucasian language they belong to the same phoneme.

It follows that phonology recognizes in the phoneme those aspects of speech sounds which—in the original sense of the term—are significant, i.e., sign-forming, or distinctive within a code. Besides these significant differences there are many insignificant ones. In English the /l/ in "light" and "feel" are produced differently; nevertheless the difference in meaning of the two words does not depend upon this difference in articulation. In Russian, however, these two forms of the same sound must be clearly distinguished, or else misunderstandings might arise. In English these sounds are different *allophones* of the same phoneme; in Russian they are two different phonemes.

In English it does not matter whether /t/ is aspirated or not. In the words "top" and "stop" the difference in the /t/ is not used as a distinguishing mark. Whereas in English the aspirated and nonaspirated /t/ are allophones of the same phoneme, in Chinese and several other languages they are two different phonemes.

The notion that a phoneme can be considered as a class or category of allophones, and a morpheme as a class of allomorphs, links up with two interesting lines of thought. One of these takes us back to Saussurian "differences and likenesses": the production and perception of sounds is channelled through a sorting device which disregards irrelevant differences and classifies sounds according to criteria which matter in the particular language. These criteria must therefore be *acquired*.

The other classification of morphemes and phonemes can be related to the *constancy phenomenon* well known in general psychology. The form constancy of a table as rectangular, however distorted it may appear on the retina, is clearly analogous. Whatever /l/ sounds like, provided it is clearly differentiated from, say, /m/ and /k/, we disregard any distortion.

Bühler's introductory example of flag signals starts from the assumption that the partners have made an agreement. We must now consider the situation of an anthropologist who visits an unknown tribe and wants to find out what variations are meaningful. In this situation, which is often referred to in the American literature, it is customary to operate with the notion of the "native speaker." A speaker for whom the language in question is the first language is asked to repeat the relevant utterances. Or the anthropologist copies him and finds out what copy is acceptable as repetition and what therefore would be tolerated as allophonic variation or, alternatively, what would constitute a change in meaning. An English native speaker would tolerate it if "right" were pronounced "roight" but he would reject it if it was pronounced "rot."

At first sight this procedure appears simple and unambiguous, but it conceals a psychological problem: much depends on the motivations of the native speaker. If he thinks he is being tested for his auditory discrimination, he will declare "right" and "roight" as different. In no way is the native speaker simply an automatic identifier of differences as he is characterized by structuralistic linguistics, which is concerned only with identities and differences. (For a further discussion of this issue, cf. Hörmann, 1976.)

A more difficult problem can be illustrated by the following example from German. Suppose an anthropologist in an investigation on the German language wants to compare "Donnerwetter" (thunderstorm) without aspirated initial /d/ with "Donnerwetter!", with aspirated initial /dh/, uttered as an emotive expression (Heavens, Good gracious) in order to find out whether unaspirated and aspirated /d/ in word-initial position are distinct phonemes or allophones. He will therefore ask his informant whether there is a difference in meaning. The answer to this question will depend upon how widely the concept of "meaning" is interpreted. This issue takes us back to an earlier point in our argument: we are reminded of Bühler's distinction between symbol, symptom, and signal or of the division into denotative and connotative meaning, and of the discussion on the distinction between language and expression.

Another aspect, illustrated by the last example, is that a phoneme is not only what we globally refer to as a vowel or consonant, but it may also be the intensity, pitch, or duration of a sound. Thus, in Italian, *fatto* must be distinguished from *fa:tto*.

By introducing the phoneme as a functional unit, phonology has effectively reduced the multiplicity inherent in the acoustic events. Yet, the complicated interplay of contrasts and identities which is at the basis of this element leads to the further question of whether the distinction between two phonemes can be made more tangible. The minimal difference is a so-called *distinctive feature*. This term originated in the studies of the Prague Circle, in particular in the work of Roman Jakobson who later lived in the United States. According to this view, a phoneme is characterized as a bundle of distinctive features. One phoneme is separated from another by at least one such feature. In this conception the distinctive features can be regarded as the atoms of linguistic structure (Malmberg, 1963). The addition, exchange or subtraction of a single distinctive feature is in effect a qualitative jump at the phonemic level: it converts one phoneme into another.

The heuristic value of this further division into distinctive features is the following: a feature which distinguishes one pair of phonemes is likely to differentiate also another pair. Thus /t/ and /d/ are distinguished by the feature voiced/unvoiced; but the same feature distinguishes also /p/ and /b/.

By comparing in a given language each phoneme with every other phoneme it is possible to work out which bundle of distinctive features forms (or better: defines) the phoneme in question. Table 1 describes such a grouping for English.

Table 1. Jakobson-Fant-Halle's analytic transcription of the phonemes of English (received pronunciation). "The phonemes may be broken down into the inherent distinctive features which are the ultimate signals" (preliminaries).

	o	a	e	u	ə	i	l	ŋ	ʃ	ʃ̂	k	ʒ	ʒ̂	g	m	f	p	v	b	n	s	θ	t	z	ð	d	h	#
1. Vocalic/Nonvocalic	+	+	+	+	+	+	+	−	−	−	−	−	−	−	−	−	−	−	−	−	−	−	−	−	−	−	−	−
2. Consonantal/Nonconsonantal	−	−	−	−	−	−	+	+	+	+	+	+	+	+	+	+	+	+	+	+	+	+	+	+	+	+	−	−
3. Compact-Diffuse	+	+	+	−	−	−		+	+	+	+	+	+	+	−	−	−	−	−	−	−	−	−	−	−	−		
4. Grave/Acute	+	+	−	+	+	−		+	−	−	+	−	−	+	+	+	+	+	+	−	−	−	−	−	−	−		
5. Flat/Plain	+	−		+	+	−																						
6. Nasal/Oral								+							+					+								
7. Tense/Lax									+	+	+	−	−	−		+	+	−	−		+	+	+	−	−	−	+	
8. Continuant/Interrupted									+	−	−	+	−	−		+	−	+	−		+	+	−	+	+	−		
9. Strident/Mellow									+	+	−	+	+	−		+	−	+	−		+	−	+	+	−	−		

From Malmberg, 1967, p. 118.

To sum up, the phoneme consists of a *complex* or bundle of features, whereas the morpheme consists of a sequence of phonemes (Lüdtke, 1961).

The hierarchical structure of distinctive features as far as the syllable is described by Jakobson and Halle in the following terms: "The distinctive features are aligned into simultaneous bundles called phonemes; phonemes are concatenated into sequences; the elementary pattern underlying any grouping of phonemes is the syllable . . . . The pivotal principle of syllable structure is the contrast of successive features within the syllable. One part of the syllable stands out from the others. It is mainly the contrast vowel vs. consonant which is used to render one part of the syllable more prominent" (1956, p. 20).

In recent years Jakobson's line of approach has been further developed in an interesting way. If we look at the table of distinctive features it will be seen that each of these qualities is two-valued: voiced/unvoiced, nasal/oral, etc.

It follows that the composition of a phoneme can be represented as a series of two-valued judgments. This observation leads to the analogy of the computer which also works with binary operations. Jakobson regards the principle of the binary opposition as a fundamental characteristic of his system. According to this theory, the perception of a phoneme can be regarded as a sequence of yes-no decisions on each distinctive feature of the bundle of features which make up a particular phoneme. The English phoneme /p/ could be described by the following properties: consonantal +, plosive +, voiced −, grave +, nasal −.

This approach lends itself particularly well to an analysis in terms of information theory. Miller (1956, p. 83 f.) has related the number of distinctive features to the channel capacity of the human; that is, the basic limitation of the capacity to cope in a given period with more than a restricted number of stimuli. An increase in the number of distinctive features would inevitably lead to a slowing down of speech. The number of distinctive features which differentiate neighboring consonants is regarded by Saporta as a compromise between the speaker's striving towards simplicity of articulation (he does not want to change the position of his vocal apparatus too frequently) and the demands of the hearer for the largest possible number of differences in order to be able to choose with greatest ease.

The characterization of phonemes as bundles of distinctive features was introduced into phonology by Jakobson. There are relatively few such elementary features, and the variation in phonemes evolves from the different combinations of such elementary units. This approach plays an important part in psychology generally and in psycholinguistics in particular. One assumes here that complex visual or cognitive phenomena can be analyzed in terms of the elementary features, e.g., "round/angular," "horizontal/vertical," "bent/straight," but also in semantic terms "animate/inanimate," "solid/liquid," etc.

Later, when we discuss psychological semantics, we will have to examine this issue in some detail. A good introduction to this topic can be found in Neisser (1967).

From the morpheme, the unit of Martinet's first level, we have moved to the next smaller unit, the phonemes, and finally to the distinctive features. If we now return to the first level, it is also possible to turn in the opposite direction, towards larger units. We first come across the *syllable* which stands in a peculiar relationship to the morpheme. Both generally consist of several phonemes, but the syllable is not clearly related to meaning. In the syllable, the possible sequences of phonemes are restricted by rules (Lüdtke, 1961). The word "tigers" consists of two syllables "ti-gers" which separately contain no distinct meaning. But the same word also consists of two morphemes: tiger + s both of which, by definition, have meaning (e.g., "s" means plural).

We therefore now turn to those structures which regulate the order of appearance of morphemes. In a given language how can morphemes be put together into meaningful utterances?

The answer to this question is the object of *grammar;* that is, the combinations of language. Within grammar the distinction is made between morphology and syntax.

Morphology is concerned with combinations below the level of word, while syntax deals with those above it. Morphology and syntax are closely connected with each other, because the syntactic structure of a sentence influences the morphological structure of the words in the sentence.

We thus come to the peculiar problem of the role of the unit *word* in linguistics. The nonlinguist is inclined to regard the word as the most obviously defined linguistic unit because there is the evident discreteness manifested in the written form. Here it should be pointed out that in all linguistic and psycholinguistic studies it is taken for granted that there is not necessarily a consistent relationship between speech and written language. In contrast to the layman, the linguist, who is equally interested in languages, written, for example, in syllabaries and ideographic scripts, has great difficulties in finding a definition of the word which is equally applicable to all languages.

The first attempt which is nearest to the popular view is to define the word semantically or by its content, i.e., to identify the word with the concept which it designates. This leads quickly into those difficulties which can best be characterized by a remark made by Sapir, according to which there is a word in Nootka which must be translated, "I have been accustomed to eat twenty round objects (for example, apples) while engaged in (doing so and so)" (quoted from Carroll, 1955, p. 40). It would hardly be possible to treat this meaning as a unit.

It is therefore better to attempt once again a formal definition. A common one is Bloomfield's: "A word is a minimum free form." This means that what can stand on its own is a "free form." For example, "child" is a free form. Although "-ish" is meaningful—it indicates "relating to," "befitting"—it cannot be used independently; it is a bound form: "childish" is therefore a word, because it cannot be divided any more into parts *each* of which is both meaningful and independent. Although this definition has wide application it, too, runs into difficulties. For example, "je" ("I" in French) would not be a word according to Bloomfield, because it is not a free form. It is always used with a verb. If "I" is to be used independently, "moi" is employed.

Another quite serviceable definition is the formal one offered by Lüdtke (1961), according to which a word is that smallest unit which is at once a complex of syllables and of morphemes. "Tiger" is a word because the division into morphemes (one morpheme) coincides with the division into syllables (two syllables).

The principles of classifications in morphology are also formal. Whatever has the same distributional value within an utterance is placed in the same class. Identity or difference of distributional value is established by tests of substitution and interchange.

From the perspective of psycholinguistics, syntax is of greater interest than morphology. Syntax is the study of the relationships of signs to each other, of the role of word categories within a sentence; it is that "part of grammar which determines the order of elements" (Engel, quoted by Lewandowski, 1975).

The syntactic unit is the sentence. It is the all-encompassing linguistic unit, which depends only relatively indirectly, but not unimportantly, on the broad context surrounding it. (This would be the case, for example, where previous mention of a name leads to the use of a pronoun in a subsequent sentence.) Within a sentence, smaller linguistic units of varying levels are organized according to particular rules, and interlaced with each other. Thus the sentence is the playing field of grammar.

We are here approaching the concept of grammar "from the bottom up" as it were, i.e., beginning with the smaller units. Hence the emphasis on classification and combination of units within a sentence. On the other hand, the sentence can also be viewed as a primary unit itself, which in turn determines the role of its individual components (subject, predicate, in the accusative). In a way the sentence is, therefore, starting point and end point of linguistic analysis. Later we will introduce the notion that grammar represents that system of knowledge that permits the generation of all grammatically correct (and none of the incorrect) sentences of a language.

For now let us stay with the combinations of elements. In its usual form, grammar describes each individual sentence by identifying, labeling, and classifying the linguistic elements within the sentence as well as the relationship of these elements to each other. It is a kind of classification system (v. Johnson, 1965) for the description of the elements as well as defining the relations which are present between the elements in the particular sentence. The fact that grammar is in a certain way the nucleus of the study of language has long been recognized by linguists. For example, Glinz expresses it as follows:

> "Language is . . . mental organization within a community. It is based on the fact that mental concepts and attitudes to experience are defined by being linked with characteristic sound patterns. But this mental organization, however pervasive its effect, is in general not consciously experienced by the language user. Grammar, since its beginnings in ancient Greek times, sets itself a threefold task. It makes the user conscious of this common mental organization; it elaborates its structural laws and fundamental units, and it elucidates its overall organization down to the *minutiae* of each determining quantum, if one may use this analogy from physics" (Glinz, 1965, p. 47). Weisgerber expresses these ideas in a similar vein: "The task of grammar as one of the most ancient studies of humanity borders almost on the impossible: it attempts to create an awareness of a mental condition of human existence. Not only is the range of this condition beyond our grasp but its inner workings are also impenetrable" (1962a, I, p. 403).

Our first encounter with the concept of grammar occurred via the route of examining the problems of linguistic units. Here the sentence appears to be the encompassing unit, which obeys its own rules. A logical next step leads to the question, What are the *psychological* effects and implications of the combination of *linguistic* units? We will examine this in the next chapter.

For now we shall once more focus on the concept of grammar, this time guided by a somewhat different frame of thought. After all, a grammar not only describes how linguistic units may be combined, it also *prescribes* how they *must* be combined. In other words, grammar is a set of rules which the sentences of a language must obey in order to be accepted as correct. The predominant goal of modern linguistics is to evolve a system of rules that is able to fulfill these requirements. This goal can also be formulated in terms of a question: What does one have to know about a language in order to generate all of the sentences which a native speaker of that language would accept as grammatically well-formed, and not those which the native speaker would reject as being not well-formed?

This is the formulation of the key question on grammar by the so-called "generative grammar," which since the mid-1950s has become the most influential school of linguistics. Let us consider what is meant by this. Every native speaker has an intuitive knowledge of his language which enables him to generate and understand well-formed sentences. Undoubtedly this knowledge cannot consist of stored descriptions of all of the possible sentences in that language. If that were so, it would no doubt be simple to conceptualize the production in terms of simple selection, but this theory would be unable to explain how sentences which have never been heard before can be generated and understood. The fact that language is creative rules out the assumption that we carry within us a catalog of complete sentences.

If it is not possible to conceive of grammar as an enumerative description of all grammatically well-formed sentences, it becomes necessary to view it as a system of rules, according to which *all* grammatically well-formed sentences (and *only* those) of a language may be *generated*. The native speaker then has an intuitive knowledge of the rules according to which grammatically well-formed sentences are generated in his language. It is the goal of Chomsky, who founded the school of generative grammar, to develop a rational model which reflects this intuitive knowledge. Because this type of linguistics has had a decisive influence on psycholinguistics (and beyond that on other areas of psychology), we shall examine it in more detail below.

Chomsky characterizes this intuitive knowledge of the native speaker by using the following example. The sentence,

Colorless green ideas sleep furiously

appears perhaps somewhat strange, but it is nevertheless correct in the sense in which the following word order is incorrect:

Green sleep ideas furiously colorless.

This intuitive ability to differentiate between a "well-formed" and a "not so well-formed" sentence (more correctly between a well-formed sentence and a not well-formed string of words) must now be transformed into a system which functions without intuition, but can make the same distinction as the intuitive knowledge.

By contrasting the two lines above we can see that the grammatical well-formedness, which Chomsky is trying to systematize, has nothing to do with "meaning." (This is one of the targets for criticism of generative linguistics; but for the moment we do not need to explore that further.) In order to transform intuitive knowledge into a rational system, Chomsky introduces an important conceptual distinction: competence and performance.

Competence refers to the knowledge possessed by an *ideal* speaker/ listener about his own language, which permits him to differentiate between grammatical and ungrammatical (not well-formed) sentences. It is important to note that the concept of competence represents an idealization. "Linguistic theory is concerned primarily with an ideal speaker-listener in a completely homogeneous speech-community, who knows his language perfectly and is unaffected by such grammatically irrelevant conditions as memory limitations, distractions, shifts of attention and interest, and errors (random or characteristic) in applying his knowledge of the language in actual performance" (Chomsky, 1965, p. 3).

This speaker/listener, who is of interest to the linguist and whose knowledge is referred to as "competence," is, as we see, a fairly abstract construction. In contrast, performance is closer to reality. It could be defined as "competence plus human weaknesses," or as that which occurs in the verbal behavior of a real speaker/listener. The hierarchy of competence and performance is unambiguous for the generative linguist: "investigation of performance will proceed only so far as understanding of underlying competence permits" (Chomsky, 1965, p. 10). In this way generative linguistics takes a position vis-á-vis everyday verbal reality, which can easily lead to confusion and/or difficulties. A competence theory cannot be challenged either on the basis that sentences generated by it are not acceptable to a "real" native speaker, or on the basis that sentences which it does not generate are acceptable to a "real" native speaker. In either case the source of incongruity can be attributed to performance, which is of course subject to error (for further discussion of this problem, see Hörmann, 1976). This calls into question whether a competence theory can be empirically validated and the extent to which the theory can make predictions about actual verbal behavior.

What, then, constitutes the competence of an ideal speaker/listener of a language? The standard model, proposed by Chomsky, consists of a base-component and a transformational component based on the former. This dual formation is introduced in order to facilitate differentiation of two levels of language, deep structure and surface structure. The following sentences have similar surface structures, but totally different deep structures:

John is easy to please.

John is eager to please.

The structural meanings such as subject-of are anchored in the deep structure which is generated by the basic component of the model. This is then followed by the action of the transformational component of the model which produces the surface structure by reordering the elements in the deep structure, as is required in such transformations as negation. Transformations such as negation, passive voice, question form, etc., generally leave the deep structure of a sentence more or less unchanged, but they are responsible for the apparent modifications which one deep structure may undergo, as is the case in the following sentences:

Fritz sells a car to Franz.

A car is sold by Fritz to Franz.

Is Fritz not selling a car to Franz?

The surface structure of the sentence, which already contains information about the order of the words, is finally subjected to the third component of the model, namely the *phonological* component which provides the necessary program for the proper articulation (Fig. 10).

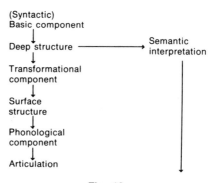

Fig. 10

If we now raise the question, How does the meaning of the sentence enter into the model? the answer is, not at all. Chomsky says that the deep structure is semantically interpreted by means of a process that he does not specify. The perfunctory treatment of semantics has naturally led to criticisms and corrections of the standard model that we have just described. But before we discuss these, let us look in greater detail at the implications of the standard model. In attempting to analyze a sentence within the framework of generative linguistics, the search will likely center first on the transformations which the sentence has undergone in the process of being generated, until one arrives at one form which approximately corresponds to the deep structure.[2] It is then analyzed in terms of its constituent parts according to what are called "rules of phrase structure." For example, the sentence, "A child fears the dog," is composed of the constituent parts shown in Fig. 11.

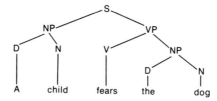

Fig. 11. S = sentence; NP = noun phrase; VP = verb phrase; D = determiner, e.g., article; N = noun; V = verb.

Thus the sentence is analyzed according to certain substitution or rewrite rules, in order that its immediate constituents become apparent:

$$S \rightarrow NP + VP$$
$$NP \rightarrow D + N$$
$$VP \rightarrow V + NP$$

$$N \rightarrow \text{Stove, chain, dog, wool, child} \ldots$$

[2] Strictly speaking, it is impossible to express deep structure in words.

From our example we can see that the VP contains a second NP as a dependent part. The rewrite analysis terminates in a lexicon (dictionary) which is articulated in terms of grammatical categories (N, V, D, . . .), which is also part of the competence, i.e., the knowledge, which a speaker has about his language.

Thus we see that generative grammar is a phrase-structure grammar to which is attached a transformational component. This combination results in a very parsimonious system which, from this point of view, is also psychologically interesting. For example, if someone has learned the transformation required for negation he is then in a position to convert any affirmative sentence into a negative one. He does not need to learn or even generate an affirmative and a negative form for each sentence.

> Brown has pointed out that there is an analogy to the above mentioned transformation of a sentence in the so-called conditioned reaction investigated by Lashley. A rat can learn to select from the two signals △ ▽ the triangle which stands on its base. It can also be trained to accept the reversal of this meaning if the triangles appear against a striped background ▲ ▽ . The stripes transform the total meaning and therefore function in an analogous manner to the above mentioned negation.

"A generative grammar is a system of explicit rules that assign to each sequence of phones, . . . a structural description that contains all information about how this sequence of phones is represented on each of the several linguistic levels—in particular, information as to whether this sequence of phones is a properly formed or *grammatical* sentence and if not, in what respect it deviates from well-formedness" (Chomsky, 1961, p. 220).

From this programmatic claim of the generative linguists we can tell what they are willing to undertake, but it also shows what they do not intend to undertake. The grammatical description of a sentence should contain the structure of *linguistic* information, where linguistic is synonymous with syntactical. A sentence is grammatically correct (i.e., well-formed) if the words that constitute it are placed in the proper order according to their particular word-class (noun, adjective, verb). Syntax dominates grammar.

In contrast let us make quite clear that *psychology* of language addresses a much broader problem area. Here we are not just interested in the emergence and the effects of syntactical well-formedness, but also in determining the conditions and the functions of the use of speech in general. Let us return once more to the standard model of Chomsky that was discussed above. Based on this model, an analysis of the sentence

A child fears the dog

would make sure that a noun appears at that point in the sentence where it is required according to the rules of the English language. It does not, however, assure that a noun which fits in terms of its meaning has been selected from the large lexical class N. If every member of the class N is equally entitled to appear in the relevant place in the tree diagram (and therefore in the sentence), then we are unable to avoid sentences like

A stove fears the dog

(and, of course, this would also be true for "colorless green ideas sleep furiously"). Chomsky's standard model is willing to put up with *semantic anomalies* of this kind. Meaning, that which differentiates between "stove" and "child," is added later, by an additional step, called semantic interpretation. However, all we know about this semantic interpretation is that through it the sequence of constituent parts is to be assigned meaning.

> But it is difficult to draw a line between a grammar which is essentially identical with syntax and a content-oriented semantic. Bühler has pointed out that in German compound nouns it is meaning which determines how the vaguely indicated syntactical relationship between the parts of the compound is to be understood. As an illustration he points out the change in syntactical function of the morpheme "back" (German for "bake") in such compounds as "Back-ofen" (an oven for baking), "Back-stein" (brick: a stone which has been fired or baked), "Back-huhn" (a roasting chicken: a chicken which can be roasted), "Back-pulver" (baking powder: powder with which one can bake). Thirty years later Putnam wrote, "The reason that we would add a category to our grammar is mainly that it enables us to note a larger number of regularities. If these regularities concern only a very restricted class of sentences, we prefer not to call them grammatical regularities; but if they apply to a large number of sentences or to the use of important classes of morphemes, e.g. pronouns or articles, it is traditionally more acceptable to call them grammar rules. From this point of view it is more a matter of usefulness and convenience and certainly not a genuinely theoretical question where to draw the dividing line between grammar and semantics" (Putnam, 1965, p. 1120).

The most important modification of Chomsky's standard model arises from the very fact that the dividing line between a syntax-oriented grammar and a meaning-oriented semantic cannot be drawn clearly. Katz and Fodor (1963) describe a framework for a semantic theory that would fit into a generative model but that would also augment it in several places. These authors also try to develop a system of rules which would enable the competent speaker/listener to distinguish between well-formed and not-so-well-formed sentences. The modifications they suggest must be made to the model in those places where it gets into difficulty because it totally ignores matters of content.

At issue are three points: (a) semantic ambiguity, (b) semantic anomaly, and (c) paraphrase. An example of semantic ambiguity is the sentence, "The bill is large." The listener, even if he knows the grammar, does not know how to interpret this sentence. Does it describe a request for a large amount of money, or does it refer to a big beak? Here we can see that a grammatically (syntactically) correct, unambiguous sentence can be semantically ambiguous. A semantic theory must therefore make provisions that enable the speaker/listener to resolve such ambiguities. Semantic anomaly is another factor that may prove difficult for the competent speaker. Here again we have a sentence that is perfectly well-formed according to grammatical criteria. Chomsky already referred to this problem by means of his well-known example of the furiously sleeping green ideas. For purposes of the discussion here, let us take the sentence:

The paint is silent.

The listener who is competent in the English language (and not just familiar with its syntax) will judge this sentence to be somewhat strange or anomalous, in any case, less well-formed than the sentence:

The paint is wet.

"The paint is silent" represents a semantic anomaly because "silent" generally refers only to living things and cannot be attributed to paint.

Finally, the third point at which a syntax-oriented grammar has to be supplemented by a semantic component is paraphrase. The model must include provisions which lead to the recognition that the following two sentences have the same meaning:

There are two chairs in this room.

There are two things in this room both of which are chairs.

(Of course, these two sentences have the same meaning only in one respect, but at this point we shall not enter into a discussion of a differentiation of the concept of meaning.)

How is a semantic theory going to deal with these three goals? Katz and Fodor suggest that the structure of the lexicon (which for Chomsky was articulated only grossly into classes like noun, verb, determiner), could be further differentiated by dividing the meaning of each word into *elements of meaning*. The specific constellation of these elements (semantic markers or features) would, so to speak, define the word. A componential analysis of this kind is not new in the field of semantics. Lounsbury, for example, compiled the words:

man, woman, child
stallion, mare, foal
bull, cow, calf

in order to articulate the dimensions of meaning for "masculine," "feminine," "child-like" or "human," "horse-like," and "cattle-like."

Katz and Fodor attempt to define the semantic markers in such a way that the meaning of a sentence evolves from the summing or integration of these elements of meaning of the words of which the sentence is composed. Their approach is modeled after phonetics, where the phonemes are defined as bundles of elementary distinctive features. According to this approach, the meaning of the word "man" can be defined in terms of the following series of semantic characteristics:

physical object
animated
human
adult
male

The markers which serve to identify "man" also serve along with other features to identify other words in the lexicon. That is to say, the semantic features form the dimensions of the lexicon, which is the store for the vocabulary of the speaker. Each word is then defined by the dimensions on which it is localized. It seems reasonable to relate the concept of the lexicon structured in this manner to the similarly structured memory. One may ask whether the structures of our memory are identical to those structures which the linguist proposes for the lexicon. We are going to look at these and similar questions in some detail later on.

Let us for the moment return to Katz and Fodor and their goal of constructing a semantic theory which would fill the gaps in the purely syntactic theory of Chomsky. How can semantic ambiguities be resolved, how can semantic anomalies be prevented? The answer is as follows:

Attached to the semantic markers of the word are certain prescriptive conditions, the selection restrictions. Associated with the feature "inanimate," for example, is the selection restriction that it cannot be combined in a sentence with words which carry the label "animate." "Silent" has as one of its semantic features the marker "animate" and therefore cannot be combined with the word "paint" to form the anomalous sentence, "The paint is silent," because "paint" carries among others the feature "inanimate." By using these selection restrictions attached to the semantic markers, Katz and Fodor guarantee that a given sentence will contain only syntactic combinations of such words as are compatible with respect to their meaning. In doing this, however, they do make the assumption that the semantic features of a word are fixed in the lexicon of the competent speaker once and for all; and that therefore the combination of incompatible features in a sentence *must always* result in a semantic anomaly. Thus the fact that we are able to understand a metaphoric phrase like, "the smiling spring meadow," without the slightest feeling of anomaly is an important objection to this approach (cf. Hörmann, 1973). Neither Chomsky's model nor Katz and Fodor's modification contain provisions which assure that a metaphor is not analyzed according to the normal rules, thus becoming labeled an anomaly.

In the same way, most so-called idioms would not be correctly analyzed if they were processed according to the Chomsky-Katz-Fodor model. The sentence, "John had to bite the dust," is a typical example. Analyzing this sentence in terms of nominal and verbal phrase, etc., one finally reaches the lexical entries for "dust" and "bite" with their respective semantic features, which would not lead to a comprehension of the true meaning of the sentence. *In this case* the constituent parts of the sentence must not be understood separately, and the individual words must not be analyzed in terms of their semantic features, if one wants to comprehend the real meaning of the sentence, namely that "John had to die." Chafe (1970) presents an excellent analysis of this problem.

Pursuing this difficulty further, it becomes evident that it is necessary to assume yet another factor beyond grammar or syntax respectively. This factor determines whether, and how far, the analysis must be continued to assure comprehension of the sentence. This factor, which is also involved in distinguishing between anomaly and metaphor, was described in terms of the concept of "sense constancy" by Hörmann (1976). We find, on the one hand, that Katz and Fodor do attempt to include a semantic component in a generative theory of language, but this component is simply added to a basically syntax-oriented model. On the other hand, the school of "generative semantics," while retaining Chomsky's distinction between deep and surface structures, conceptualizes the deep structure in a way that is to a large extent semantic, or, more precisely, lying at a point prior to the differentiation of syntactics and semantics. Fillmore (1968a), for example, points to the fact that in the case of the sentence, "The man cuts the bread with the knife," it would be less appropriate to see it as a chain of subject, verb, object or as NP + VP, (that is true of innumerable other sentences as well), than to single out the predicate (to cut) and to determine the various roles (the so-called cases or arguments) which are implied by it. If there is talk about "cutting" we can expect to hear about an agent (the man) and a patient (the bread), and possibly an instrument (with the knife).

Depending on which and how many arguments belonging to a predicate are realized in a given sentence, they, together with certain prepositions, assume various positions in the surface structure of the sentence. For example, if in the case of the verb "cut" the role of the agent and of the instrument are to be filled, then the noun belonging to the instrument must carry the preposition "with": "The man cuts with the knife." If the agent role is vacant then the instrument can take the nominative role (the knife cuts).

This "generative semantics" becomes psychologically interesting because it attempts to analyze the basic structures of a sentence in terms of a few characteristic relationships between things and events. These have a great deal in common with the cognitive relations which man as a user of language sees between himself and the objects and events in the world. Is it possible that the basic structures of linguistic expression are the same as the basic structures of human perception and action?

We will encounter these and similar questions frequently later on in this book. For now we conclude our description of the linguistic tools that are required in order to examine the relationships between linguistic and psychological events and structures.

CHAPTER 4

Language, Information, and Communication

The concept of information—Code—Information value and uncertainty—The bit—Utilization of the communication channel—Classification and identification—The motor theory of speech perception—Analysis by synthesis—Interference in the speech channel—The concept of channel capacity.

In the previous chapters we first introduced the concept of sign and then dealt with the concept of linguistic unit. We learned that linguistic expressions can be viewed as chains of signs or instructions which direct the selection of particular units. All this brings us closer to the concept of information, as it was first defined by Shannon in his information theory. Since 1948 this concept has been widely adopted within psychology, and particularly within psycholinguistics. We now turn to this concept, even though in most recent times it has become apparent that it is not the universal key to psycholinguistics as was assumed at first.

In order to see the place of this concept in psycholinguistics in the right perspective, let us briefly remind ourselves of the argument which was presented in the Introduction. We noted an area of indeterminacy between the spontaneity of the organism and its vital space. The imbalance between the two poles "self" and "world" appeared to us as the generator which keeps the business of life going. As human life is characterized by the existential fact that *world,* to a large extent, is represented by other persons, this imbalance between them generates language. There is first of all an imbalance of intent, and secondly an imbalance of information. A knows more than B; A can transmit to B what B lacks.

The concept of information has the function of making quantitatively measurable what it is that must be transmitted so as to remove uncertainty. "The idea of transmission of information is based upon the polarity between transmitter and receiver" (Schmetterer, 1960, p. 156).

An act of communication, e.g., a telegram, a letter or a speech, *is* information or *contains* information. It is the "or" in the preceding sentence, as v. Weizsäcker (1959) has shown, that is a particularly good starting point for an introduction to a discussion of the concept of information. The following remarks present the main lines of v. Weizsäcker's argument.

Is the telegram information or does it *contain* information? Do we mean by information the printer's ink on the telegram form, i.e., something objectively given, or is it the content of consciousness which develops as the telegram is being read, i.e., something subjectively experienced? It is, in fact, neither. The printer's ink did not come through the cable. What the sender wrote is not the same stuff the receiver of the message holds in his hand. And it may also be assumed that the content of the mind of the sender is different from that of the receiver. Neither printer's ink nor mental content have been transmitted. "Information is not a particular act of consciousness, but something that the act of consciousness 'knows', something that is held in common by the two persons, however different their minds may be. We are getting accustomed to looking upon information as a third thing, different from mind and matter. This discovery is an old truth in a new guise. It is the Platonic *eidos*, the Aristotelian form, dressed up in such a way that even man in the twentieth century can get a glimmer of it" (v. Weizsäcker, 1959, p. 44 f.).

The notion of information belongs, therefore, to the area of abstraction in which the concepts of language or of grammar are located also.

Information is structure. Carrier of this structure may be printer's ink, sound waves, or electric impulses. The telegram, sent by cable, and the telegram, read over the telephone by the operator, contain the same information.

With this proposition the concept of information is already narrowed down. Supposing I live in Toronto and receive a long-distance call from New York and hear that it is cold there, then information in the sense in which it interests us here is contained in this message. But what I hear contains yet another kind of information. The voice tells me something about the speaker: it is the voice of a woman who must have lived in New York for a long time; she also sounds rather bored. The sound spectrum, the speed of utterance, and characteristic pauses, etc., may lead me to the conviction that the speaker is my aunt Mathilda.

In this sense a communicative act contains information if and only if, by means of this act, uncertainty is removed or reduced in the receiver. Thus if I come into the house shivering and I am told, "It is cold outside," I have received no information, because I, as the receiver of this message, was not in a state of uncertainty with regard to its content.

> It should be added that the uncertainty of the receiver must be matched by the unambiguity of the message. v. Weizsäcker has elucidated this point with the following illustration, "The sentence of Heraclitus 'The father of all things is war' can be a profound truth, only because it contains no information, and it can contain no information because the words 'father' and 'war' in it are not unambiguous. If they referred to what they normally mean, the statement would indeed be nonsense. It cannot even be said that they have simply been redefined, so that they could be considered as speculative concepts in the

philosophy of Heraclitus. It should rather be assumed that it is in the nature of genuine speculative concepts not to be unambiguous'' (1959, p. 48).

Information, then, in the sense in which the term is used here presupposes a state of uncertainty in the hearer and unambiguity of the message. If we toss a coin, it is uncertain whether it will come down ''heads'' or ''tails.'' If someone looks and then says ''heads,'' the hearer receives information, for the unambiguous message has removed uncertainty. The amount of information, the information content of the message, equals the amount of uncertainty that has been reduced through the transmission of information.

The same facts will now be considered from a slightly different point of view. Shannon, the initiator of information theory, characteristically served as a mathematician to the Bell Company, the large telephone and telegraph concern. His basic problem was to produce, at the output end of an information-transmission system, a message which at the input end had been selected for transmission. (It will shortly be seen that the formulation ''selected for transmission'' is of some importance.) The meaning of the transmitted message is of no concern to the communications engineer— another statement which is important for our discussion. The information content of a message must not be confused with the meaning of this message. Once a tossed coin has come down it has a definite content of information, i.e., one bit, regardless of whether the result of the toss might mean a man's death or paying for a round of drinks.

Shannon attempted to find an exact quantitative term for what is transmitted in a given communications system so as to be able to make an exact statement about the efficiency of the system. The communications engineer wishes to understand the utility of a transmission system.

In precise terms, therefore, what we are concerned with is not so much a theory of information as a theory of information *transmission*.

The basic model assumes that at the input end *one* message, out of several possible messages, is selected for transmission. If a coin is tossed, two messages are possible: heads or tails. Before the message reaches the output end of the channel, the receiver is in a state of uncertainty as to which of the two messages will reach him.

This has very important consequences: the receiver must know in advance which messages are possible. In other words, the receiver must have at his disposal the same repertoire of possible messages as the transmitter who selects from it the message to be sent (Fig. 12). This repertoire of possible

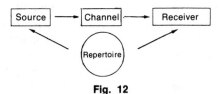

Fig. 12

information or available signs with their assignments of meaning is defined as *code*.

It may happen, however, that transmitter and receiver do not draw on identical repertoires, because the events which have led to the development of the repertoires are different in the biographies of sender and receiver. This situation can be represented by the diagram in Fig. 13.

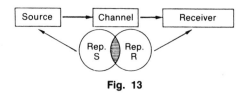

Fig. 13

In this case a communication is only possible to the extent to which the two repertoires overlap (based on Moles, 1963).

> Let us briefly digress once more to relate this to the organon model of Bühler (see pp. 21 f.). At first sight one would tend to assume that information is what is called the representational function in this model. But are "symbols" transmitted in a communication system? What is transmitted are "signals," i.e., instructions for action by the receiver, selection orders or commands according to which a receiver is to choose from his repertoire.
>
> Yet, the conclusion that information theory is concerned with the signal function of the linguistic sign would not be quite accurate. The behavior of the receiver, which is guided by *signals*, consists in the selection of *symbols*. In other words, the sharp division that Bühler makes between signal and symbol function (or between expression and representation) cannot be maintained here.

This fact has implications for psycholinguistics as well as for information theory. Information is certainly not identical with language. It presupposes language. Or to put it more precisely in the terms in which v. Weizsäcker has expressed it, "Anyone who talks about language must not forget that language can be used for information, and anyone who talks about information must never forget that language as information is only possible against the background of knowledge that language cannot be transformed into unambiguous information" (1959, pp. 52 f.).

This brings us to an important problem which currently is frequently neglected. If one views transmission of information as translation into a certain code (e.g., the translation of thought into a code of linguistic signs), then this process can function only if there is implicit agreement between speaker and listener concerning the prerequisites for the codification. One needs to know under what conditions a certain encoding rule is to be followed, and under what conditions it is not to be followed. But these rules for application of (encoding) rules principally cannot be part of the same code. Garfinkel (1972) carried out an ingenious study, showing that agreement concerning codification rules presupposes comprehension of the goal orientation of speaker and listener.[1]

This fact has far-reaching consequences. An explanation of linguistic events *must not* start with a description of a code of signs which are to be combined according to certain syntactical rules. Quite the contrary, every explanation of linguistic events must in a way begin "prior" to the code, it must reveal the tool-like character of the code. The code is an arsenal of tools which is put into action in a stream of events which is already in progress, and in this action responds to the more general demands of these events.

Let us now return to the basic model of information theory. The information about the face of the coin, i.e., which of the two possibilities has occurred, reduces to nil the uncertainty in the receiver. If two coins are tossed in succession four messages are possible: both heads; first heads, then tails; first tails, then heads; both tails. The uncertainty is greater than in the first example, so that the message when received, because it removes a higher degree of uncertainty, possesses a higher information value.

If the information value equals the uncertainty which is removed by the message, we go on to ask what determines the amount of uncertainty. The answer is: it is determined by the number of possible events. When a coin is tossed two events are possible; when a die is cast, there are six. The message concerning a coin contains less information than a message concerning a die.

Although these reflections may seem simple, they have far-reaching consequences. From them we can infer that, in the analysis of linguistic events, we must take into account not only what happens, but also what does *not* happen but might have happened. The amount of information depends on the relationship between the actual event and all other possible events. The question therefore arises whether perhaps the number of possible events might be used as a measuring unit of information. Accordingly, tossing a coin where two events are possible would yield two units of information. Two coins would produce four units. If three coins are tossed there are eight units. The number of units rises steeply. It would be more convenient to operate with a unit of measurement which increases at a uniform rate; in this case this is the logarithm.

The measuring unit for information is called "bit," an abbreviation for binary digit. It is the power to which two must be raised in order to obtain the number of equally likely possibilities. The information on the fall of the tossed coin removes the uncertainty with regard to which of two possible events has occurred. The message contains one bit of information; for $2^1 = 2$.

Another example may further illustrate the use of bit as an information measure. There is a well-known party game in which the players agree upon an

[1] There is little sense to speak here of meta-language. For a discussion of this problem, see Hörmann, 1976.

object which has to be discovered by a player who has, meanwhile, been sent out of the room. On his return this player is only allowed to ask questions in such a way that they can be answered by yes or no. To illustrate this, let us assume that, instead of a concrete object one of the 64 squares of a chessboard has been selected (Fig. 14). The questioner is supposed to find out which square has been chosen, and the object of the game is to do so in the most economical way, in other words, with the smallest number of questions.[2]

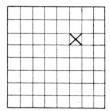

Fig. 14

How many questions are needed to reduce the questioner's uncertainty to nil? The answer is precisely six.
  1. Is it a square in the upper half? (Yes)
  2. Is it a square in the left half of the remainder? (No)
  3. Is it a square in the lower half of the sixteen remaining? (Yes)
  4. Is it a square in the right half of the eight remaining? (No)
  5. Is it one of the two right ones of the four remaining? (Yes)
  6. Is it the lower one of these two? (No)
Six yes-or-no decisions are needed to specify 64 equally probable possiblities. Six bits of information are required to reduce the uncertainty contained in this system to nil, for $64 = 2^6$.

In general terms: if the number of equally probable possibilities of a system is called m and the amount of required information H bits, then $m = 2^H$. Or expressed in another way, the number of bits equals the logarithm of the number of possibilities to the base of 2.

> *Logarithmus dualis* (logarithm to the base of two) means that in contrast to the usual logarithms it is not the figure 10 but 2 which is used as a base. This is an arbitrary decision; it is also possible to work in information theory with a decimal system. But the binary system has a number of advantages: apart from the one already mentioned that, with the doubling of the possibilities, uncertainty increases by one bit, one should mention above all the advantage in terms of communication engineering. The binary system which knows only yes or no or only the figures 0 and 1, is most convenient for communication engineering: if the current is *on*, this can represent 1, and if it is *off*, 0. The human nervous system seems to operate in a similar way: firing or no firing.

[2] It should be remembered that what interested Shannon was precisely a measure of the economic capacity of a communication system.

So far we have talked about systems in which each possibility is equally probable. In the tossing of an unbent coin heads or tails have equal probability p, viz, 1 divided by the number of possibilities m: in this case $1/2 = 0.5$. In the chess-board example each square had equal probability of having been selected, viz, 1/64. To express it in more general terms, the probability p of the appearance of a particular possibility is 1, divided by the number of possibilities m, or

$$p = \frac{1}{m}.$$

Therefore

$$m = \frac{1}{p}.$$

The content of information H had earlier been defined as $H = \log_2 m$, which can be rewritten as

$$H = \log_2 \frac{1}{p}.$$

This is now to be generalized to such cases where the various possibilities have different probabilities of appearance.

Since previously all possibilities were regarded as equally probable, we were able to summarize them in a single measure H. If now all possibilities are no longer equally probable, each requires its own measure of information: h_i is the information which results from the appearance of the possibility i. This is represented by

$$h_i = \log_2 \frac{1}{p_i}.$$

One example: a bent coin is tossed, which in 90 percent of tosses shows heads, and in 10 percent tails. The probability that it is heads is therefore $p_{Hd} = 0.9$; the probability that tails is uppermost is $p_T = 0.1$. Accordingly, the information which is contained in the message "heads" would be

$$h_{Hd} = \log_2 \frac{1}{0.9} = \log_2 1.11 = 0.15 \text{ bits.}$$

The information that is contained in "tails" is

$$h_T = \log_2 \frac{1}{0.1} = \log_2 10 = 3.22 \text{ bits.}$$

These two messages, therefore, do not contain an equal amount of information. This is quite easy to understand: in the bent coin we expect a priori "heads" in 90 percent of the throws, the message that it is "heads" is therefore not surprising; it removes little uncertainty. However, if it is "tails" we are very surprised.

We next inquire after the average information in a long series of tosses with the bent coin. Each message "heads" will contribute 0.15 bits to this average, whereas each message "tails" will contribute 3.22 bits. Now "heads" is likely to appear very much more frequently than "tails," because the probability of "heads" is 0.9, the probability of "tails" only 0.1. This fact must be taken into account in working out the average: "heads" must contribute nine times as much as "tails."

$$(0.90 \times 0.15) + (0.10 \times 3.22) = 0.47 \text{ bits}$$

This average value is again designated as H.

If this average value of 0.47 is compared with the information value of straight coins (1.0 bit) it will be seen that the tosses with a bent coin on the average yield less information than those with a straight coin. The results of tosses of a bent coin are less uncertain.

At this point we can find an interesting link between information theory and thermodynamics, especially with regard to the concept of "entropy." A system has maximal entropy when all its possible states are equally probable. In this situation uncertainty is at its maximum. In a system with less than maximal entropy some states are more probable than others and therefore their occurrence has lower information value.

What was calculated as average value here was based on the formula:

$$H = p_1 h_1 + p_2 h_2 + \ldots + p_x h_x$$

H is therefore the sum of all products: p multiplied by h;

$$H = \sum^{i} p_i h_i,$$

where i designates each possibility.

Earlier, h was equated with $\log_2 \frac{1}{p}$. In the above summation formula $\log_2 \frac{1}{p}$ can take the place of h. This yields the following:

$$H = \sum^{i} p_i \log_2 \frac{1}{p_i}.$$

In order to avoid fractions one can write:

$$H = -\sum^{i} p_i \log_2 p_i.$$

This is the well-known Shannon-Wiener measure of information.

The above presentation of the mathematical side of information theory (which leans heavily on the excellent introduction by Attneave, 1959) is sufficient for our purpose.

Let us remember that in order to employ concepts related to information theory we must know the sign repertoire (i.e., the code), the rules for employing the code, and the probability of the occurrence of the events which are to be symbolized by the signs of the code. It is unfortunately true that such concepts from information theory are employed in many psychological and sociological investigations, without meeting this prerequisite.

As a first step from pure information theory towards its application to psycholinguistics, let us now resume the arguments first developed in Chapter 3 where it was shown that our mechanism of perception classifies acoustic sounds as phonemes.

Information theory is applicable to discrete events. The die must fall on one of its six sides; in a wire the current is either on or off; there are no gradual transitions. Language, looked at from a linguistic or psycholinguistic angle, consists of such discrete events. A sound either is or is not in a certain class of phonemes. A graphic symbol is to be pronounced as a voiced or unvoiced sound. Viewed in this way the operations of information theory may be applied to language.

However, these facts look quite different from the point of view of the acoustician. If linguistic utterances are recorded, for instance, by means of an oscillograph or a spectrograph, no clear differentiations can be made between voiced and unvoiced or between "a" and "non-a." The acoustician describes the speech sound through a series of measurements, and these measurements are not discrete choices of an "either-or" character, but are variations on a continuous scale.

In the perceptual system of the receiver, the continuous input is analyzed into discrete events. The same process occurs in reverse order when we speak: the articulation process transforms the discrete sequence of inner events into the continuous variables of the acoustic phenomenon.

This process of transformation was described in such detail because psycholinguistics operates both with acoustic concepts, which describe continuous variables, and with linguistic ones, which describe discrete events. The processes of encoding and decoding are transformations from one to the other. The information the speaker transmits to the hearer is the command to adopt a certain state of mind or to switch his system into a particular state, e.g., either [i] or [e].

The next question is, How *complicated* can the command or message which is transmitted through the communication channel linking speaker and hearer be per time unit? The complexity of the message to be transmitted per unit of time depends upon the distinctions which the mechanism of perception is capable of handling in processing the sound signals which carry the message. That is to say, the answer to the above question is a task for information theory and psychophysics.

This can be made clear by an analogy from the field of vision. How much information can be transmitted through flag signals? Different flags could, among other distinctions, be varied according to size. This means that as many distinctions can be made as the visual apparatus can handle. The observer would not be able to distinguish two flags, one of which measured 1030 cm² and the other 1029 cm²; hence difference in size cannot be used to transmit different messages with these two flags. Color and shape, besides size, could have been used as distinguishing features.

It is accepted that the sound event can be analyzed according to frequency, amplitude, phase and duration. Frequency is measured in cycles per second, abbreviated cps, i.e., the number of vibrations per second. The concert pitch has a frequency of 440 cps. Psychologically, the pitch of a heard sound corresponds to the physical "frequency" variable.

Corresponding to amplitude is the loudness of a sound. It is generally measured as intensity or sound pressure. It is the relation of P_x, the pressure to be measured, to a standard intensity P_0. This standard pressure P_0 is conventionally fixed at 0.0002 dyne per square centimeter. The unit of measurement, customarily employed in acoustics, db or decibel, is defined as 20 log P_x/P_0, i.e., the logarithm, multiplied by 20, of the relation between the pressure in question P_x and the standard pressure P_0. The low whisper of a person 5 feet away has approx. 20 db, the noise of a cinema audience about 45 db, the noise in a department store approx. 60 db, while a train passing through a subway station registers approximately 100db.

The discriminatory capacity of the ear for frequency and amplitude (ignoring for the moment the other two dimensions) is not equally good over the whole range of these dimensions, as can be represented by Fig. 15 (based on the work of Stevens and Davis).

Frequency is indicated in cps on the x-axis, amplitude on the y-axis in decibels. The curves link points of equal discriminatory power. It should be noted that the most sensitive area for the auditory organ lies between 1500 and 3000 cps and between 80 and 120 db. Therefore, within this range the hearer can receive a maximum of information.

We will now attempt to answer the question asked previously, How complex a message can be sent per time unit over the communication channel and can be received by the hearer? The human ear can distinguish intensities between 0 and 125db[3] and frequencies between 10 cps and 20,000 cps.

But how sensitive is the power of discrimination along these two dimensions? How close together may two stimuli be so that the human ear still recognizes them as two, i.e., as differing from each other? Can we distinguish a sound of 1000 from one of 1001 cps? According to Rosenblith (1963),

[3] At about 125 db is the upper limit beyond which pain and possible lesions may occur.

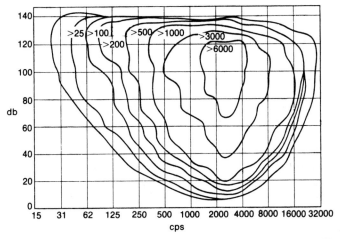

Fig. 15. The curves link points of equal discriminatory sensitivity. The peak of the "mountain range" lies between 80 and 120 db and between 1500 and 3000 cps. Within these ranges the ear is capable of the most delicate discriminations. (Based on Rosenblith, from Moles and Vallancien, 1963, p. 69)

whose presentation we follow here, the threshold of discrimination for intensity amounts to approximately 0.50 db, for frequencies it amounts to approximately 20 cps. Thus a sound of an intensity of 20 db is perceived as louder than one of 19.5 db; a sound of 1020 cps is perceived as higher than one of 1000 cps. The dimension of intensity which extends from 0 to 125 db yields, therefore, 250 possible distinctions, the dimension of pitch approximately 1000. Each of these 1000 sounds varying in pitch could again be perceived in 250 degrees of intensity, so that our hearing should be able to distinguish approximately 250,000 different sounds—"chiffre fantastique comme nous le verrons" (Rosenblith, p. 70).

Human speech uses approximately 50 different sounds, i.e., the phonemes of each language. What explains this discrepancy, this inadequate use of the channel of communication?

In order to answer this question we must once more examine the approach to the problem we have just outlined. It is true that the hearing—as psychophysical studies of thresholds have shown—can distinguish closely neighboring stimuli when they are presented closely together. But speech sounds are not normally offered so as to be distinguished from each other, but in such a way that they must be identified independently. The question is not, Are these sounds alike or different? but, Which sound is this? Investigations by Pollack (1952, 1953a,b, 1954) illuminate particularly well this aspect of the capacity of hearing. Subjects were given pure tones with the instruction to identify them. It was found that subjects can distinguish or identify a "high," "medium" and "low" tone; they can even operate with a five-point scale (very high, high, medium, low, very low), but beyond more than five different degrees they had difficulties.

> The object of this investigation is similar to what is often referred to as *perfect pitch,* but Rosenblith has rightly pointed out that perfect pitch is customarily tested with a piano which does not produce pure sounds. Musicians do not do better than others in the Pollack experiments, and even a preliminary practice phase has little effect on performance.

Along another dimension, e.g., intensity, the results are again similar. Subjects can reliably identify between five and seven different intensities. People tend to assign similar phenomena, objects, etc., to approximately seven categories. No matter how large the variation of the stimuli along the particular dimension, the person perceiving them assigns all of them to one or another category and perceives them as being classified in this manner.

"Perception involves an act of categorization . . . we stimulate an organism with a suitable input, and the organism reacts by sorting the input into a class of things or events" (Bruner, 1957b, p. 123).

It is clear, then, that in the study of the capacity of speech perception we meet once more the same process of classification that we came across before.

In Pollack's investigations which have so far been mentioned, subjects were asked to identify sounds for single dimensions, either frequency or intensity. If in each of these dimensions seven absolute judgments are possible (in contrast to the relative distinctions of "more" or "less" in the above mentioned threshold studies), in the combination of two dimensions we reach a figure of approximately 50 absolutely distinguishable sounds, whereas in the case of distinguishing thresholds a figure of 250,000 was calculated. However, Pollack has shown experimentally that even this calculation does not do justice to reality. If sounds are to be identified for pitch and loudness simultaneously (e.g., "This sound was medium-high and very loud") the subject is not capable of identifying 50, but only about 8 or 9. If we take more than two dimensions, it is true the number of identifiable sounds increases, but the rate of increase steadily declines.

In other words, one dimension can carry about seven distinctions or—to speak in terms of information theory—2 or 3 bits. If a stimulus is assessed simultaneously for six dimensions, each of the six dimensions has only 1.2 bits of information content, and altogether they have about 7 bits.

"What happens in speech perception is an identification which does not take place on the basis of a single dimension, it is an identification of several simultaneous aspects on the basis of several distinctive features" (Rosenblith, 1963, p. 73).

This leads us back once more to Jakobson's theory, discussed in Chapter 3, according to which a phoneme is a bundle of distinctive sound features, each of which is binary. According to Rosenblith's and Jakobson's views, linguistic perception is roughly as follows: Each input signal is received with the binary questions, Vowel or nonvowel? Voiced or unvoiced? etc. Choices are made upon as many alternatives as are needed for the recognition of the particular signal.

Speech perception, therefore, functions in a manner which exploits only a fraction of the possibilities offered by the communication channel.[4]

One might feel tempted to ask a purely teleological question: What is achieved by this "inadequate" exploitation of the channel capacity? The answer is: *certainty,* i.e., certainty of the effectiveness of communication. Speaking is facilitated because it is not necessary to hit a definite sound but only a class of sounds, i.e., a certain phoneme. Likewise, comprehension is eased. The listener does not have to analyze a sound in minute detail, but only to the point that he can classify it without danger of confusion. Often a minor part of the qualities of a sound sequence is enough to classify this event and to recognize it, for example, as a case of /i/.

This classifying process must proceed with extraordinary rapidity. Approximately ten phonemes are uttered per second (Flanagan, 1965), i.e., on the phonemic level alone 10 decisions have to be made every second. Can this mechanism which leads so rapidly to absolute judgments be further elucidated? Beginnings of such an explanation are to be found in the investigations by Liberman and his associates, to be described in the following paragraphs.

It is possible with the help of a pattern playback (see Chapter 3) to produce an acoustic event which is perceived by the listener as a definite phoneme, i.e., distinguished from other events. If this same acoustic event, the identical piece of magnetic tape, is cut out from the linguistic context and offered as part of a nonlinguistic noise sequence, the listener can no longer distinguish it without difficulty from other events in this sequence. A given acoustic event or signal is perceived by the listener correctly as a particular phoneme only if the input mechanism is tuned for language. This tuning-in of the apparatus of perception is therefore needed from the start so as to turn an acoustic event into a speech event.

Further information on the way this process operates is provided by the investigations of Liberman et al. (1963). Fourteen synthetic speech patterns were selected in such a way that small stepwise variations led from /b/ via /d/ to /g/. In the first part of the experiment these stimuli were presented to the subjects singly and in random order; subjects were asked to identify them as /b/ or /d/ or /g/. In this experiment again subjects were offered an acoustically almost continuous variation; but perception turned it into three sharply

---

[4] It has already been mentioned that, in addition, a sound event may yield "ecto-semantic" information, e.g., information about the age of the speaker or whether he has a cold. This, however, in no way affects the above arguments.

divided categories; within a category no gradual transitions were perceived. The alteration of the acoustic variable is perceived only at the boundary between two phonemes.

In the second part of the experiment the stimuli were presented paired, and the subjects were asked to state whether they noticed differences between the stimuli. This procedure showed that the power of discrimination is more acute in the vicinity of the phoneme boundaries than in the middle of a phoneme category (Fig. 16).

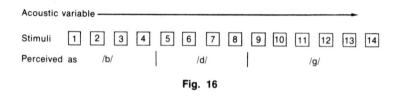

Fig. 16

The difference between stimuli 4 and 5 is noticed with greater frequency than the objectively equal difference between 2 and 3, or 5 and 6. Acoustically equal differences are perceived more easily near the boundaries of the phoneme than within the phoneme category, although the subject has a set for acoustic discrimination and not for linguistic distinction. This phenomenon was so marked that the authors came to the conclusion that the hearer can only distinguish the sounds when he identifies them as different phonemes, or in other words, when he assigns them to different classes.[5]

This experimental finding, it would seem, has important and far-reaching implications. First of all, it demonstrates that, even at this basic level, below the stage of meaning, perception of the world around us is dependent upon the language we have learned to speak. As Humboldt said, it is only through language that world is recreated as mind.

Second, this finding is of interest from the point of view of *learning*. The phonemes are linguistic units which the hearer masters. Since there are no phonemes-in-general, but only phonemes of Arabic, English, or German, etc., the phonemes, or more precisely, phonemic differentiations, are acquired. Hence there must also be an element of learning in the capacity to make differentiations at phoneme boundaries.

There are two possible explanations for this. It may be argued that originally all acoustic stimuli of these speech events were equally distinguishable as is now true of only the most clearly differentiated ones. Subjects have learned to neglect distinctions which are unimportant for communication: this is called *acquired similarity*. It may also be argued, alternatively, that acoustic stimuli were originally all equally difficult to distinguish. Man learns to discriminate more sharply where this is important for comprehen-

---

[5] Incidentally, these results only apply to consonants, not to vowels.

sion, namely at phoneme boundaries. This would be the case for *acquired distinctiveness*.

Liberman is of the opinion that what is learned are the subtleties of discrimination at critical points; in other words, he argues for acquired distinctiveness.

It will be recalled that the mechanism of perception functions according to the principle of absolute judgments. The question now is, How is it that this mechanism can make clear discriminatory judgments at these points while elsewhere it can only make absolute judgments? According to Liberman, this is made possible through a feedback mechanism from speech articulation to speech perception. The discriminatory power is acquired as a combination of heard sounds with the articulation necessary for the production of these sounds. Since in the hearer the incoming acoustic stimulus triggers off the tendency to produce this sound himself and this tendency is perceived by the hearer as a preparatory set in the appropriate muscles, it is possible to make use of these proprioceptive stimuli as additional criteria of discrimination.

This argument has quite far-reaching consequences. It suggests that the process of perception is determined less by the physical nature of the linguistic stimulus than, above all, by the articulatory processes which are needed to produce this linguistic stimulus and which the hearer imitates subvocally. Hitherto it was customary to symbolize the sequence of a speech event as in Fig. 17: the articulatory response R_A forms a stimulus S_P which has to be described in acoustic-physical terms and which in turn leads to the perceptive response R_{Per} in the hearer. A correction of this model as described in Fig. 18 is now indicated.

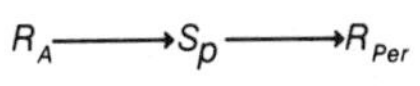

$$R_A \longrightarrow S_p \dashrightarrow R_{Per}$$
$$\downarrow \qquad\qquad \uparrow$$
$$R_{A'} \longrightarrow S_{pro}$$

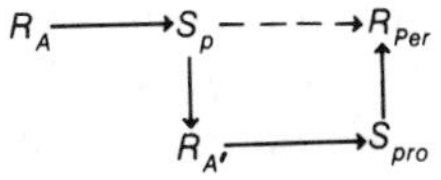

Fig. 18

$$R_A \longrightarrow S_p \longrightarrow R_{Per}$$

Fig. 17

The articulatory response R_A of the speaker forms a physical stimulus S_P which leads to a nonmanifest articulatory response $R_{A'}$ in the listener. The listener, as it were, repeats in a sketchy way what the speaker must have done to produce the speech stimulus S_P. The articulatory innervations and movements, produced by the hearer ($R_{A'}$), are experienced by him proprioceptively as a definite stimulus pattern (S_{pro}). And it is only this stimulation, produced, so to speak, as an echo, which leads to perception R_{Per}. Because the detour via $R_{A'}$ and S_{pro} is below the level of awareness, the listener projects the starting point of the perceptual event directly onto R_A via S_P.

This, in essence, is the central proposition of Liberman's *motor theory of speech perception*[6] to which we had already drawn attention before (see p.

---

[6] On this point see also Lane (1965).

37). This theory stands so clearly in contrast to the usual and obvious view, according to which speech perception has more to do with the acoustic stimulus than with the necessary articulatory processes in the speaker, that a whole series of supporting experimental evidence is needed if this view is to carry conviction. The investigations will be briefly reported below with examples.

The first experiment shows that in certain cases a continuously varying perception corresponds to a discontinuous variation of the acoustic stimulus which in turn corresponds to a continuous variation of articulation; thus, in these cases audition parallels articulation. Fig. 19 shows the spectrograms of the consonant-vowel sequence [di/de/d...] and [gi/ge/...]. In the [d] series the direction and course of the transition of the second formant are different according to the variation in the subsequent vowel, but all these transitions start out from identical frequency positions, i.e., 1800 cps. Because of this acoustic invariance, the same consonant is perceived before each vowel.

It is quite different in the case of [g]. For the vowels [i] to [a] there is again an invariant point of departure leading to the transition round 3000 cps. But the acoustic picture—and only the *acoustic* picture—completely changes for [ɔ], the vowel which is closest to [a]. Again one hears [g] before a subsequent vowel, and the speaker *produces* a [g] as before, but *acoustically* the [g] looks quite different. From the point of view of articulation and perception [gi/ge] to [gu] forms a continuous series—only the properties of the acoustic stimulus mediating between articulation and perception display discontinuity at one point.

The result of an experiment by Lane (1962) can be regarded as a confirmation of the Liberman theory. In this investigation it was shown that changes in the amplitude, duration or spectrum of a vowel appear larger to the speaker than to the listener. The speaker can perceive smaller differences than the hearer, although the latter receives the same acoustic stimulus. But

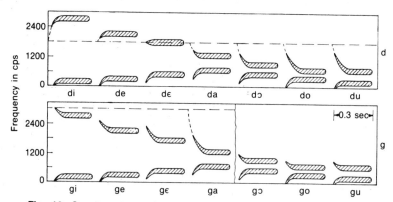

Fig. 19. Spectrograms of consonant-vowel sequences. (Based on Liberman, from Saporta, 1961, p. 149)

the speaker has at his disposal, in addition, the feedback which results from the proprioceptive stimulation resulting from his own articulation.

In summary, it may be said that the Liberman theory rests on three groups of findings: (a) acoustically *similar* stimuli, which were produced by *different* patterns of articulation, lead to *different* perceptions; (b) acoustically *different* stimuli, which were produced by *similar* patterns of articulation, lead to *similar* perceptions; (c) if both articulation and acoustic stimulation are continuously varied, changes in perception correlate most highly with those of articulation.

However, the objections that have been raised against the Liberman motor theory of speech perception should also be mentioned. Jakobson reports the experience that in certain Caucasian languages he could distinguish their numerous phonemes, without being able, in spite of all his efforts, to produce them himself. Parallel to that, he noted that he was able to read these languages but not to write them. Similar phenomena are of course generally observed in the learning of a foreign language: it is easier to understand than to speak and this has no doubt other causes besides the difference between an active and passive vocabulary. Bay regards the fact that the expressive aspect of language presents greater difficulties than the receptive one as an essential feature of language.[7] This is shown above all in the acquisition of speech in the child, where, for a time, the understanding of language is clearly in advance of its productive use. Lenneberg (1962) describes a case in which learning to speak was impossible because of a pathological defect, and yet this did not affect the development of speech comprehension (cf. Studert-Kennedy et al., 1970).

> If we want to consider whether the learning processes through which articulation participates in speech perception, operate through a loss of unimportant distinctions or the emphasis of important ones (acquired similarity *versus* acquired distinctiveness), an observation of child psychology mentioned by Langer is important: "In a social environment, the vocalizing and articulating instinct of babyhood is fostered by response, and as the sounds become symbols their use becomes a dominant habit. Yet the passing of the *instinctive phase* is marked by the fact that a great many phonemes which do not meet with response are completely lost.
>
> "Undoubtedly that is why children, who have not entirely lost the impulse to make random sounds which their mother tongue does not require, can so easily learn a foreign language and even master several at once . . ." (1963, p. 122). Looked at in this perspective it appears likely that acquired similarity is more important than acquired distinctiveness, because the number of various sounds declines.

The discussions about this problem have benefited greatly from the experiments carried out by Molfese and Freeman (1973) with preverbal infants.

---

[7] Bay, 1964, p. 140.

Like older children and adults, these infants already responded with differentiated brain wave patterns when listening to various sounds. Speech sounds (single phonemes and words) elicit a stronger wave pattern in the left than in the right brain hemisphere. These babies, in contrast to adults, do not show the predominant response from the right hemisphere to nonverbal sounds.

These findings not only throw new light on the question of acquired similarity vs acquired distinctiveness referred to above, but quite generally provide evidence against a simple motor theory of speech perception. Although these infants are clearly not able to generate (articulate) any speech, they are, nevertheless, apparently prepared to perceive specifically verbal sounds.

In attempting to determine the explanatory value of a motor theory of speech perception by means of evaluation of positive and negative findings, two problem areas must be considered: A large number of Russian studies have shown that physiological processes take place within the *hearer* which are akin to those phases observed in speech *production* (cf. Smirnow, 1960; Sokolow, 1971; Leontjew, 1972). During certain phases of memory storage an articulatory coding of the material takes place (cf. Locke, 1970).

If one looks at such varied sources, the border between a narrowly defined motor theory and a more general analysis-by-synthesis model becomes blurred. The first postulates that speech perception requires a perceptual phase during which a "copy" of what is heard is articulated. The latter, which in principle was introduced into psychology as early as 1951 by Bruner's hypothesis-testing model, states the following: The organism generates an hypothesis about that which is to be expected. The actual stimulation is then tested for consistency with the hypothesis. A model of this kind was applied to speech perception by Halle and Stevens (1959). In their theory, too, a preconstruction is necessary in the organism in order to identify the impinging stimulation in a comparison process as fit/no fit. In contrast, however, to the motor theory, this approach does not assign this construction to the phoneme-articulation level.

Meanwhile, Neisser (1967) and a number of other investigators have suggested that prior to such a process of analysis-by-synthesis, the perceptual process must undergo at least one more phase consisting of purely analytical processes. Massaro (1972) introduced a theory of speech perception which, unlike Liberman's, does not postulate the phoneme to be the basis of the perception, but assumes a more comprehensive linguistic unit about the size of a syllable to take on this function. Because these units are in a memory store, available to the process of analysis for a longer period, this theory does not need to take recourse to articulatory processes as carriers of information.

By the way, of course, analysis-by-synthesis models are based on the ability of the organism to organize subjectively that which is perceived, a fact which was emphasized primarily by Gestalt psychology. Arnheim (1947) defined perception as arising from the application of perceptual categories to perceptual events, which are activated by the structure of the particular stimulus configurations. The presence of such categories is the indispensable prerequisite for understanding that which is perceived.

Every conception of this kind implies the importance of the listener's expectation to that which he hears. We can see now why knowledge about the probabilities of occurrence of linguistic units is a decisive factor in linguistic communication. We will have to look at this again, later on.

The transformation of experience into conceptualization, which was discussed on p. 11, is made possible by the fact that the symbol as a store and generalizer is not just received passively by the hearer, but can at any moment be actively seized by him and conceptualized. In the last resort, language is perhaps such a specifically human creation not because we can yield to it passively, but because in order to grasp what we receive we must first of all make it actively our own.

Speech perception is geared more towards a high degree of security of communication than towards a maximum exploitation of channel capacity.

The certainty of communication reaches a high level if only a portion of the possible distinctions is sufficient to identify a speech event as belonging to the class of signal x. The certainty we thus attain will prove its worth particularly under conditions when the communication is far from the ideal we have so far assumed.

In the ideal channel of communication the input of the source reaches the receiver undiminished, undistorted, and without the addition of a disturbing noise. In reality such an ideal channel hardly ever exists. Thus the air vibrations of speech on their way from the speaker to the hearer are deviated by obstacles and distorted, e.g., fewer high frequencies occur behind the speaker than in front of him; the intensity of the air vibrations declines with distance; the channel, because its width is restricted, transmits perhaps only a part of the signal; and, the most important source of disturbance, extraneous sound events and signals which do not originate in the speaker penetrate into the channel.

For the purpose of our discussion these disturbances may be divided into omissions, distortions and additions.

If most of the qualities which can be distinguished in an acoustic event are not exploited, it must be possible to deprive the event of a considerable part of these qualities without impairing the linguistic message and without disturbing the transmission of information.

Investigations in this problem area have been carried out, among others, by French and Steinberg (1947). The spectra of the utterances coming from a speaker were artificially modified by inserting filters into the channels which allowed only high or only low frequencies to pass through. If a high-pass filter is used, for example, a filter which allows all parts of a speech event above 1000 cps to pass through, only 85 percent of syllables are intelligible. If only frequencies above 3000 cps are allowed to pass, comprehensibility goes down to 30 percent. The effect of a low-pass filter, which only lets through frequencies below a certain level, is correspondingly similar; if, for example, all speech components above 300 or 400 cps are filtered out, it is almost impossible to understand anything (Fig. 20).

The point of intersection of these curves at approximately 1900 cps indicates that, if only the frequencies above this figure are used as signal carrier, approximately two thirds of the syllables are intelligible; the same result is obtained if only the frequencies below this figure reach the listener. In other words, it hardly matters *which* frequency bands are used as signal carrier: communication occurs as long as in the total spectrum there is a margin for variation, an area which allows for those distinctions which carry information.

As one would expect, the exact position of these curves is a function of the sex of the speaker. Carterette and Møller (1963) obtained similar results for different subjects, a different context, and in a different language—which suggests that fundamental characteristics of the mechanism of perception are involved.

In the experiments we have just discussed the frequency spectrum of the language was selectively filtered out. Other investigations have left intact the frequencies of the acoustic event but have selectively varied amplitudes.

In the simplest case the peaks of amplitudes are cut off; having done this we can transmit to the listener either these peaks or the remaining center portions of the wave. Licklider was able to demonstrate that intelligibility of speech is hardly affected if the peaks are omitted, whereas in the case of the omission of the center portion of the wave and the exclusive use of the peaks intelligibility is nearly down to zero.

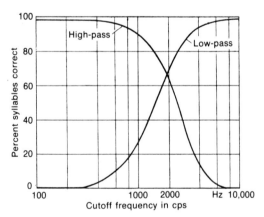

Fig. 20. Dependence of discrimination on the frequency range. (Based on French and Steinberg, 1947, from Miller, 1951a, p. 64)

How can this result be explained? There must be signals which are characterized by the following qualities: they have very high intensities; yet they can be omitted without affecting intelligibility; at the same time they have not enough information content to transmit messages without a center portion. Such signals are the vowels. Clipping wave peaks affects the vowels, but the consonants hardly at all, since only vowels have such high intensities. The finding confirms that consonants carry more information than vowels because the number of consonants is greater. As was explained above the amount of information transmitted by a signal depends upon the number of possibilities from which the signal has been selected (Fig. 21).

From quite a different point of view the example of Arabic can show that the loss of vowels affects the intelligibility of a language less than the loss of consonants: in Arabic script it is customary to write only consonants; for beginners in the language and also wherever it is regarded as important vowel signs are placed above or below the consonant.

So far we have discussed the effect of disturbances on communication when the signal on its way from the source has been mutilated in its acoustic band-width and, as a result, has probably been distorted. More important from a practical point of view are those cases in which something is added to the signal on its way. On the telephone one hears a speech event which is not only reduced in its frequency spectrum, but to which are added electrical disturbances and perhaps also a conversation on another line. The listener in this case receives a mixture of desired, genuine information and of noise, i.e., misinformation from a source of disturbance.

The problem the listener faces is, How can the genuine information which comes from the speaker be picked out from the mixture?

There are two aspects to this problem: one mathematical, which has been thoroughly investigated by Shannon and which will not be treated here, and the other psychological in a narrower sense: how much is perception of

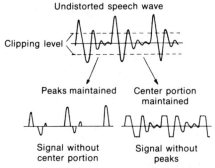

Fig. 21. Two kinds of distortion of the wave form produced by amplitude selection. (Based on Miller, 1951a, p. 72)

speech sounds affected by competing acoustic events or *noise*? In this context, noise is defined as all undesired information.

One of the concepts which is frequently used in this context is that of *masking*. In experiments on masking or covering up of the 'real' information, it is customary to use a random mixture of all audible frequencies. In analogy to white sun light, which is a mixture of all visible wavelengths, this random swishing noise is called *white noise*.

If the disturbing effect of this white noise on speech perception is to be studied, a measure for the intensity of the noise is needed, because this intensity is the independent variable in the experiment to be described below. The measure is the decibel already defined on page 66 above.

By way of introduction to such experiments, it may be helpful to remind the reader of the fact that the sensitivity of the human ear is dependent upon the frequency of the sound to be perceived. As can be seen (Fig. 22), the threshold of detectability is lowest for sounds of 2000 to 3000 cps; here the sound needs the lowest intensity to be perceived.

If the audibility threshold is to be determined not only by transmitting the tone to be detected but also white noise, the diagram in Fig. 23 results.

Even noise of 30 db requires a rise in the threshold level for tones around 2000 cps; in order to detect these tones their loudness must be increased beyond the point which would be necessary without white noise. If the white noise has an intensity of 50 to 60 db, all frequencies are affected.

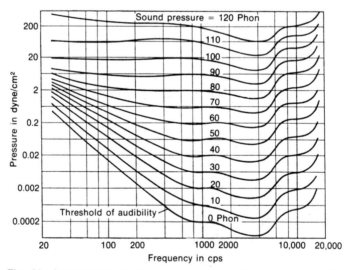

Fig. 22. Curves of identical loudness in binaural hearing as a function of frequency and sound pressure. Frequency is plotted along the abscissa and pressure along the ordinate, both on a logarithmic scale. At 1000 cps the phone scale corresponds to the decibel scale. (Based on Fletcher and Munson, from Rein and Schneider, 1964, p. 688)

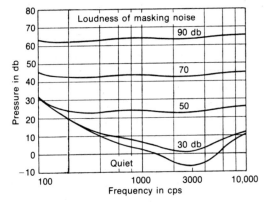

Fig. 23. Threshold for pure tones when masked by white noise: the parameter is the level of the masking noise. (Based on Hawkins and Stevens, 1950, from Miller, 1951a, p. 55)

For the sake of simplicity, we have so far confined ourselves to the masking of pure tones; of greater interest is the question to what extent noise affects speech perception.

As Fig. 24 shows, the detection of speech occurs if the noise level is not higher than 17 db above speech. The *comprehension* of speech is dependent upon a number of other factors still to be discussed.

The masking effect of the interfering noise depends not only on its intensity, but also on the spectrum. The more the spectrum of the interfering noise is similar to the spectrum of speech the more affected is the perception of speech.

To explain the masking of tones by noise, Miller now reasons as follows. Suppose that the signal to be detected has a component of 1000 cps and that

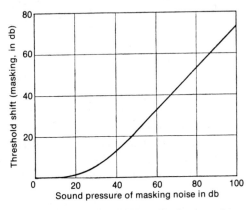

Fig. 24. Shift in the threshold of detectability for speech as a function of the intensity of white noise. (Based on Hawkins and Stevens, 1950, from Miller, 1951a, p. 62)

accurate discrimination of this component is decisive for the perception of the signal. If noise is present (assuming it is white noise) it will also have a component of 1000 cps. As noise is produced randomly, it is not possible to say whether the 1000 cps component is in phase with the signal and added to it or if it is out of phase so that the 1000 cps component of the signal and the noise cancel each other. The addition of noise to the 1000 cps speech component would add a certain fuzzy effect, but an exact determination of this component is not possible. If the area of fuzziness is large, large changes of the corresponding signal component are needed, so as to perceive these changes as such and not as accidental fuzziness. In other words: the smaller the *signal-to-noise ratio*[8] the fewer distinctions of the signal can be detected by the receiver, i.e., the fainter is the possibility for him to receive information.

Suppose now a language employs many delicate distinctions, these could perfectly well be detected over an undisturbed channel, i.e., in the quiet, and would permit a very high rate of information transmission per time unit. But under conditions of noise, communication operating with such delicate distinctions would soon break down.

While the study of masking by white noise gives information on quasi-physiological processes in the peripheral sectors of perception, the studies which use a second interfering event for masking instead of white noise probe the interaction of the stimulus on the one side and the characteristics of the organism at more central sectors of perception on the other. These last-named investigations have of course also a greater practical application; and for this reason we shall describe them in somewhat greater detail.

To what extent is the perception of a speech event disturbed by the simultaneous occurrence of a second speech event? Broadbent whose research on this question has been of particular merit has carried out the following basic experiment. The subject receives a piece of squared paper. The squares are numbered and within each square are signs, e.g., a cross or a circle. The subject hears through headphones such questions as, "Is there a cross in square two?" If the answer is yes, the subject has to record this on an answer sheet. A second voice comes in over the same headphones, asking similar questions. The result is that subjects have great difficulties when both voices ask these questions simultaneously.

One might be tempted to explain these difficulties in purely sensory terms: the two questions mask each other, are overlaid in the hearing and can therefore not be understood. That this view is not at all correct, and that therefore the masking is not a peripheral event is shown by the following variation of the experiment: one voice is called A and the other B and the

---

[8] The relationship between the intensity of the speech signal and the intensity of the interfering noise is referred to as "signal-to-noise ratio."

subject is instructed to pay attention only to the questions asked by A. In this case the second voice (B) hardly interferes at all.

It is true that the subject must have the instruction to pay attention only to A *before* the input of questions. If he is asked afterwards to answer only the questions of A, the subject finds it just as difficult to do so as if he had the task of answering both A and B. The prior instruction "Answer only A's questions" sets in motion a selection mechanism which annuls part of the incoming information, i.e., B's questions, and thus enables the subject to receive undisturbed the messages coming from A.

What can we learn about the central selection mechanism? To clarify this question let us again look at some further investigations by Broadbent and his collaborators.

Two simultaneous messages may be understood if they contain little information. If the information content increases, a point is soon reached where comprehension can no longer keep up. It follows that the capacity for registering and handling messages is limited with regard to the *quantity* of information it can process. If the message contains little information and a second message with equally little information is added, the limit of this capacity is not yet reached. If the number of bits is raised at input (i.e., what the listener receives) the number of bits at output (i.e., what he records as having understood) is also increased. If one of the messages, however, already contains a great deal of information the rise in input is no longer followed by a corresponding rise in output. The channel capacity, i.e., the capacity of the receiver to handle information, is transcended (Fig. 25).

In the previously mentioned experiments, in which the listener simultaneously receives two messages only one of which, according to instructions, is relevant, it is all the easier to exclude or filter out the irrelevant one, the more clues are present for a distinction between the two messages. If one of the messages comes from the left and the other from the right, or if one is spoken by a man's voice and the other by a woman's, a separation is easily possible.

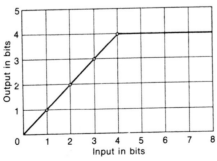

Fig. 25. Schematic representation of the limits of channel capacity.

It was just pointed out that the irrelevant message would be "filtered out," "suppressed," or "not registered." This demands some further elucidations which will at the same time explain how the selection mechanism functions. If the "irrelevant" speaker repeats the message of the "relevant" speaker but with a delay of ten seconds, the subject is enabled to concentrate entirely on the relevant message without even noticing that the irrelevant voice after a delay of ten seconds repeats the message. However, if the delay of the second message is reduced to four seconds, the listener suddenly notices that the two messages are identical (Cherry, 1957).

This has two implications: the relevant message must leave a kind of trace for about four seconds; and the irrelevant message, it appears, is not simply discarded; the apparatus of perception in a certain way takes cognizance of it. This suggests that the selection mechanism has a kind of store at its disposal. How this storing device works can be seen from certain experiments by Broadbent. Messages are heard over separate loudspeakers each of which begins with a call signal: "This is Fred speaking," "This is Bill speaking." The subject is instructed to pay attention only to what Fred says. Both signals are simultaneous. The responses of the subject show that both signals and both channels are received and then a decision is made which of the two voices should be listened to. The filtering-out process of the irrelevant one must be imagined roughly as follows: the receiver listens only to one channel but if he realizes that it is the irrelevant one, he can switch to the other channel and can find in it what has just recently occurred. It must be remembered that the event in channels one and two are objectively speaking strictly simultaneous. The events which lead to an acoustic input are definitely preserved for a brief span of time. If it is decided that the input is irrelevant, it is not passed for further processing and is quickly forgotten.

The effect of this store, which is set before the selection mechanism, can be demonstrated by the following experiment. The subject hears over the left headphone the figure 723 and simultaneously over the right one 954. Subsequently he is instructed to repeat all the numbers he has heard. He says "723954" or "954723," i.e., the response consists of *all* the information transmitted over one channel followed by all the information on the other channel. The subject cannot proceed in any other way; he is incapable of uttering the sequence which objectively occurred.

> This experiment shows that in the course of the process of acoustic perception (and accordingly also in the process of speech perception) memory enters into the formation of units. The process of retention demands the formation of such units or chunks, as Miller has proved. According to Miller (1956), the number of such chunks may under certain circumstances be the decisive variable for retention, not the information content of what has been retained. (Compare on this point also Ehrlich, 1961). This relationship between perception (where the *information content* of the term matters) and retention (which is determined by the number of items) must also be considered in psycholinguistic research.

It had previously been observed that two simultaneously heard messages would only be understood if their information content was not too high. We can now add a further restriction: the information content must not exceed the channel capacity except for a short spell of time so that this excess can be stored until it is processed. Such storing is possible so long as the input in the seconds immediately following is not too high. Broadbent's *filter theory* which is based on these and numerous other results need not be considered here in greater detail.

This theory has been supplemented, and in part extensively modified, by a number of investigators, such as Treisman, Morton, and Norman, to name a few. Through this work, a particular problem has become apparent that relates to the fact that semantic factors, i.e., the meaning of the linguistic signs employed must function as criteria for admission to the "central processing mechanism." But how can meaning, which is surely stored in long-term memory, be effective in those preliminary phases in which, according to the model, the input has not yet reached the central store? The integration of this problem with those arising from the analysis-by-synthesis models represents a research area which is of common interest to workers in the field of perception, memory, and psycholinguistics.

CHAPTER 5

Frequency and Probability

The role of hypotheses in perception—Frequency and expectation—Diversification of the vocabulary—Formulas of readability—Possibility and probability—The concept of redundance—Joint and transitional probabilities—Approximations to genuine speech—Lexical units and logogens.

In the previous chapter we discussed the capacity of the communication channel, connecting the speaker and the listener, in terms of information theory. It was proposed that the informational content of a message is closely linked to the number of possible signals and the probability of their occurrence. As we have seen, this knowledge of what can be expected plays an important role in linguistic communication. We now turn to those effects which are psychological in nature.

As an introduction, a study by Miller, Heise and Lichten (1951) is particularly useful. In this inquiry the subjects were given the task of identifying words heard under conditions of noise. In each case the size of the vocabulary from which the words were chosen was exactly known. It comprised 2, 4, 8, etc., words respectively. For example, when the vocabulary consisted of eight words, the subjects knew that what they would hear through their headphones could only be one of these eight words (Fig. 26). The larger the vocabulary from which the test words are selected the greater must be the intensity of speech with which the words are uttered relative to the noise in order to ensure that an equal percentage of words is understood correctly. Figure 27 gives a second result of the same investigation. It appears that digits (0–9) are understood by far the best; next follow words in sentences, whereas nonsense syllables even under a much more favorable signal-to-noise ratio yield lower scores. The digits have, of course, the lowest information content, because there are only 10 possibilities. Words in sentences contain very much more information, whereas the information content of syllables is particularly high, because here almost anything is possible.

The percentages of items recognized correctly in these three series—digits, words in sentences, and nonsense syllables—are different, but the content of information, received at a given signal-to-noise ratio, is fairly

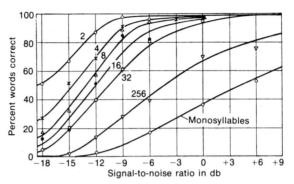

Fig. 26. Percentage of words correct for test vocabularies of different sizes; the bottom curve, "monsyllables," was obtained with a vocabulary of approximately 1000 monosyllabic words. (Based on Miller, Heise and Lichten, 1951, from Miller, 1951a, p. 77)

constant: in the case of the digits many items are understood but they have little information content, while in the case of nonsense syllables few have been correctly heard but they have a very high information content.

How can this result be explained? When the listener hears digits he needs only few acoustic clues of the incoming message in order to decide that it can only be "five" if he hears /fai/. In the case of a meaningful word the listener must of course receive more acoustic clues, but even if a few are drowned by the noise, he can supplement these missing clues by his previous knowledge of common sound combinations in his language. Isolated words at a given

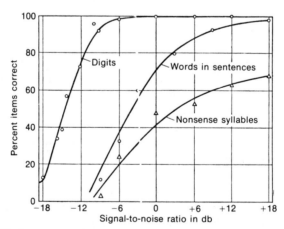

Fig. 27. Percentage of items recognized correctly for different signal-to-noise ratios for digits, words in sentences, and nonsense syllables. (Based on Miller, Heise and Lichten, 1951, as reported by Miller, 1951a, p. 75)

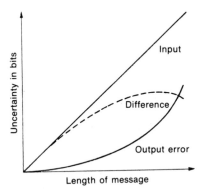

Fig. 28. Schematic presentation of information received. The information received is equal to the difference between information input and the information loss, i.e., output errors. (Adapted from Pollack, 1953a, p. 430)

signal-to-noise ratio are less clearly understood than the same words at an equal noise level in sentences, for the sentence structure already gives a clue as to which word is possible in a given position.

Let us recall the hypotheses theory of perception, referred to above; the more limited the listener is in his production of hypotheses, ("the next item must be a digit . . ."), the more he will be able to establish a correspondence between the stimulus input and this hypothesis and thereby "perceive" the stimulus.

Pollack (1953a) attempted to find out the relative influence on the extent of information loss of two variables: the number of items in the message (i.e., the length of the message) and the number of possibilities per item. He transmitted to his subjects messages of a given number of items; each item in turn was one of a definite number of possibilities. The immediate result was that per message item the loss of information is greater the larger the number of items in the message and the larger the number of possibilities per item. If the length of the message (i.e., the number of items) is held constant, the percentage of information loss is independent of the number of possibilities per item. In other words, if the number of possibilities per item is great, some items will certainly not be received, but the items which have been registered yield a great deal of information because in every case they represent one of many possibilities. Figure 28 represents a model of these relationships.

If the message is short, the information received by the listener is equal to the information transmitted by the source: there is no information loss. If the messages are a little longer the size of the error is small; but this means that the information content received rises. At a medium length of message the difference between input and output is roughly constant; a certain amount of information transmitted is always lost. If the message is very long the loss of information rises steeply, more steeply than can be compensated for by the increase in transmitted information.

It follows that for each number of possibilities per item there is a definite length of message which allows comprehension of a maximum of information. If a shorter message is transmitted, less information than would really be possible is sent; if longer messages are sent, the loss of information rises disproportionately. In other words, in these inquiries we again come across the notion of channel capacity which we discussed in the previous chapter.

From the point of view of information theory, understanding a message always involves more than is contained in the signal itself; it implies reference to the totality of possibilities which is available to the receiver and from which the signal in question has been selected. This totality of possibilities is by no means uniform, but has in each case a characteristic profile: some possibilities are more probable than others, and the variations in the degrees of probability influence the decoding process in the receiver.

In its simplest form this probability profile of a language is met as the average value of the occurrence of a certain unit—and unit may be taken to mean an element on a certain level, e.g., phoneme, letter, syllable, word, etc. Such average values can be calculated by counts of fairly large spoken verbal products, such as lectures, telephone conversations, etc., or of written verbal products, e.g., newspapers, letters, or books. Such frequency counts of linguistic units have been undertaken in Germany by Kaeding (1897) and Meier (1964) and in America by Thorndike and Lorge (1944) and Zipf (1949).

Meier grouped into 14 levels the frequencies of the words in the texts he analyzed, which consisted of a total of 10 million words. Table 2 illustrates the astonishing result which in all such investigations has been found again and again. The 30 most frequently occurring words in German constitute almost a third of all texts. One half of the texts consists of 200 of the most frequent words of the German language, or to express it in another way: not quite one percent of the different words makes up half the texts. Against this, the 15,477 word types on frequency level 10 (6 percent of all different words) constitute barely two percent of the texts. Which are the thirty most frequent words occurring in German? They are: die, der, und, in, zu, den, das, nicht, von, sie, ist, des, sich, mit, dem, daß, er, es, ein, ich, auf, so, eine, auch, als, am, nach, wie, im, für.[1]

Zipf goes one step further: he compares the frequencies of occurrence of different words by relating graphically the rank order of frequency with the

---

[1] *Translator's note.* Approximate English equivalent of these are: the (and various other case forms), and, in, to, not, of, they/she, is, himself (and similar reflexive pronouns), with, that, he, it a/an, I, on, so, also, as, at, towards/after, how, in, for.

Table 2

Level	Number of word types at each level	Percent of word types	Number of word tokens representing these word types	Percent of all word tokens
Ia	30	0.01	3,468,082	31.79
Ib	70	0.03	1,670,379	15.31
Ic	107	0.04	791,693	7.25
II	305	0.12	925,035	8.48
III	510	0.20	695,265	6.37
IV	995	0.39	690,029	6.32
V	1278	0.50	488,995	4.48
VI	1396	0.54	341,669	3.13
VII	3303	1.28	469,057	4.30
VIII	5221	2.02	369,338	3.39
IX	12,391	4.80	386,882	3.55
X	15,477	6.00	209,515	1.92
XI	38,633	14.96 ⎤	404,838	3.71
XII	178,457	69.12 ⎦		
Total	258,173	100.00	10,910,777	100.00

Based on Meier, 1964, p. 53.

frequency of occurrence of a particular word. Zipf's famous law is represented in Fig. 29.

In order to understand this diagram correctly it is important to explain the coordinates: the rank sequence n of the words in terms of decreasing frequency is plotted on the abscissa: the most frequent, the second most frequent, the third most frequent word, etc. The ordinate records the actual frequencies P_n in a given text. Both scales are logarithmic. The resulting straight line indicates that the product nP_n is constant.

Curve A resulted from a count of James Joyce's *Ulysses,* curve B from a count of a large sample of American newspapers.

If we want to make a correct interpretation of these curves, which have been found again and again in the most varied samples, it must be made clear that the two variables, rank and frequency, are *not* independent. Since the rank position of a word depends on the frequency of its occurrence, the direction of the curve is, at least partially, simply the expression of the mathematical relationship between the two variables; i.e., the curve cannot be higher on the right than on the left because a word with a low frequency cannot occupy a higher rank position than a word with a higher frequency. But if all words were equally frequent the curve would be nearly horizontal; and if there were only some very frequent words and some very rare, it would be nearly vertical. Between these two extremes the shape of the line is, therefore, determined by

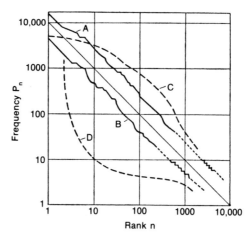

Fig. 29. Rank frequency of words. **A** James Joyce's *Ulysses*; **B** American newspapers; **C** and **D** hypothetical curves. (Based on Zipf, from Cherry, 1963, p. 141)

the empirical facts. Our next question is, How are we to interpret this strange finding (nP_n = constant)? What conditions must be present to produce it?

According to Zipf, human behavior in many spheres is founded on the *principle of least effort*. The organism strives to maintain as low an average level of exertion as possible. Not only does word frequency obey this principle, but it applies equally to the relative size of cities in a country or to the arrangement of tools at a work bench. According to Zipf, language—from the speaker's point of view—would be at its simplest if the speaker had only to utter the same word again and again, or, in other words, if the language consisted only of a single word. From the listener's point of view, on the other hand, the language would be most rational and most convenient if every distinctive meaning had its own word. To put it differently, in language two tendencies confront each other: one to say things as economically as possible, and the other to be explicit. Zipf names the first the tendency of unification and the second the tendency of diversification.[2] Zipf's law can therefore be viewed as the equilibrium between these two tendencies.

A flatter curve (*C*) would result if the speaker would use common words not quite so frequently, and rare words not quite so rarely, so that the tendency to diversify would predominate and therefore language would be used in a way which the hearer desires. Conversely, a steeper curve (*D*) would indicate the tendency of unification or a certain egocentricity in the speaker. The linguistic products of schizophrenics appear to be characterized by a greater steepness of these rank-frequency curves.

[2] Jespersen noted similar dynamics in language, particularly so in lexical choice: a maximum of effectiveness with a minimum of effort.

Of course, we should not neglect to mention that a number of authors (notably Herdan, 1960) have stated important objections to the "lawfulness" of Zipf's and similar formulas. But we cannot examine this further here.

A clearer picture than that of the relative steepness of Zipf's curves is presented by individual preferences of frequency classes relative to a norm, on the basis of Meier's *spectrum* (Fig. 30). The "language of prescriptions" (*B*), for example, is syntactically somewhat reduced; this is indicated by the decline in frequency of those very frequent words which in "normal" texts predominate. Equally, in an investigation by Kelchner (1929), a letter of a young female factory worker, analyzed under *C* in Fig. 30, confines itself to a very general vocabulary. Meier describes texts of this type as *lexically-restricted*. Meier's use of this concept offers an example of a content analysis from a formal point of view.

Meier demonstrates that lexically restricted spectra emerge in moments of genuine stress. Such regression to the most usual words can no doubt be related to the well-known psychological observation that stress leads to increased rigidity of thought and to a reduction of creative ideas. Spectra with a wide lexical spread are found in descriptions, in scholarly papers, in reports of lexically specialized character, such as on the sports page or the fashion page, or in ironical discourse. The analysis *D* in Fig. 30 represents a police warrant.

Other lines of thought lead from Zipf's results to certain other interesting problems. One of these is the determination of the *size of the vocabulary* of an individual. The spoken and written texts produced by a single person can be considered a sample of the total universe of words at the disposal of this person. Howes (1964, p. 57) is of the opinion that, however large the sample, it can never exhaust the total vocabulary; if the size of the sample is further increased, new words—according to Zipf's formula—will continue to appear. A numerical comparison of the vocabularies of different persons is

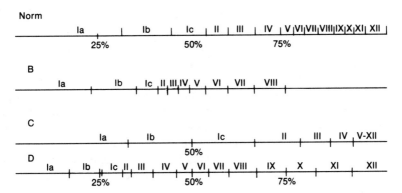

Fig. 30. Comparison of different frequency spectra. (Based on Meier, 1964, pp. 54, 58, 66, and 112)

therefore only of little value; what can be compared are the parameter values of their Zipf functions.

> We can relate an observation from psychopathology to this argument. Goldstein has observed that in many cases of aphasia the patient has special difficulties in finding abstract words and in carrying out abstract thought operations, whereas the use of concrete words is less affected. From this observation Goldstein has derived a well-known theory of aphasia, i.e., that aphasia is a pathological shift from abstract to concrete levels of behavior, or a loss of the capacity to abstract. Against this view, Howes argues that Zipf's law applies even in extreme cases of aphasia; only the parameters are shifted. There is no genuine loss of vocabulary; in a sample of a given size the patient tends to use only fewer different words than a healthy person. If the size of the sample is sufficiently large, he can also use all the words that are at the disposal of a healthy individual. Since abstract words are normally already less frequent than concrete words, they are especially affected in aphasia through the shift of parameters; but those concrete words which are equally infrequent suffer the same deficit; i.e., aphasia is not concomitant with a loss of the capacity of abstraction.[3]

The thoughts which relate Zipf's law to individual vocabularies tend to contribute more to a psychology of individual differences than to general psychology. Whereas Zipf himself strives to discover average word frequencies in the language generally, vocabulary studies are intended to discover differences among members of different social, age, or intelligence groups. Such comparisons are more suitably made with the help of the so-called type-token ratio (TTR) than with the individual or group parameters of the Zipf formula. The type-token ratio, which was introduced by W. Johnson following Carroll (1938), is based on the relationship, already referred to earlier, between the number of different words in a text and the number of running words in that text. In type-token ratio studies the basic unit is the word, whereas Zipf functions can be established with reference to all other possible units. In a text which comprises 65 words in which one word occurs four times, 5 words three times each, 9 words twice each, and 28 words once each, the type-token ratio would be 43 : 65 or 0.66.

There is a significant relationship between the TTR score of a text and the intelligence of its author, as indicated in Fig. 31.

A weakness of this ratio lies in the fact that it declines with the increasing length of a text, but this decline unfortunately happens in an irregular manner and therefore cannot be compensated for mathematically. On page one of a novel a writer need hardly repeat himself in the choice of words (the TTR would therefore be high) but after a few hundred pages he must necessarily reemploy words he has used before. By means of suitable sampling this defect can be obviated in the case of very long texts.

---

[3] Brown (1958a) offers an excellent discussion on the whole psycholinguistic problem involved in the concepts, "concrete" and "abstract."

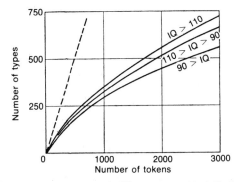

Fig. 31. The average number of different types is plotted against the total number of words used (tokens) by children of different intelligence levels. (Based on Chotlos, 1944, from Miller, 1951a, p. 123)

Lexically restricted or lexically elaborated spectra, respectively, and the just mentioned relationship between TTR on the one hand, and social class or intelligence, respectively, on the other hand are problems extensively investigated by a sizeable group of sociolinguists. Based on the work of Bernstein (1958, 1962) it was assumed that a restricted speech production would be found among the "lower" classes, while an elaborated production would be found among the "higher" classes. The term "restricted" as used here is very similar to what the term "low TTR" implies. However, what was viewed in the beginning as simply a meagerness of the vocabulary employed soon had to be conceptualized in a more differentiated manner.

Whereas Zipf, as well as Carroll and Johnson, the "inventors" of the TTR, aimed at finding functional relationships within language, Thorndike aimed at straightforward description. Together with his student Lorge he made the attempt to count which words in the English language occurred frequently and which occurred infrequently. The sample consisted of many millions of words in periodicals.

A similar count had already been made before the turn of the century by Kaeding who in 1897—98 produced, as a private publishing venture at Steglitz near Berlin, a frequency dictionary of the German language. This work served as a basis for Meier's *Statistics of the German Language* (*Deutsche Sprachstatistik (1964)*) already referred to, the imposing work of a lone scholar who had recognized earlier and more effectively than many linguistic scholars the necessity and value of statistics in linguistic inquiries. If in the following remarks the less complex Thorndike-Lorge studies are treated in greater detail, this is done only for one reason: Thorndike-Lorge has had considerable influence on psychological research, which can hardly be said of Kaeding and, not yet, of Meier.

Thorndike was prompted to undertake his count by the necessity to grade quantitatively the difficulty of reading matter employed in schools. The less frequently the words in a text are used in everyday language, the more difficult is the text.

The Thorndike-Lorge count has become the basis for two trends of development, one of which is more practical and the other more theoretical in its orientation. The first is concerned with the systematic study of the *readability* or *intelligibility* of texts. The other trend has expressed itself in the use of frequency indices, worked out by Thorndike and Lorge, for the purpose of systematic variation of verbal materials in psychological experiments. Both trends will be briefly discussed in the following paragraphs.

Some documents are written in a way that makes them difficult to understand, whereas others manage to express complicated thoughts in easily intelligible language. For example, legal language is so unintelligible to the layman that a good portion of a lawyer's time is spent in explaining what it "really" means. What causes this lack of intelligibility? What makes one novelist harder to read than another? Both, after all, write grammatically correct sentences.[4]

If a series of texts is ranked for readability by different judges, it is found that easily readable texts consist of words which—according to the Thorndike-Lorge lists—occur very frequently in the language. Texts which are difficult to follow contain many rare words. Short words make a text more readable than long ones. It should be remembered that, according to Zipf, short words are more frequent than long ones. Short words, at the same time, are those without prefixes or suffixes. The use of short and frequent words without pre- or suffixes leads to a low TTR. In other words, these different statistical indices correlate highly with one another.

Next to frequency of use of common words in a text, another factor influencing comprehension is, of course, sentence length. According to Meier's statistical analysis of the German language roughly half of all German sentences have in general a length of less than eighteen words. In scientific texts, however, sentences of this length constitute only about a third of all sentences; in sermons they constitute 60 percent.

In addition a number of other factors influences readability. One of the best and most commonly used formulae for quantifying readability is that developed by Flesch (1946).

In Germany, "readability" of texts has been investigated primarily by Langer and Schulz von Thun (1974). Groeben (1972) examined the theoretical problems of text comprehension and has published a review article in 1976 dealing with the issues within this area.

The exact measurement of readability in quantitative terms is no doubt of great practical significance—and not only in advertising. Of much greater scientific interest, however, is the use of Thorndike-Lorge frequency scores

---

[4] *Translator's note.* The author here contrasts two German novelists, Musil as a difficult writer and Heinrich Böll as a more readable one.

in experimental psychology. Many investigations make use of verbal material, e.g., studies of perception, learning, or memory. Previously almost the only variation in the verbal material had been the distinction between meaningful and nonsense materials. The inclusion of the frequency aspect has made it possible to relate the psychological events of perception, learning or memorizing to the frequency or probability structure of the verbal material.

Let us now attempt to review the theoretical outcome of this series of studies which stretches from Miller-Heise-Lichten via Zipf to Thorndike-Lorge. During decoding the receiver goes through a sequence of discrete states. Which state comes next is partly determined by what is received as a signal, but partly also by what has the greatest probability for the receiver. The world with which we enter into contact is not amorphous; it has a probability profile. This enables us in perception to go beyond the information given. If we hear /si/ and expect figures, the next state that clicks is "six." This click occurs because this state has the greatest probability of occurrence on grounds of acquired verbal habits, of expectancy, and also on the basis of the stimulus that has occurred.

This feature of going beyond the information actually given is basic to all higher processes of perception and cognition. Bruner (1957a) has written a well-known article on this subject, whose main arguments will now be discussed because they summarize, to a great extent, much of what has been alluded to in various contexts in the earlier sections of this book.

A first form of this going beyond the available information consists in the process of assigning an object, as it presents itself, to a class of objects; i.e., the thing is understood as an exemplar of a certain class. We have already met this kind of process once, in our discussion of the discrimination of phonemes; it will be encountered again at a later stage in connection with certain psychological thoughts expressed by Brown. In principle, the mechanism involved in this process of classification is clear: the class is characterized by a number of qualities; if parts of the characteristics of a new object are identical with the defining characteristics of the class, this object is treated as an exemplar belonging to this class. Nevertheless the apparent ease of this ordering process has remained on a restricted and purely formal level. The inductive step from the individual thing to the class is often already taken when only few characteristics are available—e.g., in the case of verbal material when only fragments of the word are heard—so few that "it is positively irresponsible" to make a decision on class membership ("That's six"). It is not the weight of the argument of actually noted characteristics of the object which acts as a driving force; the class is like a magnet that pulls the object towards it, and this "magnetic force" is all the greater the more frequently the class has previously occurred. This can well be illustrated by the dynamics which exist between two neighboring phonemes: here it is not a process of gradual weighing of one quality against another, as if a gradual shift occurred from one phoneme class to another; on the contrary at the point of maximum uncertainty ("Is it still /g/ or already /d/?") we find a strange but most ingenious built-in "tipping" device.

The same process, interpreted somewhat differently, is called *closure* by Gestalt psychology; what is needed to complete the configuration is added. Hebb's explanation of closure in empiricist terms, different from "Gestalt" psychology (the phase sequence, corresponding to the complete gestalt, can be set in motion by any part), could be most helpful in accounting for the processes we have just outlined.

Of course, this peripheral reference to Gestalt psychology makes us aware that this probabilistic approach requires further expansion. Perception, retention, and comprehension is not just determined by that which has occurred frequently, but also by the tendency to form a *meaningful* whole (even if this whole is unusual). One must not reduce that which is meaningful to that which is expected. We will return to this point later. For the moment, let us once again emphasize the most important points.

It must be recognized how very much this tendency towards a biologically meaningful economy permeates all behavior and experience. It begins at the lowest, almost physiological level, with what in general psychology is known as constancy phenomena. A table is perceived as rectangular—regardless of whether it is viewed from above or obliquely from the side. It is seen as rectangular, as one constant object; the various views are, as it were, separate examples of the single class which alone matters, the class "this table."

And at much higher levels we again meet this tendency towards a biologically meaningful economy in the area of social psychology as prejudice or stereotype. As soon as we identify someone as Chinese, Catholic, a Southerner or a Communist, characteristic features for each class are immediately available. That this reduction of variety frequently does not have a desirable result, is perhaps caused by the fact that—to put it crudely—culture has complicated nature and thus it is no longer possible to rely on the energy-saving device of prejudice.

William James, as early as 1890, stressed the importance of this classification process when he said that cognitive life begins when it is possible to exclaim, "Hollo! Thingumbob again."

Placing an individual event into a class of events is one form of going beyond the information given. Another closely related form occurs when we complete missing elements on the basis of present data and the total array of various likely possibilities. In the word PXYCHXLINGUXSTICS the missing elements are supplemented without difficulty. What we meet as an "event"—as we have already learned, for example, from the investigations by Miller, Heise, and Lichten—does not only go with other actual events, but also with other unrealized possible events. Thus, in a concrete speech event, one part of a network of possibilities offered by the structure of the language is lifted into reality. Our perception and behavior are determined by this network as much as by the external stimulation that impinges upon us. The acquisition of this network of probabilities, the knowledge of the probable sequence of events A and B indicate that we have abstracted rules from the continuous sequence of real events—a fact to which Heider (1957) has drawn attention. These formal schemata lie on a higher plane of abstraction than the concrete events. Their acquisition is called *coding* by Bruner. The acquisition of coding systems is probably the most important learning process in the construction of language and cognition.

Looked at from the point of view of language, one of the most decisive problems of the psychology of learning is: How can anything be abstracted, learned and retained from a concrete event or from sequences of events which are in essence unrepeatable? Among the concepts developed by learning theory to come to grips with this problem are the notions of "generalization" and "transfer"; but, we must ask, are the mechanisms denoted by these terms powerful enough to account for these processes? Is successful transfer perhaps less a prerequisite than a consequence of the formation and use of a coding schema? More specifically in terms of language, verbal habits, on the one hand, are the foundations from which to go beyond the information given, but, on the other, the formation or learning of a verbal habit is already a going beyond the concreteness of individual events in the direction of an abstract, general rule. As v. Allesch put it, we grasp generalities *in* things and *by means of* things.

Thus, man faces a world which is not ruled by wild chance, but structured by probabilities. Man is not oriented toward expecting anything and everything that is possible; he anticipates certain possibilities more than others. It is in this area of probability that the regularities which psycholinguistics explores are found. These regularities become evident on the level of concrete reality, but the laws themselves are statements about probabilities. The rules describe the profile of possibilities, and concrete events follow its contour. One objective of a psychology of language is to gain access through concrete events to the probabilistic structure of linguistic processes. By allowing language to happen, man as a speaker or listener makes use of his freedom to link the randomness of reality with the laws of probability.

We must presuppose that man has an organ to be sensitive to this world of latent possibilities. Indeed, what we have described could be interpreted as another expression of the ingeniously designed interaction of organism and environment which has been mentioned repeatedly. What good would it be—to put it in starkly teleological terms—if the events of the world were ordered and lawful, but if the organism were incapable of deriving such order and lawfulness from these events and of taking them into account in his own behavior?

It should be added that we speak of "organism" here quite deliberately and not, for example, of "human intellect," because this "coding" process or

abstracting of rules from events does not occur only in humans, and in humans
not only in conscious activity.

There is no more impressive illustration of this ingeniously designed
relationship between world and organism than the subtle to and fro between
the order which we derive from events and the order which we impose upon
them. Are the classes into which we sort concrete events something we find
in the world or something that we invent *for* the world?

That the linguistic realm possesses a particularly distinct probabilistic
structure may be due to the fact that it is built up of discrete elements. In the
selection and combination of such elements statistical regularities can manifest themselves with particular clarity.

We meet the probabilistic structure of language in its simplest form in the
average values of the appearance of certain items, which add up to millions
of word sequences. These are the values which Zipf and Thorndike have
made use of in such a profitable way.

So far we have spoken globally of the probability with which a particular
word x in the English language is likely to occur. In the following section we
will, so to speak, interpose a kind of more powerful magnification; or, to put
it differently, we will adopt a more dynamic point of view. We are now no
longer concerned with the probability of the appearance of word x in general
in a given language, but with the probability of the appearance of word x
supposing it was immediately preceded by word w.

Whereas in the previous part the probability in general of the appearance
of d in this language, regardless of context, was evinced, we are now
concerned with probabilistic relationships within certain sequences and the
consequences of such relationships, or to put it in more general terms, we
are studying the effect of certain states or events upon later states or events
in a sequence.

Such effects can be noted already in very simple events, which prima facie
would appear to be determined entirely by their physical, i.e., acoustic,
structure. In the description of vowels it was pointed out that a vowel is
determined by the position of its formants; this is a fundamental principle of
phonetics. An investigation by Ladefoged and Broadbent (1957), however,
shows that this view is oversimplified. These two authors asked the question, Does the identification of a vowel depend upon the absolute values of
its formants (this is the commonly accepted view), or does it depend on the
relationship of these formant values to the values of other vowels which the
hearer has already heard from the same speaker?

The experiment was conducted in the following manner. The subject hears
a synthesized, i.e., artificially produced, introductory statement: "Please say
what this word is," followed by the test word: "bit," "bet," "bat," or
"but." The introductory statements are distinguished only by the formant
structure of their vowels, i.e., one, for example, might sound a little
"darker" than another. The result is that, for example, the test word A is

identified by 87 percent of the listeners as "bit" if it is preceded by version one of the introductory statement, but the *same* test word *A* is identified as "bet" by 90 percent of the listeners if it is preceded by version two of the introductory sentence.

The results of this experiment indicate two things. First, the listener adjusts his program of analysis so to speak to the general sound patterns of the (preceding) auditory events. Second, later events or conditions of a sequence are perceived in a way which is determined by the perception of previous events and states of the sequence. Thus linguistic events are conceptualized here as though they were structured according to a Markov process.

> A Markov process is a stochastic process, i.e., an event which proceeds according to laws of probability. The probability of the occurrence of a certain state in the future can be fully predicted from the present state. This prediction cannot be improved upon by additional information on the past of the system (based on Kendall and Buckland, 1960, p. 174). A Markov model is therefore a so-called finite-state model.

Linguistic expressions, sentences consist of structured sequences of individual events. From this perspective, and under the impact of information theory, it appeared reasonable to conceptualize the nature of grammatical rules that characterize and determine a sentence as Markov chains. Saying it differently and more crudely, what the linguist describes as grammatical rules, should be viewed theoretically by the psychologist as transitional and joint probabilities of the elements of a sentence.

This assumption served as an impetus for many of the investigations which will be discussed later in this chapter. In anticipation, however, let us point to the weaknesses of this model. The model attempts to describe the linkage of units in probabilistic terms, and then proceeds to explain linguistic phenomena in terms of such associations. But the units to which it refers are always members of the same set or level; they are either phonemes *or* letters *or* words. The unit that is selected is then used for the analysis of the entire sequence. As we discussed extensively in the previous chapter, however, grammatical structures consist of hierarchical relationships between units of *different* sets, e.g., nominal phrase, substantive, in the accusative, in the plural. In historical retrospect, it is easy to say that a total reduction of grammatical structures to probabilistic ones is doomed to failure. Nevertheless this approach has come amazingly far. (One of the weaknesses of the grammatic-syntactic models, which dominate today, is that they totally ignore probabilistic determinants.)

It was just noted that linguistic events consist of structured sequences. This can be expressed in another way by saying that linguistic events are redundant or contain redundancies. Redundancy is not a characteristic of a single event but of a sequence of events. If the degree of redundancy is zero, all possible events have equal probability of occurrence. Suppose we write each letter of the alphabet on a separate piece of paper, put all the pieces into a hat, then pick one at random and after copying the letter put it back, the sequence of letters we will thus make up will have zero redundancy, e.g., ZSBKBJPGXEVAOOWGAS. In such a sequence the knowledge of one letter has no predictive value for the next; a maximal degree of uncertainty remains. Each letter has the equal probability of occurrence of 1 over 26. In other words, each letter has an information content of approximately 4.5 bits $(26 = 2^{4.5})$.

But supposing now that individual letters or definite sequences of letters (or also of other units) appear more frequently than others, the average information content in each unit decreases. The extreme case would be 100 percent redundancy in which events succeed each other according to a fixed rule, so that if one event is known all subsequent ones can be predicted. A sequence AAAAA . . . is completely redundant, but so is the sequence XFKXFKXFKX . . .

Linguistic sequences have a redundancy degree between 0 and 100 percent. The more redundant a language is, the more individual events or single symbols are needed to transmit a message.

Taking a telegram as an example, let us analyze it at the word level (i.e., with the word as the unit of analysis). It reads: "I am arriving on Monday, the 4th of February, 1963, at 12 o'clock noon." This telegram contains redundancies. As soon as one has read "I" the subsequent verb form must be "am" with the verb "arriving," and likewise "am arriving" can only go with "I." The message that the 4th of February, 1963, is a Monday is also redundant, because a calendar can establish this. And if one assumes a 24-hour clock, the message that 12 o'clock is noon would be equally redundant.

An economical sender could shorten this message by cutting out redundancies. Redundancy is therefore the noneconomical element in the transmission of information.

We came across a similar phenomenon previously when we noted that the information capacity of the human voice was only exploited to a small degree. Just as it would be possible in the case of vocalization to manage with a smaller number of intensities and frequencies, in the present case far fewer words, and far fewer symbols would be sufficient if all of them had the largest possible information content and if therefore all would be equally probable. In both instances, instead of extreme economy, preference is given to safety of communication. In a message which contains redundancies it does not matter if one or the other mistake occurs; it does not affect the sense or create a misunderstanding: I UM ARIVING ON MANDAY 44 EEBRUARY 1963 AT 112 O'CLOCK NOOM.

Up to this point we have discussed joint probabilities, i.e., the probability of the simultaneous occurrence of two or more events, and conversely, transitional probabilities, i.e., the probability of the event y occurring, when *x* has previously occurred. The concept of redundancy has also been defined in a general way. Now let us attempt to show, by reviewing empirical studies, the manner in which these concepts can be used to explain psychologically the linguistic processes occurring in the listener (speaker). To do so we must first introduce the idea of approximation to natural language: zero-order approximation, first or second order approximation, etc.

We mentioned earlier a sequence of letters in which the 26 letters of the alphabet have equal probability of appearance. Such a completely random sequence is a zero-order approximation to English. Following the principle of Thorndike-Lorge it can be stated how often each letter of the alphabet appears in a very long text in a language. A table with such values for German is presented in Table 3.

If we put into a hat from which we want to draw random sequences of letters quantities of letters corresponding to the frequencies indicated in the table (and not as in a zero-order approximation all letters in equal quantities) a first-order approximation can be drawn. A German example is: NTDE SWNIKRUTARH ENIAS. An English example of a first-order approximation would be the following letter sequences: OCRO HLI RGWR NMIEL-WIS EU LL NBNESEBYA etc.[5]

With the next step we want to study the occurrence of two-letter sequences or digrams in English and German. A technique which is frequently employed in such studies is the following. A two-letter sequence is picked first, e.g., LE. Then the next occurrence in the text of E is looked for and the letter immediately following, for example, G. Subsequently we pick the next G in the text and the letter after it. The following item might, for example, be a space. A second-order approximation to German, produced in this way, looks as follows:

LEG OMSOFER ZE AN MEMENEIT SES KLACH

An example based on an English text would be:

ON IE ANTSOUTINYS ARE T INCTORE ST BE S DEAMY etc.

An illustration of German third-order approximation or trigram is:

NICH UND EIN WARTE TICHEN

English third-order approximations are:

IN NO IST LAT WHEY CRATICT FROURE BIRS GROCID etc.

What has been done so far on the level of the letter symbol can equally be done with the unit ''word.'' The zero-order approximation consists of words

---

Table 3. Mean frequency of occurrence of letters in a German text comprising one million lexical items.

Interval	151490
E	147004
N	88351
R	68577
I	63770
S	53881
T	47310
D	43854
H	43554
A	43309
U	31877
L	29312
C	26733
G	26672
M	21336
O	17717
B	15972
Z	14225
W	14201
F	13598
K	9558
V	7350
Ü	5799
P	4992
Ä	4907
Ö	2547
J	1645
Y	173
Q	142
X	129
Total	999985

Based on Zemanek, 1959, with modifications from Steinbuch, 1965, p. 42.

picked at random from the dictionary. A first-order approximation contains words proportional to their general frequency as determined in the Thorndike-Lorge manner. Approximations of a higher order are commonly developed in the following way: the first person is given a word, e.g., "come," with the request to add a word which might follow. A subject responds with the word "with." The next subject is given "with" and might write "sugar," the following subject adding to "sugar," writes, for example, "or." This yields as a second-order approximation sequence: "come with sugar or."[6]

This procedure, which goes back to Shannon, uses verbal habits to arrive at statements on the structure of the language or to study the relationships between this structure and the psychological processes involved in speaking and hearing.

Approximations of the various orders at the word-unit level lead to the following English examples taken from Shannon. First-order word approximations (chosen independently but with the appropriate frequencies): REPRESENTING AND SPEEDILY IS AN GOOD APT OR COME CAN DIFFERENT NATURAL HERE HE THE A IN etc.

Second-order word approximations: THE HEAD AND IN FRONTAL ATTACK ON AN ENGLISH WRITER THAT THE CHARACTER OF THIS POINT IS THEREFORE ANOTHER METHOD etc.[7]

As the order of approximation rises the influence of preceding elements on a subsequent item steadily increases. At a fourth-order approximation at word level, each individual word is determined by three preceding words. The context—this is in the nature of redundancy—produces certain constraints, but not an absolute compulsion, as to what may or may not occur in this context.

This series of approximations to genuine language is regarded by Miller as a continuum starting with "nonsense" at one pole and moving more and more towards meaningful utterances at the opposite pole. In other words, Miller regards the difference between meaningless and meaningful utterances not as strict alternatives but as a finely graded dimension.

This is just one possible way to define meaning and many linguists are not going to accept it, despite the fact that they cannot propose a generally acceptable alternative. If, however, it is heuristically profitable to equate the series of approximations with the dimension of sense/nonsense, it should be possible to come to grips with a problem which has troubled the psychology of learning as well as psycholinguistics for a long time, namely the problem of why meaningful material should be learned and retained more easily than nonsense material. What was and was not meaningful could, up to now, be determined only subjectively. If Miller's equation should prove true, we

---

[6] *Translator's note.* The author's German example starting from 'komme' has led to the sequence: 'komme ich bin doch . . .'

[7] The following German examples are taken from an investigation by Herrmann.

Zero-order: Beweis Ausraufung stabil Linde Stiel gemäß der . . .
              (Proof tearing-out stable lime-tree stem according the . . .)

First-order: Aus wurde Kino von über wir Thema noch Korn Grund . . .
              (Out became cinema of over we topic still corn bottom . . .)

Third-order: Arbeit gedeiht im Januar schneit es oft lieber geschwätzig als Putzfrau fegen . . .
              (Work thrives in January it snows often rather loquacious as cleaner sweep . . .)

Sixth-order: Mainz fand vorige Woche der Kongreß statt und endete mit Applaus aller . . .
              (Mainz took place last week the congress and ended with applause of all . . .)

would at least have an operational definition for an important dimension of linguistic phenomena, even if we probably should call it something other than meaningfulness.

Using words as units, Miller and Selfridge (1950) constructed approximations of different order. These were arranged in lists of varying length (10, 20, 30, and 50 words) so that there were: one set of four lists of different lengths of zero-order approximation, another set of four lists of varying lengths of first-order approximation, and so forth. Each list was recorded on magnetic tape, and subjects were asked to listen to these recordings. Each subject's task was to write down immediately what he had retained. The score was the percentage of words remembered correctly.

In Fig. 32 the coordinates are order of approximation and percentage of correctly remembered words. The parameter is the length of the list. The same results are represented in Fig. 33 with the order of approximation as the parameter and the length of the lists plotted along the abscissa.

As one would expect, the evidence shows, first of all, that the percentage of correctly remembered words declines as the length of the list increases. Second, the evidence shows—and this is what interests us here—that the percentage of correctly remembered words increases with the rising order of approximation.

What stands out is that there is no variation in retention from about the fifth order of approximation, not even with "genuine" text. Strictly speaking, all degrees of approximation are nonsense, but memory, it appears, does not function according to the dichotomy; a passage of fifth or sixth order of approximation is retained as well as genuine text. Thus, the psychologically relevant distinction is not the sharp division between sense and nonsense, but the distinction between material in which earlier learning can become

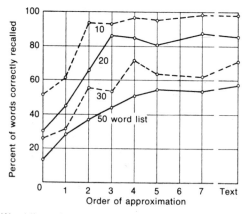

Fig. 32. Word lists of varying length were presented (10, 20, 30, or 50 words). The figure shows the percentage of words recalled correctly as a function of the order of approximation to English. (From Miller and Selfridge, 1950, p. 181)

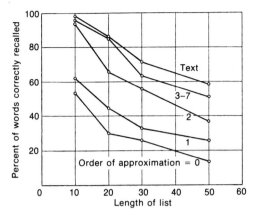

Fig. 33. Data as in Fig. 32. Percentage of words recalled correctly presented as a function of the length of the word lists for different orders of approximation (0, 1, 2, 3–7) and authentic text. (From Miller and Selfridge, 1950, p. 181)

effective and material in which earlier learning has less influence. What has been learned earlier is the structured nature of language. As language is acquired, such learning includes the transitional probabilities which lead from one event to the next. The experiment by Miller and Selfridge is designed to make the effect visible upon retention of these acquired transitional probabilities. If in the past it used to be said that meaningful material is easier to retain because it is meaningful, we can now be more precise by saying: meaningful material is easier to retain because it contains, to a higher degree than nonsense material does, the transitional probabilities of everyday language.

The investigation by Miller and Selfridge was an attempt to study the effect of a certain form of redundancy. In Miller's experiments, redundancy is a higher degree of approximation to English structure, or greater contextual determination or lowered content of information per unit. Such redundancy normally eases or improves the performance. Miller made subjects learn redundant and less redundant letter sequences, Adelson, Muckler and Williams (1955) letters in redundant and less redundant lists, Rubenstein and Aborn (1954) an artificial language of varying degrees of redundancy: in every case learning improves with redundancy. This proposition, however, is only applicable as long as the learning achievement is measured by the quantity of learned material. But as redundancy lowers the information content per unit, redundancy does not, or at least does not inevitably, increase the learning performance in terms of information theory.

The influence of order of approximation upon learning and retention of the material can of course be interpreted as positive transfer of verbal habits acquired through the use of everyday language. Whatever is in keeping with such habits does not have to be learned afresh again.

An effect of redundancy on the perception of speech was seen in a different context in the investigation by Miller, Heise, and Lichten: under conditions of noise isolated words are not recognized as well as words in sentences. Speed of reading and writing is greater in sequences of a higher order of approximation than in sequences of a lower order (Sumby and Pollack, 1954).

In such investigations the length of the sequence used plays an important part, because if the sequence is too short, the effect of context, i.e., redundancy, is hardly noticeable. Even if we make subjects guess the gaps in a text, the process of guessing is guided by the verbal habits of the subject, or by the knowledge the subject possesses of the statistical structure of his native language. Miller and Friedman (1957) found that, in sequences of eleven letter-symbols each, the first and last letter can be guessed correctly in fifty to sixty percent of cases, but the sixth letter, on the other hand, in 95 percent. The influence of context is effective in both the forward and the backward direction. If it was effective only in the forward direction, it should be possible to guess the final letter more easily than the sixth and the sixth better than the first. This finding leads beyond a pure Markov theory; and we shall, therefore, not pursue it for the moment.

From quite a different angle similar problems were already encountered before the turn of the century. According to J. McK. Cattell (1885), in the same time span which is needed to identify four or five randomly chosen letters, it is possible to read three short words containing each four or five letters. Erdmann and Dodge, whose investigations on the reading process around the turn of the century became world famous, were able to show that complete words are still readable at a distance when individual letters can no longer be identified.

What eminently practical consequences such investigations may have can be illustrated by the following study. Wallach (1963) exposed nonsense words for brief moments to fifth-grade children. These words represented varying degrees of approximation to English. It was shown that good spellers among the children were able to recognize words of a higher order of approximation significantly faster than poor spellers. From this result it can be inferred that good spellers have acquired a knowledge of the transitional probabilities common in their language and they are able to transfer this knowledge to the solution of a new task.

The probability structures, stored in the receptor mechanism, determine to a large extent what this mechanism achieves. Broadbent has expressed it in a formula: If someone is supposed to reproduce what he has read or heard, he tends to produce what he and others would have uttered, if immediately beforehand they themselves had said what has previously been uttered in the experiment. While the notion of verbal habit, a concept akin to transitional probability, has thus moved into the foreground, it must not be oversimplified. Even if the stimulus has not been correctly understood, this does not mean that the most probable state will automatically appear. If noise makes a word incomprehensible, it is still possible for the number of syllables, for example, to have a codetermining influence on the choice of what has been heard. To make this evident, Broadbent, following Treisman, assumes a series of dictionary units. Each of these units corresponds to a given word. What actually happens in this series is statistically determined by the units which have just been activated and by the kind of immediate stimulation. Broadbent illustrates this approach by this example: Someone overhears in a noisy room a political conversation and picks out the following fragment, "I think that, at the next election Mr. Carter will . . ." followed by a monosyllabic word with the sound "ite." A position of readiness is adopted by those units of the internal dictionary which correspond to verbs (to satisfy syntax) and which have political significance (because of the context). The sensory information adds to these response factors the stimulus factors which reinforce the activity of monosyllabic units of those ending in "ite." The combination of these factors produces as the most probable word "fight" and the listener will hear this word. But the decision is statistical and may be wrong; perhaps the speaker said "bite" (Table 4).

Broadbent's dictionary units are somewhat undefined formulations. The concept on which they are based was expanded by Morton (1969), who calls these units *logogens*. A logogen is a sort of counter which adds information from two sources. Via the sensory analyzer, it takes in information about the features of the auditory stimuli, but it also receives information from the mechanisms that produce the context. When the information within the particular logogen has reached or exceeded a certain threshold, the word that corresponds to it becomes available; it can then appear, for example, as a response in a perception experiment or contribute to conscious comprehension. We see that each logogen is defined, on the one hand, in terms of the semantic, visual, and acoustic attributes that it can absorb (and add) as information and, on the other hand, in terms of the word that it makes available, after reaching the appropriate level of informedness.[8]

If we wish to explain continuous reading, for example, by means of this model, or apply it to the comprehension of spoken text, then we must further assume that the countersetting of each logogen must rapidly (i.e., within 1 second) return to its base level. In those cases where we are dealing with coherent text, the base level of certain logogens will always be higher than others which are not related to the particular context. There is a linkage here to the term "presupposition," a concept which has been used extensively (in some cases overused) by contemporary text linguistics, but we are not going to explore this further.

---

[8] We cannot enter here into a discussion of the difference between this model and that proposed by Deutsch and Deutsch (1963); to do so would require an examination of the concept of attention.

Table 4

Words under consideration	Verb	Political context	-ite sound	One syllable	Total
Bite	+	−	+	+	3
Stand	+	+	−	+	3
Appetite	−	−	+	−	1
Filibuster	+	+	−	−	2
Fight	+	+	+	+	4

Based on Broadbent, in Reuck and O'Connor, 1964, p. 85.

The "unknowns" in Morton's model are, of course, the context-producing mechanisms. A more detailed analysis of the factors that are important here soon forces us to abandon the so-called left-right models (i.e., all models that are able to explain later conditions only in terms of a preceding one, and that includes the Markov models) and to introduce hierarchical structures, thereby returning once more to the domain of grammar.

It is not surprising that since the early 1960s psycholinguists have all but abandoned the questions of frequency of occurrence, probability, and degree of availability. There has been a general awareness that a probabilistic model could neither explain the grammaticality of sentences nor adequately describe the structure of events taking place within the sentence. Thus we lost sight of a determining factor (of couse, not *the* determining factor) of linguistic phenomena. Quite aside from the fact that probability components of language have important practical applications, ranging from the composition of easily comprehended text to the design of typewriter keyboards, recently it has, once more, become evident that aspects of probability must also be considered in a *theory* of linguistic events. Chafe (1970) recognized that not all utterances can be processed according to the same generative schema, e.g., an idiom must not be analyzed at the level of words. For the psychologist, this raises the question whether perhaps probabilistic factors determine which (grammatical) program of analysis is to be employed in each particular case.

Van Lancker (1975) has presented extensive data with respect to speech *production* which also support an increased need for taking probabilistic approaches into consideration in the formulation of theories. She has shown that persons with damage to the left hemisphere of the brain show little or no deficits in the production of verbal expressions that are highly overlearned, i.e., which are characterized by a high level of joint probabilities. Apparently such expressions as "how do you do?," "best regards," "good-bye" are produced in a different manner and, in any case, with the aid of a different part of the brain than those expressions which have a weaker probability of association. Such "new" expressions are much more affected by lesions in the left hemisphere than are those with high probabilities. According to Van Lancker, speech consists of groups of expressions that vary greatly in terms of their degree of automaticity. It is precisely in terms of these considerations that the probability structure of speech, which we have discussed in this chapter, gains renewed theoretical importance.

CHAPTER 6

Verbal Association and the Problem of Meaning

From a sequential to an associationist viewpoint—The concept of association—Galton and Marbe—Association experiments and everyday verbal behavior—Norms of association and their range of application— Group and personality factors in the differentiation of verbal habits— Jung's investigations and Laffal's critique—Elements of meaning— Clark—The concept of semantic field—Deese's studies of association.

The present chapter adopts a different viewpoint from the preceding chapters. This change can be made clear by referring back to Saussure. In his discussion on the arbitrary nature of symbols he says that symbols are restricted in two ways, or a speech event is determined by two groups of factors. The first group consists of the syntactical and probabilistic relationships which bind one link in the chain of an utterance with the preceding and subsequent ones. These are the relationships we considered in the preceding chapters.

But a linguistic unit has other units not only before and after but also above and below it, so to speak; each link in the sentence chain is connected with other words, images or thoughts which are *associated* with it. As soon as a word is thought or uttered, other words simultaneously appear in consciousness or on the threshold of consciousness. According to Saussure, this is the second group of factors determining the speech event.

The distinction between the sequential and associative approach can be illustrated by the following example. A sentence: This man comes from Canada is a stretch in the dimension of time. As the sentence is uttered or heard, it is as if a pointer marking each moment of the utterance moved from one block to the next. Sequential psycholinguistics seeks to find the structures which link these blocks.

So far we have limited our discussion to the effects of those probability structures that link a present element of the speech structure with a preceding element. This approach deals with manifest speech events that do not require special methods to make them amenable to investigation. From the very start the material is factual and clearly apparent.

Now supposing we stop the course of time at one point. Our question is whether in the verbal item which is just occurring there are links to latently present verbal materials in the speaker or listener (Fig. 34).

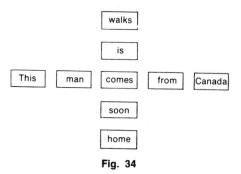

Fig. 34

The associative approach which will occupy us in the following pages also looks for relationships: not for relationships which manifest themselves in the concrete speech event, but in the relations between a manifest unit and one (or more than one) latent or covert unit.

In discourse, in the sequence of the verbal utterance, as Saussure said (Am. edition, 1959, p. 123), all elements are ordered in a linear fashion: combinations of such consecutive units are called syntagms. Outside discourse, or more precisely, between the element occurring in the utterance and the processes which simultaneously occur consciously or unconsciously in the listener or speaker, there are links of an associative character.

Syntagmatic links are relationships *in praesentia*. Associative links, on the other hand, as Saussure says, bring together concepts, *in absentia*, into a potential series.

In order to be able to discover associative structures, the latent, covert *units*—as we shall call them more cautiously than if we spoke of *concepts*—must be actualized or made manifest by means of a special technique.

A technique or aid is needed to find out whether in addition to the manifest unit (the uttered word) something else is present and possibly active in the darkness of the subconscious. Such an aid is the word-association experiment which serves to transform an associative relationship which is not immediately tangible into a sequential and tangible one.

The principle of this experiment is the following: The subject is given a single unit (a word) with the instruction to respond to this unit with the first word that comes to his mind. The underlying rationale is: if no other structure determines what should follow (e.g., the intention to utter a particular sentence or the probabilistic determination derived from a particular sequence) then what follows is linked to the particular unit by association.

The concept of "association" has certain mechanistic overtones—and for many linguistic scholars and psychologists in German-speaking countries "mechanistic" is still a derogatory expression. Anyone who has reservations of this kind (and indeed anyone with reservations about the soulless quantitative approach in earlier sections of this book) might well consider a reflection by Stenzel who as a *philosopher* of language wrote as follows: "Even the expression at the sensory level and the combination of expressions into higher linguistic configurations are governed by certain regularities which are distinct from the freely intended meaning and yet are of greatest importance for the expressive possibilities of meanings through language. These regularities can be described as the laws of association . . . An unprejudiced appreciation of the psychological study of language again reveals a basic antinomy of speech: language at each moment of its existence transcends the area of intended meaning and at the same time is still governed by the fundamentally different laws of the psychophysical plane from which it originates and from which it cannot escape. Here the power of association is the great provider of substance for expression, and objectively language, realized in the growth, life and decline of a particular idiom, is unthinkable without this primitive psychophysical foundation" (1934, p. 9).

The notion of *association* originated in Greek philosophy. Ideas, images, and thoughts are combined in such a way that the appearance of one brings to mind another *associated* with it. Such association can (according to Aristotle) be brought about in two ways.

A first factor leading to such combinations consists in the *quality* of the images or thoughts. One image is associated with others which are either similar or stand in contrast to it. The word "big" accordingly would be associated with "huge" as well as with "small." This use of the notion of similarity can lead to difficulties: we associate what is similar—but, at the same time, similar is what is associated.

The second source, from which associations may come, according to this view, is *experience*. What is experienced as simultaneous or successive is associated. If ideas *a* and *b* were once experienced as simultaneous or in close succession, idea *a* will, when it occurs in future, tend to call to consciousness idea *b*.

This view which sees the origin of association not in the inherent characteristics of the associated facts but in empirically verifiable events has remained to this day the foundation of the psychology of learning.

Above all, the English school of philosophers of the eighteenth and nineteenth centuries regarded associations as the basic mechanism of the entire psychic life; Hobbes, Locke, Hume, the two Mills, and Spencer should be mentioned here.

The attempt to comprehend the concept of association experimentally is linked—like so many important events in psychology—with the name of Galton.

Galton simply wrote 75 words on slips of paper, put these away for a few days, then picking one of them without looking at it, put it under a book in such a way that by leaning over he could read what was written on it. As soon as he saw the word, he started a "chronograph" and stopped it again the moment two ideas in connection with this word had come to his mind. He divided the ideas which came to his mind into (a) visual or other imagery of past events; (b) histrionic representations, i.e., the reenacting of an event or attitude, and (c) purely verbal ideas: names, sentences or quotations.

The frequencies with which these three classes appeared were 33, 22, and 45 percent. Basing himself on these experiments, he expressed the following reflection in the journal *Brain*: "It would be very instructive to print the actual records at length, made by many experimenters, if the records could be clubbed together and thrown into a statistical form; but it would be too absurd to print one's own singly. They lay bare the foundations of a man's thoughts with curious distinctness and exhibit his mental anatomy with more vividness and truth than he himself would probably care to publish to the world" (1880, p. 162).

This statement by Galton represents a milestone which is common to two, in other respects, very different lines of scientific development: on the one hand Freud's psychoanalysis, and on the other contemporary psychology of learning and psycholinguistics.

Galton's technique was in the first instance taken up by Trautscholdt (1883) in the first psychological laboratory, set up at that time by Wundt in Leipzig, and then, above all, by one of Wundt's American doctoral candidates, J. McK. Cattell (1886). From the beginning the studies almost always examined both of Galton's variables: first, the response made to a stimulus, and second, the time between stimulus and response. And even the instruction to the subject remained identical over the decades: "I am going to read to you (*or in visual presentation,* "I am going to show to you") a list of words. After each word please answer with the first word that comes to your mind."

What this prototype of the association experiment demonstrates is regarded—as was already pointed out—as a connection resulting either from the quality of the associated words (similarity or contrast) or as a connection resulting from an earlier experience of cooccurrence of the two words.

As can be seen, the study of association and its theoretical foundations brings psycholinguistics into the neighborhood of the psychology of learning (similarly, sequential psycholinguistics found a place close to information theory). This link with the psychology of learning will prove to be crucial because it connects psycholinguistics with many other fields.

Let us begin our presentation of the results of association studies by a relatively detailed report on some older inquiries in order to see in perspective what sort of data are produced by subjects in an association experiment.

In 1901 Thumb and Marbe published a study which to this day has remained fundamental.[1] Sixty words, one after another, were called out to the subjects; the list was made up of 10 terms of family relations (father, mother . . .), 10 adjectives (big, small . . .), 10 pronouns (I, you . . .), 10 adverbials of place (in front of, where . . .), 10 adverbials of time (when, now . . .) and the numerals 1 to 10—all these in random order. The responses of the subjects were noted as well as the time between stimulus and response.

It was found that generally terms of family relations led to answers with terms of family relations; indeed a particular stimulus-word would lead to quite a particular response. In the cases investigated by Marbe the reaction to "brother" was always "sister," to "son" generally "father" rarely "daughter" and never "brother" or "uncle." The associations called out by a stimulus-word do not consist of *any* words, but they fall into distinct classes. For each stimulus-word one can rank the frequency of occurrence of different responses. In the terminology of the psychology of learning it might be formulated as follows: if the S-R sequence in an association experiment is regarded as a habit, the habits released by a stimulus-word vary in strength. This formulation is possible, because the probability of occurrence is the principal indicator of habit-strength. Accordingly, the habit of responding to the word "son" with "father" would be stronger than the habit of reacting to "son" with "daughter."

If, in analogy to the psychology of learning, the probability of occurrence of a response is treated as an indicator of habit- or associative-strength, it is not far-fetched to inquire also into the other indicator of habit-strength, the reaction-time between S and R. Marbe found that in general more frequently preferred associations occur more rapidly than less preferred ones.

The curve in which Marbe related the frequency of occurrence of an association to reaction-time has found its place in the history of psychology as Marbe's law (Fig. 35).

Continuing our discussion we interpret the Thumb-Marbe investigations as follows:

1. Stimulus- and response-words in an association experiment are often, but not always, similar in form: kinship terms are met with kinship terms, nouns with nouns, and adjectives with adjectives. The stimulus, as it were, unlocks a certain class, or touches off a certain category which thus leads to the selection of an actual response. A definite regularity of associative linguistic behavior is thus indicated.

2. A given stimulus-word produces identical responses in different subjects to a marked degree. The relative frequency of certain associations is, therefore, an important starting point for further inquiries.

---

[1] Incidentally, this investigation was the result of a collaboration—rare in German-speaking countries—between a linguist and a psychologist. Thumb was a professor of comparative philology, Marbe a lecturer in philosophy at Würzburg.

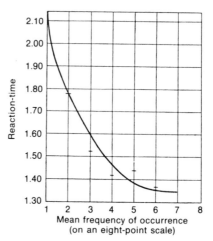

Fig. 35. Reaction time for association as a function of the frequency of occurrence. (Based on Thumb and Marbe, 1901, p. 46)

3. The delay between stimulus and response or reaction-time stands in a lawful relationship to the relative frequency of occurrence of a response. This time score, therefore, can equally be subjected to further investigation.

Historically (and logically) the first steps in the systematic advance in this area have been the following:

First, a "phenomenology" or inventory of associations is established. Which are the most frequent associations with "table," "bed," "chair," "drive," "work," "long," and "love"? With what frequency do they occur? What is the next most frequent response? In other words, the first step consists in the setting up of norms.

Second, certain questions result from these considerations: how widely do these norms apply? Do French speakers respond to the same stimulus-words differently from English speakers? Are the habitual verbal responses of, say, manual workers different from those of university students? Are there changes with the age of the subjects in the relative frequency of particular associations?

Third, how are we to interpret individual deviations from these norms? Is the fact that someone fails to react with the most common associations significant for the total verbal behavior of that individual or even his nonverbal behavior? We can put the same question for the other index of associative strength: Can any significance be attributed to the fact that in the case of a given individual certain responses appear only after·an unusually long reaction-time?

In short, our questions are concerned (1) with the general principles of organization of the fields of force underlying verbal behavior, (2) with social, cultural and developmental variants of these principles of organization and, finally, (3) with personality-specific variations which may be symptomatic only for verbal behavior, but which may also be indices of extralinguistic aspects of behavior.

Norms were established above all through the investigations of Kent and Rosanoff, published in 1910, and based on the responses of 1000 subjects. Table 5 shows the distribution of responses to the stimulus-word "needle."

This investigation shows that a small number of responses appear relatively frequently, while a large number are produced only by single subjects.

Table 5. Distribution of associations with the stimulus-word "needle." The left-hand column indicates the number of subjects who responded to "needle" with the word in the right-hand column.

Frequency in 1000 subjects	Response-word
160	thread
158	pin(s)
152	sharp
135	sew(s)
107	sewing
53	steel
40	point
26	instrument
17	eye
15	thimble
12	useful
11	prick(s)
9	pointed
7	cotton
6	work
5	implement
5	tool
4	cloth
4	darning
4	knitting
4	sharpness
3	article
3	fine
3	metal
2 each	books, button(s), clothes, coat, dressmaker, hurt, hypodermic, industry, pricking, small, sting, thick, thin,
1 each	blood, broken, camel, crocheting, cut, diligence, embroidery, handy, help, hole, home, housewife, labor, long, magnetic, material, mending, nail, ornament, patching, pincushion, shiny, slippers, stitching, surgeon, tailor, use, using, weapon. wire, woman

From Woodworth. 1954, p. 51.

The most frequent response to a stimulus-word is called the *primary response*.

These investigations were concerned with accurate *descriptions* of the associations of the experimental subjects; we now turn to the question of how these norms are changed or differentiated, if we do not deal simply with subjects in general, but with subjects belonging to defined groups. In other words, we are not now studying verbal habits as such, but the verbal habits of defined groups. The following discussion, therefore, lies on the borderline between psycholinguistics and sociolinguistics.

Thanks to investigations by Russell and Rosenzweig we are now in a position to compare American, French and German groups of students. The basis of these investigations was, throughout, the Kent-Rosanoff list of stimulus-words and their translations. Table 6 shows a part of the 100

Table 6. Stimulus-words of the word-association test, primary responses in German, French, and English, and for each response percentage of subjects.

German, French, English	% German	% French	% English
1. Tisch, table, table	29 Stuhl	53 chaise	84 chair
2. dunkel, sombre, dark	44 hell, e	45 clair	83 light
3. Musik, musique, music	9 Ton, Töne	16 note, s	18 song, s
4. Krankheit, maladie, sickness	15 Gesundheit	10 santé	38 health
5. Mann, homme, man	52 Frau	66 femme	77 woman, en
6. tief, profond, deep	49 hoch	12 creux	32 shallow
7. weich, mou, soft	39 hart	39 dur, e	45 hard
8. Essen, manger, eating	23 trinken	39 boire	39 food
9. Berg, montagne, mountain	35 Tal	13 plaine	27 hill, s
10. Haus, maison, house	14 Hof	14 toit	25 home
11. schwarz, noir, black	48 weiß	41 blanc	25 white
12. Hammelfleisch, mouton, mutton	7 Rindfleisch, Essen	25 laine	37 lamb
13. Bequemlichkeit, confort, comfort	15 Sessel	19 fauteuil	12 chair
14. Hand, main, hand	20 Fuß	25 pied, s	26 foot, (ee)
15. kurz, petit, short	53 lang	48 grand	40 tall
16. Obst, fruit, fruit	18 Gemüse	20 pomme, s	38 apple
17. Schmetterling, papillon, butterfly	12 Falter	11 fleur, s	15 moth
18. glatt, lisse, smooth	34 Eis	18 rugueux	33 rough
19. kommandieren, ordre, command	23 befehlen	24 désordre	20 order
20. Stuhl, chaise, chair	20 Tisch	24 table	50 table
21. süß, doux, sweet	39 sauer	11 dur, e	44 sour

From Russell and Meseck, 1959, p. 196.

stimulus-words with their corresponding primary responses (i.e., the most frequent associations) in each of the three linguistic groups.

In 1961 Rosenzweig compared the available data in American, German, French, and Italian Kent-Rosanoff studies; he determined the number of cases in which the associative primary response to a particular stimulus-word was equivalent in meaning with that given to the corresponding stimulus in the other language. The response to "table" in English is "chair," to "Tisch" in German "Stuhl," and to "table" in French "chaise." This suggests that there are associative structures transcending single linguistic communities.[2] The more frequently a primary response occurs in one languge, the greater is the probability that the equivalent response to the corresponding stimulus-word also occurs in kindred languages.

Even more interesting than the comparison of the semantic content of the associations is a comparison of frequencies with which certain associations appear in different languages.

If, for example, the German and French experimental groups are compared, a high measure of agreement of the frequency distribution will be found. This, of course, does not mean that "Fenster" and "fenêtre" elicit *identical* responses, the agreement refers to the degree of spread of certain associations in general. But it is here that a surprising difference occurs between the French and German groups on the one side and the American group on the other. As an illustration, let us take item 49 from Table 7 "Adler," "eagle," and "aigle" all yield as primary responses "bird" or their equivalents in the other languages, but among German and French students these primary responses have frequencies of 21 and 16 percent respectively, whereas 55 percent of all American students respond to "eagle" with "bird." Similar trends are noted with many other responses.

Thus, in the American group there is a marked tendency to react uniformly to a stimulus-word, whereas the associations elicited by the stimulus-words in the German and French groups are much more heterogeneous. Nearly a quarter of all American associations produce higher frequencies than the most frequent German association. The difference between the mean value of the two curves of distribution is significant at the .001 level.

To sum up, in content, the associations in the three languages are very similar to each other; only quantitatively there is this surprising disparity. This result provokes speculation about national psychology. Fortunately there is empirical evidence to guide such speculations.

J. J. Jenkins of the University of Minnesota, one of the leading researchers in this area, has published a comparison of earlier American association

---

[2] A somewhat more problematical comparison of word associations in the four European languages with the associations of Navaho Indians suggests a far greater degree of agreement among the European languages than between each of these and the Navaho language.

Table 7. Stimulus-words of the word-association test, primary responses in German, English and French, and for each response percentage of subjects.

German, French, English	% German	% French	% English
49. Adler, aigle, eagle	21 Vogel	16 (l')oiseau	55 bird
50. Magen, estomac, stomach	14 Darm	8 digestion	21 food
51. Stiel, tige, stem	39 Besen	33 fleur, s	40 flower
52. Lampe, lampe, lamp	36 Licht	35 lumière	63 light
53. träumen, rêver, dream	19 schlafen	17 sommeil	45 sleep
54. gelb, jaune, yellow	12 rot	11 vert	15 blue
55. Brot, pain, bread	20 essen	11 (et) vin	61 butter
56. Gerechtigkeit, justice, justice	12 Gericht	9 juge, s	25 peace
57. Junge, garçon, boy	37 Mädchen	42 fille	76 girl
58. Licht, clair, light	22 dunkel	31 obscur	64 dark
59. Gesundheit, santé, health	35 Krankheit	19 maladie	25 sickness
60. Bibel, évangile, Bible	20 Buch	11 Dieu	23 God
61. Gedächtnis, mémoire, memory	8 Gehirn	18 souvenir, s	12 mind
62. Schaf, agneau, sheep	15 Wolle	15 brebis	20 wool
63. Bad, bain, bath	18 Wasser	16 (de) mer	31 clean
64. Häuschen, villa, cottage	17 Garten (ä)	16 maison	30 house
65. schnell, rapide, swift	32 langsam	35 train	37 fast
66. blau, bleu, blue	25 Himmel	31 ciel	17 sky
76. hungrig, faim, hungry	20 durstig	24 soif	36 food
68. Priester, prêtre, priest	17 Kirche	13 noire, e	33 church
69. Ozean, océan, ocean	34 Meer	24 mer	31 water
70. Kopf, tête, head	13 Haare	11 cheveu, x	13 hair
71. Ofen, fourneau, stove	17 Wärme	19 (de) cuisine	23 hot
72. lang, long, long	44 kurz	24 court	75 short
73. Religion, religion, religion	12 Glaube	9 prêtre, s	28 church

From Russell and Meseck, 1959, p. 197.

norms with present-day norms. Schellenberg's norms for freshmen at Minnesota in 1929 are available, and in the early 1950s Jenkins and Russell produced new Kent-Rosanoff norms for Minnesota freshmen. While it was hitherto tacitly assumed that such norms are relatively stable over time, since the language remains fairly constant over a time span of twenty years, this comparison clearly revealed that this assumption was not justified. The frequency of primary answers had changed. The most frequent responses of 1929 were still the most frequent in 1952 but their frequency had increased by one third. The comparison with the Kent-Rosanoff norms of 1910 suggests that idiosyncratic responses (produced only by a single individual) become more and more infrequent. In 1952 nearly all responses are identical. If in the earlier investigation the three most frequent responses to a stimulus-word made up hardly half of all the responses, in the more recent study they constitute two thirds. In other words, the communality of responses has risen.

Other results of this diachronic comparison are: the so-called superordinate response (red—color) are replaced by more specific ones (red—white); abstract responses decrease; concrete responses increase. The question asked by Jenkins, why this change should have occurred, is of some interest, because one might say quite tentatively that it looks as if the German and French results are like the American ones of 1929. Jenkins suggests that the reason for this trend towards uniformity and "concreteness" is the growing "outer-directedness" of society in Riesman's sense, i.e., the literally overwhelming influence of the mass media, of advertising, and the standardization of school instruction. He concludes his interpretation with the words, "If the associative processes relate to thought as we suspect they do, then the age of 'group-think' is virtually upon us" (1959, p. 584).

Szalay and his co-workers (1970, 1972, 1973) also investigated cross-cultural comparisons. However, he used a more complex association procedure. His interests were the group and culture specific organization of concepts, because he perceives the linkage of various associations as an indication of the semantic field which surrounds a particular stimulus word. (We will have to examine the concept of the semantic field more extensively later on.) Szalay found, for example, that American students grouped around the word "educated" primarily words that were related to knowledge and learning while (English-speaking) Korean students assigned to the word "educated" words that characterized a social and moral leadership. Such findings raise the question whether such differences occur not only between different linguistic communities and can, therefore, be accounted for by differences between the languages in question, but also whether within one linguistic community they might not follow the boundary lines between various social groups.

Investigations on this question began shortly after the turn of the century. According to Wreschner (1907), 60 percent of university students and professors produce associations which belong to the same parts of speech as the stimulus-words, whereas only 48 percent of workers responded in the same way. In more recent times, Rosenzweig (1964) has made systematic comparisons between French students and workers and between American students and workmen. In the French group there are much greater differences between students and workmen than in the American group. Whereas in France only 40 percent of the primary responses are identical, in the United States 68 percent are alike. The responses of French students are more in accord with those of American students than with those of French workmen.

On the basis of studies in this area one is likely to find confirmation for Rosenzweig's conclusion that subjects belonging to the same language community but to different social groups may have different verbal habits. In France, where class differences between workmen and students are greater than in the United States, the differences in verbal habits are correspondingly also larger.

We started our survey on associative behavior with a description of empirical norms. We then considered the area of application of these norms, i.e., we asked ourselves whether a single set of responses or a single distribution of frequencies is adequate for a description of the associative habits of *all* members of a linguistic community. In the attempt to answer this question, we found it necessary to differentiate according to sociological groupings.

We must now add other differentiations to the differences already found within one linguistic community: viz, according to sex and age of the subject. Palermo and Jenkins (1965) compared the associations of male and female college students. Women give fewer different responses to each stimulus, respond more frequently than men with one of the four most frequent responses to a stimulus, and tend to give fewer superordinate responses.

It has been known since approximately 1915 that children have different associations from adults. But it is only in recent years—especially through the investigations by Ervin (1961a), Entwisle, Forsyth, and Muus (1964)—that more exact information has become available.

As we have seen, adults tend to respond with the same grammatical class as that of the stimulus-word. A noun is followed by a noun, and a verb by a verb; i.e., adults predominantly give paradigmatic associations. The two words appearing as stimulus or response could be substituted for each other in a sentence frame. By way of example suppose the sentence frame is "I can see a . . . ," the empty slot can be filled by "chair," or "table," as well as by "man," "woman," "light," or "difference." In another sentence frame, "The man is walking . . . ," we might add "slowly" or "along," but not "table" or "chair." In the actual speech event we select one word from a paradigmatic set (chair, table, man, woman, light, difference . . .); the mechanism involved is called *selection* by Saussure.

While adults predominantly choose paradigmatic associations, children generally make syntagmatic responses. They tend to respond to "table" not with "chair," but perhaps with "sit," "eat," or "work." The adult associates words like "running" or "standing" with "walking," while a child produces "about" or "home." In the child, stimulus and response are not related as words which can be substituted for each other in a sentence frame, but as words which in a sentence normally follow each other. The corresponding mechanism is, according to Saussure, not selection but *combination*.

Selection and combination are also considered basic linguistic processes in speech pathology. Jakobson (1955), for example, used these two concepts in a classification of different forms of aphasia.

The difference in associative behavior of children and adults, therefore, lies mainly in the fact that children produce predominantly syntagmatic associations and adults paradigmatic ones. The change from one to the other occurs nowadays mainly between the ages of 6 and 8. This observation can be further supplemented by the following interesting diachronic study: comparable data of 1916 are available in a study by Woodrow and Lowell which shows that the shift from syntagmatic to paradigmatic associations occurred between the ages of 9 and 12. Once again we will have to bear in mind that the child today, because of radio and television, is much more exposed to spoken language at an early age. But it may well be a consequence of the general acceleration of development that today the verbal habits of childhood are replaced by those of the adults at an earlier age than 50 years ago.

Riegel and Riegel (1964) investigated modifications of associative behavior at more advanced ages and found an increase in variability of responses. It is interesting to note that older subjects are more inclined to respond syntagmatically than younger ones (between ages 17 to 19); this further change has not yet been adequately explained.

Next we turn to the question of whether the word-association test might not only reveal group characteristics but also indicate *personality-specific speech habits*. Here the studies by Jung are particularly worth mentioning. Shortly after the turn of the century Jung undertook word association experiments in which he employed as stimuli words which might have a special emotional significance for the subject, i.e., words which he considered as indicative of "complexes." Jung understood a complex to be a negatively toned system of recollections, images or wishes, which can, so to speak, be activated by the particular stimulus-word—even if, as is normally the case, the complex has been repressed. In Jung's view, such complexes become evident in an association test by a number of indicators, among which the most important one is the lengthening of reaction-time. Other symptoms are refusal of a response, stimulus repetition, deviant or echo associations ("table"—"able"). To what extent the mechanism of repression plays a role, can be seen from the following procedure: if after the test a second run-through with the same stimuli is made, it is found that just those responses to the stimuli which are apparently complex-charged have already been forgotten and must be replaced by others.

Admittedly, the reliability of the complex indicators is an open question. It is by no means certain that it is just the emotional problem which leads to difficulties in association. What strikes Jung as a complex indicator, appears particularly frequently whenever there are many competing (i.e., approximately equally strong) possibilities of response. If, however, one response is dominant, association errors are infrequent.

To recapitulate, we saw that a certain equivalence in the response hierarchy can lead to delays in association and to other disturbances. This permits a first glimpse into the structure of these processes. What happens—behind the scenes of the association experiment, so to speak—can be treated as a decision process; it must be decided which of several different possibilities, activated by the stimulus-word, is to be actualized. As is known from studies in general psychology, the timing of decision processes is strongly dependent on two magnitudes: (1) on the absolute valence or strength of the separate possibilities, and (2) on the difference between the valences of the separate possibilities. The smaller this difference, and the lower the level of strength of the alternatives, the longer is the time likely to be needed for a decision. It appears valuable to interpret the processes in the association experiment with the help of this model.

A major problem for the study of association which results from what has just been described is the question of the origin of the differential response-strength.

As far as syntagmatic associations are concerned, it appears that this question can be answered without difficulty. If in normal sentences of everyday-language use word B immediately follows word A, it is to be expected that in the word-association experiment stimulus-word A is followed by response B. The syntagmatic association could accordingly be interpreted as a segment from a frequently spoken sentence of everyday speech.

The question is much more difficult to answer for paradigmatic associations. In everyday-language use the verbal sequence "table—chair" or "large—small" are hardly ever met. How do these S-R connections come about, and what determines their strength? Ervin (1962–63), in discussing earlier explanations offered by Saporta (1955b), argues approximately as follows: The receiver of a verbal message must anticipate what is likely to come next. However, this can rarely lead to the anticipation of a definite word; instead it prepares the listener for a number of possible words fitting into a sentence-frame which can be expected to complete the portion of the sentence which has already been heard. Suppose the frame is, "I can see the . . ."; the continuation might be "man," "boy," "bird," "difference," "heel," etc. Whatever is likely to occur in a particular sentence structure in the same position belongs to the same paradigm. If the sentence begins with, "I can see the smiling . . ." one might add "person" or "child," but "difference" or "heel" would no longer be possible; it would be a smaller paradigm.

What we have discussed gives us a brief glimpse of a problem which we will treat more fully at a later stage. We have tried to answer provisionally the question of what guides the choice of a particular paradigm by using the notion of "anticipation." A closer look will show us that this "anticipation" can be analyzed into two components: on the one hand there are the probabilistic relationships by which preceding sentence elements lead up to the point in question (Markov model); on the other, there are grammar rules according to which even sentence elements actualized at a later stage have a determining influence on the selection of an element at a given moment. This raises the question of the psychological reality of grammar, which will be discussed in more detail in Chapter 10.

The more frequently two words are combined in a single paradigm, the more frequently the hearer experiences a connection between the anticipated possibilities and the word actually used by the speaker. And as the frequency of this "experience" increases, so the paradigmatic association is strengthened. This is to say that the larger the number of sentence patterns into which the stimulus- and response-words might fit, the closer is the link.

Experimental investigations by Ervin (1961a) and McNeill (1963) have prima facie confirmed Ervin's hypothesis. One possibility of explaining syntagmatic and paradigmatic associations by means of a mediation model will be considered later in connection with the discussion of this model (see p. 165).

It is therefore possible to consider a pair of words from the point of view of the number of sentence patterns in which either one or the other might fit. Thus it is hardly possible to imagine a sentence in which the word "big" is appropriate where "small" might not equally have occurred. If in a concrete utterance "big" occurs, it is likely that, almost in every case, "small" is also available. On the other hand, there is hardly ever a sentence in which the choice would have been made between, say, "heel" or "sour." Accordingly, "big—small" have many sentence patterns in common, "heel—sour" hardly any. It is possible to order pairs of words along a continuum which ranges from "many sentence patterns in common" to "no sentence patterns in common." And if we ask what this continuum is, it appears prima facie as the dimension of similarity. When considered from this point of view, "big—small" are more alike than "heel—sour." This similarity, defined more precisely, can be described as *similarity of meaning.*

With this we have reached a critical point in the development of contemporary psycholinguistics, namely the problem of meaning. We see here that the central problem of language is linked with an important problem for psychology, namely verbal associations. We recall Galton's statement that associations lay bare the foundations of man's thought, the associations of a word tell us what it means. We arrived at this important point by interpreting the classical association experiment from a psychological perspective, viewing the stimulus and reaction word as mutually associated units.

For the next step we remain with the association experiment, but we no longer view the stimulus and response words as whole irreducible units, rather as constellations of single, elementary features of meaning. Here we return to an approach which we encountered earlier within a different context. Katz and Fodor (1963) proposed that the lexical items (words) listed in the lexicon of a speaker/hearer should be viewed as consisting of elementary, semantic features. How can one describe the classical association studies against the background of such a "feature theory of meaning"? Clark (1970) provides the answer: In the first phase of the experiment the subject analyzes the stimulus word which he hears in terms of its relevant semantic features. For example, analyzing the word "man" in this manner leads to the following result:

   physical object +, animate +, animal +, human +, adult +, male +.

In the second phase of the experiment the subject is instructed to give the first word which comes to his mind and is not identical to the stimulus word. The simplest way to carry out these instructions is to take the last semantic feature of the stimulus word and change it in terms of its sign, changing male + to male −. The third phase of the experiment produces the word which is characterized by the following series of features:

   physical object +, animate +, animal +, human +, adult +, male −,

i.e., the word "woman."

In this manner Clark explains why "woman" is the primary response to the word "man." But he can explain more with this hypothesis. If the response "boy" is given to the stimulus word "man," then apparently the sign of the second-to-last feature has been changed, if the response is "girl" then the sign of the last and second-to-last feature has been changed. By means of the association behavior as reflected by the relative frequency of different responses, the sequence of features by which the stimulus word is analyzed, becomes apparent.

Thus we find that an analysis of association behavior within the context of contemporary semantic theory takes us to the place which we had reached earlier, namely, meaning as association. However, now *meaning as association* has been expanded in an important way. The meaning of a word is now seen as composed of elementary dimensions of meaning, thus the similarity or the "belonging together" of words can be explained in terms of their common participation in one or more of these dimensions of meaning. Semantically "man" and "woman" belong together; they are semantically similar because they are localized on the same semantic dimensions, at least if one ignores the small difference of the sign of the last semantic feature. However, the reverse is also true. When we analyze the similarity and relatedness of "man" and "woman" we can identify which of the dimensions of meaning determine the word-meaning of "man" and "woman"; these dimensions generally interlace our lexicon along with others, which are not related to "man" and "woman." This two-fold approach to viewing and employing the conceptualization of "meaning as association," i.e., the use of a *formal* association in determining the *substantive* (semantic) reasons for the presence of this association, represents a way of thinking and inferring which is quite popular in contemporary psycholinguistics.

Against this background and with this interpretation we now turn to the concept of the "semantic field" which was contributed by German linguistics of the 1920s and 1930s.

The semantic field extends the dyadic scheme on which, at its origin at least, associationism was based. It originated in the twenties under the influence of Gestalt or holistic psychology. In 1924 Ipsen talked about the "semantic field" and understood it as a group of words which together form a semantic unit. He cites as an example the Indo-Germanic words for sheep and sheep-rearing. Such words do not necessarily belong together from an etymological point of view, nor are they inevitably linked by association. They are—contrary to holistic conceptions—viewed as close to each other like the stones of a mosaic and divide up a field of activity of the ancient Indo-Europeans into semantic areas (Ipsen, pp. 224 f.).

The field concept introduced by Trier has become even more important and more influential than that of Ipsen. In contrast to a psycholinguistic approach, Trier investigates language as *ergon* or, in Saussurian terminology, as *langue*. "Existence is given to us through the intermediate world of language" (1934, p. 428). This statement defines the position from which he starts.[3]

Trier's conception of the lexical field can best be put in his own words:

> Every language confronts reality as a system of selection of a kind which always creates a completely closed and rounded image of that reality. The manner in which language constructs its image of reality, which is a complete whole with no gaps, yet, at the same time, selecting, restricting and dividing, can best be described with the concept of structure. The linguistic substance is not simply copied from reality; instead, the ordering structure of language projects upon reality a view which creates the linguistic-conceptual forms of its wholes and parts, its links and divisions (p. 429).

Humboldt's influence is evident: language orders the world—a point of view which will be examined later. "In saying this we recognize at the same time that there is nothing isolated in language. Since structure is the essence of language, each individual item results from structuring; it is determined in its nature and function by its position in the structure, its place in the whole of language" (Trier, p. 429).

Whereas scholars who operate with the concept of association view context as a synthesis of fundamentally independent elements, Trier proceeds in the opposite direction. Following a holistic approach according to which the

---

[3] We recognize clearly the reduplication of the world to which psychology with its anti-Platonic approach is opposed.

whole is prior to the parts, he argues: "If the essence of language is a structure and organization of the whole, the field approach moves downward from the whole to the part and not upward, gathering separate items into larger units" (p. 449). "The word exists only because it is part of the organized whole of lexis. This organization of the whole determines the significance of each part. Every act of speaking and listening is orientation within this structure . . ." (p. 429).

The meaning of the word is, therefore, determined by the reality of the field as a whole which is available to the speaker and the listener.

To cite one example: "A word such as 'intelligent' certainly relates to the totality of the lexis, but not directly; in the first instance it forms part of the smaller partial group to which belong, besides 'intelligent,' such words as 'wise,' 'clever,' 'smart,' 'cunning,' 'learned,' 'experienced,' 'knowledgeable,' 'educated,' etc." (Trier, p. 430). "Fields are the linguistic realities intermediate between the single word and the total lexis" (p. 430). In this formulation, again, the individual word without the field would not be meaningful; thus the field is regarded as a reality of a special kind.

Trier's lexical field-theory, which has been upheld vigorously, has exercised a great influence on German linguistics (e.g., on Weisgerber). It must, however, be noted that this concept in no small measure derives its prestige from a rather imprecise analogy with field-theoretical arguments in physics and, as already mentioned, in Gestalt psychology. Öhman has, for example, pointed out that it is not clear what the lines or points of force are in a lexical field.

Another field concept in German linguistics developed by Porzig (1934) stands in contrast to Trier's. It is less widely known but is closer to psycholinguistics. Porzig starts out from the essential semantic relationships between verbs and nouns or adjectives and nouns. The verb "walk" presupposes "legs" or "feet"; it is therefore a predicate which implies a subject; "grasp" presupposes "hand," and "blond" presupposes "hair"; the verb "bark" implies "dog." "Evidently, therefore, all items belonging together semantically within such necessary relationships are interchangeable or could be substituted for one another" (p. 73). A Porzig field is built up from below, i.e., from the individual word, a word pair, or its interpair relations.

Thus the Porzig field can be seen as a precursor of the viewpoint represented by the so-called Generative Semantic, namely that the *predicate* of a sentence implicates particular subjects as its *arguments*. The nature of this implicative relationship with its demand characteristics and its ability to prevent inappropriate associations is to be described neither as purely syntactic nor as purely semantic. This type of deep structure occurs prior to the division of syntax and semantic. The meshing of implicating and implicated parts of a sentence was described from the psychological point of view by Engelkamp (1973).

It is quite true that, viewed from the perspective of the history of science, Porzig and the older German linguists who employed the concept of field, did not have much direct influence. Ideas about the field concept have had little impact on psycholinguistics, primarily because they were unable to offer a method that would facilitate the extraction of a certain field in a reliable and objective manner. They limited the linguist to using his intuition, his sense of history, and his ingenuity. Let us recall how the method employed in the classical association experiment advanced the solution of the problems related to "meaning and association."

We should not be surprised then that a psycholinguistically productive conceptualization of the semantic field and its structure was also determined, to a large extent, by the methods which psychologists, with an empirically precise orientation, were able to employ for this purpose. We now turn to an examination of this approach.

We shall begin with a phenomenon which, for the present, shows only the effectiveness of conventionally conceived associations in memory processes, the so-called clustering. Examples of relevant studies are those by Bousfield (1953 and later). If one instructs a subject to think of names of flowers and musical instruments, the items do not occur in random order, but relatively systematically, e.g., six flowers, followed perhaps by four instruments, then again five flowers, and so forth. In other words the subject produces clusters of related words.

The same phenomenon occurs when words in random order are read aloud to the subject and recalled by him after a lapse of time. What the subject recalls is more ordered than what he was given.

The link between these observations and the word-association experiment was demonstrated by Jenkins and Russell (1952). They selected 24 stimulus-words from the Kent-Rosanoff list along with their associated primary response-words and arranged all 48 words in random order. This list was read aloud to the subjects with the instruction to subsequently write down any words they remembered without regard to the order in which they had been presented.

The authors' hypothesis was that words which in the Kent-Rosanoff norms are closely associated as stimulus and response should also be recalled as pairs or at least in close proximity. While "table" and "chair" were separated by 20 other words in the list, as it was read out, these two words, which according to the Kent-Rosanoff norms are closely associated with each other, should have been reproduced in close succession during recall. This hypothesis was confirmed with a significance beyond the 0.001 level of confidence.

This result has meanwhile been corroborated by several studies. Rosenzweig (1957) found in a French group of subjects a correlation of 0.57 between the frequency of associations in the group and the frequency with which these words, having been heard in random order, were again clustered together in recall. Russell and Meseck (1959) obtained similar results with German-speaking groups.

These investigations have taken us beyond the field we have so far considered. While in the studies which had been reported earlier we referred to associations between a word which explicitly functioned as stimulus and another word explicitly functioning as response, associations in the reproduction phase of a clustering experiment are evoked between responses; the word "table" is uttered by the subject (and not by the experimenter) as well as the word "chair." This extension of the concept of association, which henceforth comprises not only the association between stimulus and response, but also between response and response, represents the connecting link to the field concept which we shall now discuss. Apparently there are forces at work in the clustering experiment which bring together words in reproduction from memory, which *in contents, categorically* or *semantically,* belong together, making it possible for them to surface together. Apparently such associations are formed not only by dyads but may involve well-organized clusters, networks and fields.

Deese attempts to explain the *structure* of such fields by describing the relationships which exist between the responses to various stimuli: "If the associative meaning of a stimulus is given by the distribution of responses to that stimulus, then two stimuli may be said to have the same associative meaning when the distribution of associates to them is *identical.* Two stimuli overlap or resemble one another in associative meaning to the extent that they have the same distribution of associates" (1962, p. 163). The connection between associative responses is the *associative meaning* of the stimulus concerned.

For his empirical investigation Deese selects stimulus-words in a specific manner: he chooses words which, he assumes, somehow belong together. In this way he is able to study whether his concept of associative meaning and the operational definition of this concept can make evident relationships which are known to us from a prescientific linguistic insight. If this is the case it is possible to make use of this operationally defined concept even in cases where prescientific linguistic insight has no ready answers. In the following illustration Deese uses words as stimuli all of which, according to Kent-Rosanoff norms, appeared as responses to the word "butterfly." In other words, Deese makes use of a Trier-type word-field.

These words are presented to 50 subjects as stimuli in a word-association experiment (Table 8). Afterwards the frequency of occurrence of a given word as response to these stimuli is calculated. The response "moth" is given twice to the stimulus-word "insect," once to the stimulus-word "bug," 8 times to "cocoon" and 7 times to "butterfly." The similarity of associative meaning of two stimuli is determined in the following way: Deese

Table 8. Frequencies of associates in common to 19 words based on responses of 50 subjects.

Responses (associated words)	Stimulus-words (the numbers correspond to the first 19 response-words)																		
	1	2	3	4	5	6	7	8	9	10	11	12	13	14	15	16	17	18	19
1 Moth	50	2					1	8											7
2 Insect	1	50		3				3											6
3 Wings	2		50	4															5
4 Bird			25	50	4		1	2			9						2		4
5 Fly	10	9	12	15	50		2				1						1		4
6 Yellow						50	2				1			4					3
7 Flower						2	50				1	2		1	10		1	2	2
8 Bug		24			4			50	5				1						
9 Cocoon									50										2
10 Color						5				50	6								
11 Blue				1	1	2	2			8	50			1		40			
12 Bees		1				2	2					50							
13 Summer	2							1				1	50	1	1				
14 Sunshine													1	50				12	
15 Garden						6									50				
16 Sky				1							6			1		50			
17 Nature																	50	1	
18 Spring													3					50	
19 Butterfly	1							8											50
20 Light	4				1									4		1		1	
21 Pretty						3													2
22 Ant		3			1			5											
23 Bright								1						4					
24 Airplane			4		1														
25 Feather			2	3															
26 Flight			1	2															
27 Tree				2	1									1			6		
28 Plane			2		5														
29 Red						6	1			16	13								
30 White						1				5	2								
31 Green						5	2				4		1		3		2		
32 Sun						2													
33 Beetle		1						1											
34 Spider		1						1											
35 Gold						1						1	1						
36 Black		1				1				8	2								
37 Winter													17					4	
38 Warm													3	8				1	
39 Plant							2									5	1		
40 Gray						1				1	2								
41 Brown						1				1									
42 Vacation													2					1	

Based on Deese, 1962, p. 166.

Table 9. Overlap coefficients for common associates between the 19 words in Table 8 (decimals omitted).

Stimulus-words	Stimulus-words																		
	1	2	3	4	5	6	7	8	9	10	11	12	13	14	15	16	17	18	19
1 Moth	100	12	12	12	11	02	00	05	11	00	00	02	02	05	01	01	01	01	12
2 Insect		100	09	09	17	01	01	33	10	01	01	03	00	00	00	00	01	00	13
3 Wing			100	44	19	00	00	03	02	00	00	10	00	00	00	00	03	00	12
4 Bird				100	21	01	00	03	02	01	01	10	00	01	00	01	05	00	11
5 Fly					100	01	01	08	06	01	02	06	00	03	00	02	04	00	05
6 Yellow						100	07	00	00	17	23	02	02	07	05	02	04	03	06
7 Flower							100	02	07	03	07	02	01	06	18	02	06	02	04
8 Bug								100	00	00	00	05	00	00	00	00	02	00	00
9 Cocoon									100	00	00	04	00	00	00	00	02	00	22
10 Color										100	32	00	00	01	01	08	00	00	00
11 Blue											100	01	02	02	00	00	03	02	02
12 Bees												100	01	04	03	00	04	02	07
13 Summer													100	02	02	00	01	02	00
14 Sunshine														100	05	00	02	10	04
15 Garden															100	02	00	15	04
16 Sky																100	00	02	02
17 Nature																	100	01	03
18 Spring																		100	02
19 Butterfly																			100

From Deese, 1962, p. 167.

relates the number of responses which are common to these two stimuli to the maximally possible number of common responses to the same two stimulus-words.

In Deese's study (and in Table 8) the term "implicit response" is used. It is assumed that each stimulus word first triggers itself as a response—an assumption which is suggested by the common notions about the association experiment as well as by the analysis-by-synthesis approach. In this way, the table shows the following values: "moth" and "insect" have 12 responses in common: the response "moth" occurs 50 times in response to the stimulus-word "moth" (this is the implicit response), and twice in response to the stimulus-word "insect." Therefore two responses are common. The response "insect" is given once to the stimulus-word "moth" and 50 times to "insect" as stimulus-word; one response is common. The response-word "fly" occurs 10 times with "moth" as stimulus-word and 9 times with the stimulus-word "insect"; accordingly 9 responses are common. The two stimuli "moth" and "insect" have 2 + 1 + 9 = 12 common responses. The maximally possible number of common responses would be 100; it would occur if each of the stimulus-words would evoke only the other as response. The coefficient of similarity of the associative meanings of these two stimulus-words in this case amounts to 12/100 or 0.12. Deese calls this value the "overlap coefficient."

After these values have been entered on a matrix, they are subjected to factor analysis to find out mathematically how many factors can account for these relationships (Table 9). The resulting factor loadings have been set out in Table 10.

It is evident that the separation into factors has been fairly successful; approximately half the words have positive loadings on Factor I and nearly zero loadings on Factor II; the results are reversed for the other half. Factor I appears in words which suggest animal creation: moth, insect, wing, bird, fly, bug, cocoon, bees, butterfly. Factor II loadings refer to non-animate items: yellow, flower, color, etc. Factor III has zero loadings on the non-animate words and appears to order animate items on a bipolar dimension: positive loadings on such words as wing, bird, fly and bees, and negative ones on bug, cocoon and moth. Factor IV makes a bipolar split of the nonanimate words: summer, sunshine, garden, flower and spring on the one hand, and, on the other, blue, sky, yellow and color.

A comparison of factor profiles for pairs of words is particularly instructive; e.g., "blue", and "yellow." Both are alike in that they share common loadings with summer, sunshine, color, etc. On one factor they diverge: in factor V "blue" goes with sky, butterfly, wing and bird, while "yellow" goes with insect, fly, bug and bee.

The result of factor analysis, therefore, is a division of the lexis into lexical areas—exactly what Trier had attempted to achieve with his field concept. But whereas Trier invents a purely subjective, intellectualistic structure,

Table 10. Rotated centroid factor loadings of stimulus overlap coefficients presented in Table 9 (decimals omitted).

Words	I	II	III	IV	V	VI
			Factors			
Moth	44	03	−27	−01	−03	−32
Insect	50	01	−33	01	−34	11
Wing	52	01	45	01	29	−07
Bird	52	02	46	01	29	−07
Fly	48	03	32	01	−28	−03
Yellow	01	44	−03	34	−32	−02
Flower	01	39	−03	−32	03	44
Bug	41	01	−34	00	−14	37
Cocoon	40	01	−35	00	25	02
Color	−02	42	−04	44	04	−04
Blue	−02	57	−04	52	23	−04
Bees	36	04	34	−02	−30	00
Summer	−01	31	−03	−34	−02	−34
Sunshine	02	37	−04	−33	−03	−35
Garden	00	35	−02	−34	−03	44
Sky	−01	41	−03	43	38	−07
Nature	04	31	29	−02	01	34
Spring	−01	35	−03	−37	−02	−36
Butterfly	48	06	−29	−01	26	01

From Deese, 1962, p. 169.

Deese's procedure is based on the actual verbal behavior of an entire group of speakers.

Now the question arises, What is the relationship between the factorial structures found by Deese and the semantic structures of the lexicon which we encountered in our discussion of Katz and Fodor, and which are similarly found applied to the psychology of the association experiment in the case of Clark?

To answer this question we have to recall that with every factor analysis of this kind, that which is called a factor is largely determined by the selection of the stimulus words. For example, in this case, if "moth" had not been presented and analyzed in the same experiment with "insect," "wing," "sky," etc., but had instead been presented with "grandmother" and "train," the factors would look quite different. Therefore the semantic dimensions found by Deese cannot be dimensions of a lexicon which is part of the competence of the user and therefore stable over time, i.e., which remains constant. Saying it more cautiously: Deese's dimensions are not congruent with the commonly accepted concept of the lexicon where each word has *its* assigned meaning. Rather, they are dimensions which are activated in *the particular situation,* i.e., under the influence of the words which are used in the experiment, within and by means of the stimulus word.

Such indetermination, however, stands in contrast to the linguistic concept of the lexicon. For the linguist, the lexicon consists of fixed content which is anchored in the competence of the speech user, and thus takes on defining characteristics. At best, what may change is the use which is made of this lexicon.

This ambiguity about the nature of the lexicon—Does it actually always remain the same? Does it change, depending on the particular task? Or is it only the use made of it which changes?—is, of course, only the start of an approach which could have far-reaching consequences. The psycholinguist will have to decide whether he can investigate the structures of the internal lexicon independently of the various ways in which the speaker/listener uses it.

This ambiguity can also become apparent when methods other than those used by Deese are employed to investigate the structure of the lexicon. While Deese proceeded in a relatively indirect way (i.e., via the "overlap coefficient" of the associative response of the words), more direct methods have been developed recently. Here the subject is instructed to scale words according to their similarity, or to sort them into groups. Procedures of this kind were used extensively by Fillenbaum and Rapaport (1971). As an example, we will present an analysis of the field representing designations of various kinship terms.

This analysis shows, for example, that "grandfather" and "grandson" are judged as fairly similar. This supports the view of the anthropologists Romney and D'Andrade (1964) that the field of kinship terms shows, among others, the dimension "reciprocity." But it contradicts the position of Wallace and Atkins (1960) that the number of intervening generations is the deciding factor.

If we find, however, that concepts that differ only with respect to gender, e.g., son/daughter, are judged to have the highest similarity, can we conclude on the basis of this that "gender" is an apparently unimportant dimension in this semantic field? Again this would raise the question whether the scaling method employed reflects *the* structure of the internal lexicon, or whether we would get quite different results, i.e., find a different structure, if the subject's response set were changed. The studies by Miller (1971) also show how much the results of such scaling based on similarity of meaning depend upon the concrete formulation of the task. He presents the subject with nouns like "cook," "doctor," "umpire," "mother." The subject is instructed to sort those that belong together into as many groups as he needs. This is based on the notion that in order to assign two words to one group, the subject must ignore, so to speak, the semantic features which distinguish them. The fewer the features which have to be ignored and the less important they are, the higher is the probability that the subject will assign the words to the same category. In this way Miller obtains structures which can be intelligibly interpreted. For example, more subjects assigned "female persons" to a single category than "persons" because for the latter grouping the feature "female" must be abstracted.

However, if the *same* words are presented as verbs for the sorting experiment, i.e., "to cook," "to doctor," "to umpire," etc., the results are completely different, and to date have not been interpretable. Apparently the function of the words plays a decisive role in determining their semantic content within the context of the task. It is impossible to scale or sort words in isolation. At most they must be words that play a particular functional role. But what determines this role? Does it depend on the function within the sentence, within the predicate-argument-structure, within the text, or on some, as yet undefined communicative function between speaker and listener?

Meaning as association more and more appears to be a rather superficial explanatory model. It inevitably leads to questions that neither linguistics nor psycholinguistics can answer by themselves. The questions relate to the philosophical bases of the attempts to elucidate the problem of meaning. We shall now turn to these philosophical principles to learn more about the sources within the history and philosophy of science which gave rise to contemporary linguistics and psycholinguistics.

CHAPTER 7

The Philosophical Background to Modern Psychology of Language

Meaning as natural bipolar connection—The designating function of language—*Adaequatio rei et intellectus*—Language and meta-language—Empiricist criteria of truth—Pragmatism and operationalism—Between-world of meaning—Meaning as context—Role of language user—Morris—Meaning as behavior—Wittgenstein's language game—Searle's speech acts.

"The fundamental change in the relationship between philosophy and language," which distinguishes "the twentieth century from previous ones, might well be said to consist in the fact that language is no longer treated purely as a subject for philosophical inquiry. For the first time in history, language is viewed as the prerequisite which makes philosophy possible. 'Philosophy of language' is no longer simply a philosophy *of language* . . . Instead, it does today what, after Kant, epistemology had done once before. It has taken the place of ontology. In a way, linguistic analysis has pushed the Kantian critique of knowledge to its radical conclusion as a critique of language" (Apel, 1964, p. 22).

The present chapter is not intended to describe this development in full detail or in historical sequence. Instead, by highlighting a few decisive moments we merely want to indicate the horizon within which modern psycholinguistics has studied the concept of meaning. As we shall make several overlapping approaches to psychology from the standpoint of "pure" philosophy, a certain amount of repetition can hardly be avoided.

> Among recent German writings on linguistic philosophy the work of Apel is most noteworthy; the following presentation is largely based on it.

The first concept of importance for our discussion is that of *logos* in Greek philosophy. What we regard today as the confusing ambiguity of this concept—broadly speaking, "word" *and* "true idea"—is in Greek thought a unity which guarantees that language is "right" or "true." But this self-evident view soon gave way to a question: how can language be "true," i.e., "mediate" an external world? A first superficial answer to this question is: because words and sentences mean something, i.e., have a reliable relationship to the objects in the extralinguistic world. The next question is: how does this relationship to the extralinguistic world come about? In philosophy this raises the problem of linguistic truth and in psychology the problem of the acquisition of linguistic meanings.

The Platonic answer to this question is that there is a natural and necessary link between linguistic and nonlinguistic facts. In *Cratylus* we find that names are not conventional but natural; they are equally true and right for Greeks and barbarians, and they transcend individual languages. The truth of language, therefore, lies in the sound pattern of individual words. In this conception truth means that names follow things.

> This conception is reflected in linguistics in the treatment of onomatopoeia and popular etymology, and in psychology as 'word magic' and sound symbolism. It is rejected by General Semantics (cf. Chap. 12).

The view that words are naturally (*physei*) related to things outside language implies a very simple structure of that relationship which can be called "meaning": linguistic and extralinguistic facts are naturally and necessarily linked without any intervening psychological mechanism. Meaning is a bipolar or dyadic relationship which has come into being naturally without human beings having any part in it. Such arguments can be found down to the present era; as late as 1960 Gadamer said that things speak for themselves, and language, in the last resort, is the language of things (Gadamer, 1962).

The Aristotelian conception is quite different. The link between language and extralinguistic reality does not consist in factual necessity (*physei*) but is put there by man (*thesei*). Man can grasp the world or the way things are apart from language. Things, which thus are already known to man, are afterwards named by him with the help of arbitrarily chosen words. This conception of the designating function of language reaches from antiquity via Ockham and Scholasticism right into the present era. The decisive characteristic of this view is not the appropriateness of the sound pattern but the unambiguousness of the designation. In this approach the demand that language should be true becomes much more problematical than in Plato because the order of language must now reflect the order of the world. As early as the twelfth century attempts were made to link grammar, i.e., the structure of language, with the structure of reality. According to Bacon there is only *one* grammar for all languages—*licet accidentaliter varietur.*[1] In Scholasticism there was much discussion of the theory of supposition, i.e., of the relationship between the word and the object designated by the word. The triad particularly noted was *supponentia* (designations), *supposita* (the designated objects or individuals) and *supponere* as a process (i.e., the act of substituting designations for things).

[1] It is interesting to note that Chomsky makes a similar claim, although it takes on a different form. The nature and the interpretations of grammar are language universals. This was pointed out by Marshall (1970) in an extensive study.

This implies that man participates in establishing the meaning relationship and that it is, therefore, inherently arbitrary.

The discussion of the various *modi significandi* leads from a dyadic to a triadic scheme of the meaning relationship in the work of Morris. The idea of supposition, i.e., the substitution of the designation for the thing, becomes of renewed modern interest as the problem of verification in logical positivism and in the conditioning theory of meaning of Watson and Pavlov.

In contrast to the scholastic procedure the mystics attempt through contemplation to enter into direct contact with this world and the transcendent world, undisturbed by the arbitrariness of words invented by man.

If the Aristotelian-Scholastic view is adopted as a basis, then truth is the *adaequatio rei et intellectus,* the agreement between things and mind. The structure of a language can, if it is logically correct, reflect the structure of the world. But how can one be certain that language is logically right and that the *adaequatio rei* has been reached?

A further question was later added: what happens when *res* and *intellectus,* thing and language, are not regarded as independent of each other, i.e., when, in contrast to the earlier assumption, language is said to influence our view of reality? This is the issue which Humboldt, Sapir, and Whorf have discussed.

In Ockham's conception the *adaequatio rei et intellectus* is, moreover, guaranteed by the fact that the world of things in its whole qualitative richness is treated as the effective cause of our propositions (cf. on this point Apel, 1963).

In modern scholarship a similar cause-effect relationship reappears in the philosophy and psychology of language as a stimulus-response connection as, for example, in the work of Ogden and Richards, Bloomfield, and Skinner.

Another approach which has been attempted to reach *adaequatio* and, thereby, to guarantee the truth-function of language reduces to syntactical relationships the whole qualitative and intangible substance. It is in this way that Leibniz has come to view words as tokens and to operate with them according to the rules of a formal calculus.

> In the use of language it must also be considered that words are signs for things, and that we need signs not only to convey our thoughts to others, but also to help us to think. For just as in large centers of trade, in games, and so on, one does not always pay with money, but instead makes use of slips of paper or tokens, in the same way the mind uses representations of things . . . The mind is content to put the word in place of the thing . . . And just as a master of arithmetic who refuses to write a number which he could not carry in his mind would never complete his calculation, in the same way we would have to speak very slowly or remain silent, if in speech or even in thought we attempted to use a word without forming a clear picture of its meaning . . . That is why words are often used as cyphers or counters in the place of images

of things, until step by step the sum total has been attained and thus only at the logical conclusion the thing itself is reached (translated from *Unvorgreifliche Gedanken* as quoted by Stenzel, 1934, p. 62).

In a similar manner Hobbes does not see the truth or untruth in the agreement between judgment and reality but in the use of words, i.e., the relation between the signs. Accordingly, we read in *Leviathan*: "verum et falsum attributa sunt non rerum, sed orationibus."

From this position a direct line leads to logical positivism. For example, Carnap, too, ignores the content; his aim is to construct a logical syntax of language in general, without recourse to meaning, as a kind of algebra of language. In general terms, it is a basic tenet of logical positivism that language cannot communicate substance but only structures; it is up to the receiver to put substance to the signs or, in other words, to interpret them according to the situation.[2]

Information theory is, in a certain way, akin to these views. Also Mowrer's thesis belongs here: according to Mowrer, during speech meanings are not carried from one person to another, but within one person from sign to sign. The importance of interpretation is particularly stressed in the work of Ogden and Richards.

The logical structure of language as a guarantee for the capacity of language to be true is found again in Bertrand Russell's work and even in Wittgenstein's *Tractatus*: "The configuration of objects in a situation corresponds to the configuration of simple signs in the propositional sign" (i.e., in the sentence) (3.21).

New difficulties—and consequently a further development—can be seen in Russell's well-known contradiction of the lying Cretan. A Cretan says: "All Cretans are liars." If this sentence is true the speaker must also be a liar; consequently, the sentence is false if it is true. Russell solves this contradiction by proposing a logical principle: if a judgment is made about all judgments which belong to a certain class, this judgment no longer belongs to this class. This theory of logical classes is the so-called theory of types.

General Semantics would distinguish here judgment$_1$ from judgment$_2$. According to this view sentences on the logical form of language could not be expressed in the language itself but would be formulated in a language of a higher order, a meta-language. In meta-language, statements can be made about language, in the meta-meta-language, statements about the meta-language.

The separation into language and meta-language is called into question by the empirical observation that in everyday language meta-linguistic components occur, e.g., such phrases as "Do you follow?," "What do you

---

[2] Chomsky's generative grammar, which in other respects is not positivistic, also ignores all content.

mean?," "Have I made myself clear?." This is done to ensure that both partners use the same code (on this point cf. Ammer, 1961, pp. 63 ff.).

If we do not want to continue to apply the notion of meta-language ad infinitum, we face the necessity, as Carnap has done for instance, to use in the construction of a logical syntax of a language some basic concepts already formulated in that language, such as "and," "not," "if . . . then."

Probably the most exacting investigation regarding this problem was carried out by Garfinkel (1972). He found that the application of a code *always* presupposes that in order to decide whether or not to apply a certain rule to the code, the encoder requires a sphere of freedom which cannot be completely and explicitly defined. Within this sphere he obeys the intentions but not the letter of the code. We recognize here a problem which is more likely to be obscured than resolved by the handy distinction between language and meta-language.

If recourse to meaning cannot be avoided, even for the construction of a logical syntax, and more generally for the use of a code, then it becomes clear that the (syntactic) structure of language cannot be regarded as reflecting the structural order of the world.

The consequence is that the "decision on the criterion of meaning has shifted from the realm of logic to an empirical critique of everyday language" (Apel, 1965). This question of empirical verification is in the center of neopositivistic thought on the analysis of language. Thus Schlick points out that verifiability by immediately available empirical data is a criterion for regarding a sentence as meaningful.

But what constitutes "immediately available empirical data"? When does a sentence truly represent a record of experience? This question can no longer be answered by referring to a criterion which in the last resort is metaphysical, such as the thesis of the reflection of the structure of the world in the logical structure of language. In the last resort, all that remains in order to decide this issue is the "consensus of recognized scholars"[3] or the confirmation through use in everyday language. Wittgenstein in one of his later writings says: "Asking whether and how a proposition can be verified is only a particular way of asking 'How d'you mean?' The answer is a contribution to the grammar of the proposition" (*Philosophical Investigations,* § 353). "Grammar tells what kind of object anything is" (§ 373); i.e., grammar is the totality of rules, according to which the given word or given sentence is normally used in practice.

[3] Here we should mention the extremely interesting ideas of Ajdukiewicz (1934, 1935). He speaks of an "inner compulsion to consent" as constituting meaning, in his own words "constituting sense." Someone who speaks the English language must be ready, when he is in pain, to recognize the expression "it hurts." This readiness to acknowledge an expression in a particular situation anticipates Wittgenstein's conception of the language game as part of a form of life, as well as Searle's definition of the speech act.

Thus, a completely new position on the concept of truth is reached. Truth is now no longer something of absolute validity to be expressed through language. Instead, regarding the external world as given means that a decision has been taken to speak a certain language because of its usefulness (Carnap, 1950). The designating function of language—since Aristotle the leitmotif—is abandoned. Language is no longer the means of representing a preexisting world already previously perceived by other means. Symbolizing is no longer an act of grasping an existing "sense," but an act of establishing sense.

Here we clearly see the influence of Wittgenstein: "To understand a language means to be master of a technique" (§ 199). "The meaning of a word is its use in the language" (§ 43, 1958).

The beginning is *not* the symbol followed by its use; instead, it is everyday behavior from which gradually—to use the linguist's abstraction—symbolizations are formed. Wittgenstein introduces the notion of the language-game, which is intended to emphasize that "*speaking* of language is part of an activity, or a form of life" (*Philosophical Investigations,* § 23). "We may say: only someone who already knows how to do something with it can significantly ask a name" (§ 31). In linguistics Leisi, for example, on the basis of Wittgenstein's philosophy, compares language with custom. The description of the word-content is an indication of the conditions under which the use of a verbal form or, more precisely, the performance of the verbal utterance is possible and appropriate (Leisi, 1961).

The development which has just been broadly outlined has been summarized by Apel in these terms: "At the beginning, the logical order of the world was explicitly used as the theoretically given yardstick of all linguistic order, and the dependence of the categorial world order upon language was disregarded. At the end of this historical evolution, we find Wittgenstein's philosophy of analysis of language which claims to find, in the pluralism of language-games and their approach to situations, a guide to problems of logical categories" (Apel, 1962, p. 205).

It must be remembered that the search for a guide to all "problems of logical categories" is only one factor in the historical trend which is of interest in this connection. Another is the pragmatic view and mode of thought which was established by Peirce.[4] We now follow the second line of development in the evolution of present-day linguistic philosophy. American pragmatism has led to an intensification of interest in questions of linguistic philosophy. While logical positivism was more interested in logic, mathematics and physics, pragmatism leans more towards biology, physiology and sociology (cf. Neubert, 1962).

According to Peirce a scientist understands meaning as follows: if a

---

[4] It should be remembered that we are not concerned with exact priorities of chronological sequence in the history of philosophy; it is, for example, very likely indeed that the later works of Wittgenstein would not have been possible without the preceding work of Peirce.

definite instruction for an experiment is possible and is executed, it will be followed by a definite experience.

This is a statement of decisive importance for the whole of modern psycholinguistics.

Meaning, as interpreted here, is a process. The meaning of a sign, or a word, lies in what happens in terms of stimuli and responses in its environment—the real events, which precede the utterance of the word, and the real events which follow the utterance of the word. The decisive thing for the pragmatist is the practical effect elicited by the symbol within an interpersonal context (Neubert, p. 61).

Here is also the basis for the operational mode of procedure and definition, initiated by Bridgman, according to which a concept is defined as an instruction to carry out a given set of procedures; e.g., a rat is "hungry" if it has not been fed for 48 hours.

Even prior to the formulation by Bridgman this technique has achieved its greatest success in Einstein's theory of relativity. This theory was the outcome of the consistent pursuit of the question of which measuring operations could define the concept of simultaneity.

In this connection language appears as the continuation of action by different means. Bridgman himself sees the difference between language and experience in the fact that "language separates out from the living matrix little bundles and freezes them" (1964, p. 24).

This view is close to Bloomfield's conception according to which "acts of speech" are elicited by "practical events" and lead to "practical events." If reliability of communication matters, the verbal bridge linking practical events is reinforced by the addition of further speechless occurrences. The more the demand for reliable communication increases, the more it is necessary to add nonverbal operations. This reciprocal relationship is also expressed in Weizsäcker's proposition on language and science: "Precision in the object permits imprecision of language" (1960, p. 139).

Accordingly, linguistic meaning is closely connected with human activity and with the situation in which the particular word is uttered.

The inclusion of situational context means, among others, a decisive rejection of the traditional dyadic model, according to which meaning is the relation between word and object; for in this relationship the situation is of no importance. Let us now go back once more and follow up the third strand, the development of the dyadic model, to the point we have just reached, i.e., up to the inclusion of the situational context in the interpretation by the sign-user.

Saussure's scheme was still entirely dyadic, but it was no longer a crude juxtaposition of words and things. The sign (*signe*) constitutes a firm link between *signifiant* (the sound pattern) and *signifié*. And *signifié* is not the object itself but the idea or concept of the object, nor is *signifiant* the actual physical event, but the idea of this event (cf. Malmberg, 1963).

Ullmann, in a similar way, contrasts "name" and "sense," where "name" is the acoustic shape, and "sense" the mental content. Weisgerber, equally, speaks of "concept" in contrast to the "sound pattern."

What for a long time has been a stumbling block to psychologists becomes particularly evident in Weisgerber's views: "One of the most important results of human self-consciousness is the understanding of the separation of the world of the mind from the world in which we move physically. The world of real life in all its wealth and fullness cannot enter consciousness directly" (1962a, p. 38). Instead, it enters a 'mediating sphere' (*Zwischenwelt*). Where we meet verbal manifestations we can "in every case assume a mental mediating sphere" (1962a, p. 58). This separate existence of a world of meanings can also be found in Stenzel's writings: "The meaningful signs of verbal expression acquire in turn objectivity which stands between the consciousness of the speaker and the signified object . . . separating them . . . and yet making the connection between them possible" (1934, p. 35).

In this conception the world is duplicated so that we have a world of objects and, connected with it, an intermediate world of meanings. This conception no doubt has a Platonic element: a word or thought can be communicated and in the course of a conversation can retain its identity; the word and its meaning cannot be a purely subjective construct; it must have an existence of its own.

In contrast to this view, most psychologists, because of their somewhat anti-Platonic outlook, have certain hesitations to hypostatize such abstract intangible entities.

At this point it is appropriate to cast a glance at psychology. Here, too, we find a bipolar scheme retained for a long time. For Titchener: "Meaning, psychologically, is always context; one mental process is the meaning of another mental process if it is that other's context. And context, in this sense, is simply the mental process which accrues to the given process through the situation in which the organism finds itself" (1910, p. 367). For Titchener this second added mental process is the image. The word "dog" has meaning because the perception of the word evokes the image of a dog. Titchener himself was known for his extraordinarily vivid images. Hearing or reading the word "cow" elicited for him an image of a longish rectangle with a particular facial expression depicting "exaggerated pouting." On the other hand, there were equally well-known psychologists who when listening, reading, or thinking observed quite different images or no images at all.

The researcher who wants his statements to be unequivocal and precise is therefore likely to object to the "private" and introspective character of one side of the dyadic meaning-relation, that represents one point of origin for behaviorism.

It is further questionable whether general, categorical images are at all possible. An image of my spaniel Jimmy is no doubt possible, but what image goes with "dog" or, at a more general level, with "animal" or "creature," does it have fur or feathers and so on? Psycholinguists, and unfortunately psychologists generally, today use the terms "idea," "concept," and "thought" as carelessly as the term "image." As late as 1961, Leisi felt obliged to warn that "we have even less knowledge of the psychological facts and there is danger of circular definition, e.g. 'thoughts and images = elements of consciousness', 'consciousness = the totality of thoughts and images' " (1961, p. 11).

The reference to images, ideas and thoughts or, in more general terms, to states of consciousness, which dominated psychology around the turn of the century, gave rise to three opposing trends: (1) Gestalt psychology, because it mistrusted the mechanism of association linking states of consciousness; (2) psychoanalysis, because it could not find in the conscious states a common motivational thread and searched for it in the unconscious; and (3) behaviorism, because it rejected, on epistemological grounds, introspection as a method, and the appeal to states of consciousness as an explanation of psychic phenomena; but both psychoanalysis and behaviorism retained the mechanism of association.

Of these three "revolutions" the first—Gestalt psychology—has had relatively little direct effect upon psycholinguistics, because it paid less attention to learning than to perception, and language was viewed as being acquired by learning.

It should, however, be pointed out that indirectly Gestalt psychology has contributed a great deal to modern psycholinguistics by uncovering the weaknesses of orthodox behaviorism and thus forcing it to develop further.

The second revolution, depth psychology, has yielded as its most brilliant contribution to psycholinguistics Freud's analysis of slips of the pen and tongue.

The third, the behavioristic revolution, became decisive for the more recent developments in psycholinguistics.

Thanks to behaviorism, the endless search for the inner processes or states corresponding to verbal utterances was abandoned; as Brown (1958a, p. 93) expressed it, Watson mercifully closed the bloodshot inner eye of American psychology. "From the behaviorists point of view," writes Watson, "the problem of 'meaning' is a pure abstraction. It never arises in the scientific observation of behavior. We watch what the animal or human is doing. He 'means' what he does. His action shows his meaning" (Watson 1924, p. 354).

By his rejection of mental phenomena which are accessible only through introspection, Watson arrives at a point which is similar to that reached by one branch of the philosophy of language, albeit motivated by totally different considerations.

It was the rejection of Titchener's notion of meaning, i.e., meaning as an association between word and image, that led to behaviorism. But in other ways behaviorism retains the basic dyadic ideas, particularly as they relate to the notions of the genesis of the association between sign and object signified. A sign operates as stimulus for the same behavior that originally was elicited by the object signified. The origin of this substitution is quite simply explained by Watson through Pavlovian conditioning theory. If a conditioned stimulus (i.e., a sound pattern) is perceived several times in temporal contiguity with an unconditioned stimulus (i.e., the object), the conditioned stimulus will soon evoke the same behavior as hitherto the unconditioned one.

This view of the replacement of objects by signs or words has of course not originated with Pavlov or Watson; it can, for example, already be found in Swift's *Gulliver's Travels*.

> Gulliver visits an Academy and asks for an explanation of the research projects of the Faculty of Philosophy. One of these projects aims at the abolition of words. As speaking diminishes the lungs by corrosion, the professors made the following proposal: since words are the names for things it would be better to carry about the things needed for discourse. Unfortunately foolish women protested against this scheme, yet several most learned men adhered to it so that Gulliver was able to report that he saw some of these sages almost sinking under the weight of the packs they carried, going to debates where they opened their sacks to converse with the help of the objects they laid out.

The point that is made here is that the transition into the verbal medium is less troublesome and requires less effort (cf. Gehlen, 1950). The same point is made in the following illustration by Brown (1958a); we will have occasion to refer to it again later.

Suppose someone is quite familiar with the phenomenon of *rain* but has no name for it. If he is outside when it starts raining, he may open an umbrella or look for shelter. If he is at home when the rain begins, he is likely to put a coat on or, perhaps, decide not to go out. When this person learns that this event is called "rain," he will in future behave at the sound of the word "rain" as if he had felt or seen the rain. His "rain behavior" which so far was evoked by the stimulus rain is now also evoked by the stimulus-word "rain"; what has occurred is the characteristic transfer of behavior from one stimulus to another, which is familiar as the essence of the conditioning process (Brown, 1958a, p. 94).

The key position accorded to conditioning in this theory has formed the focus of a decisive critique which will be referred to in detail later in this book.

Conditioning theory as the basis for the origin of the sign is also part of Osgood's model, but he uses it more cautiously and with greater differentiation.

Behaviorism's emphasis on behavior is also recognized by linguistics, but for a different reason and in a different way, where it goes beyond the dyadic model. We find this in the development of pragmatism, to which we have referred and to which we now return after our excursion into behaviorism.

Building on Peirce, Ogden and Richards went beyond the dyadic model. Their book, *The Meaning of Meaning* (first published in 1923), was very influential from a philosophical, linguistic, and psychological point of view. The starting point for their critique is the view, implicit at least in the dyadic scheme, that a word has always only one fixed meaning: the relationship to the corresponding object or the connection with the one corresponding idea. From this view has originated, since the beginning of mankind, the argument about the "true" or "genuine" meaning of words. What is the real meaning of "God"? What do "freedom," "democracy," "love" or "happiness" *really* mean? Copernicus and Galileo were threatened with ultimate penalties because they questioned the traditional meaning of the word "earth," i.e., earth as the center of the universe.[5]

The conviction that every word must have *one real* or *true* meaning, driven to its logical extreme, leads to the appearance of "word magic." The practice of many magic formulae and incantations originates in the primitive opinion that the name *is* the thing, and even in the fairy tale there is someone who is happy that no one knows that his name is Rumplestilskin.

In contrast to these views Erdmann, around the turn of the century, already remarked: "Everywhere there are bitter fights which would soon be found to be completely futile if a few preliminary terminological questions had been settled" (Preface). "Words are signs for rather vague complexes of ideas which are more or less loosely connected . . . The boundaries of word meanings are blurred, vague and fluid" (p. 5). Therefore, ". . . the boundary of the meaning of a word can figuratively only be represented by a network of lines" (p. 8).

Let us compare with this view Wittgenstein's words about the concept of a game, written 35 years later: "Can you give the boundary? No. You can *draw* one; for, none has so far been drawn" (*Philosophical Investigations*, § 68). General Semantics has as its great mission to show that meanings are arbitrary or man-made and that they must be recognized as such, if we want to be guided by reality and not by language.

Ogden and Richards reject every fixed name-object relationship. Their conception is much more dynamic: what meaning really is can only be grasped if the process which occurs during a verbal exchange is understood. Words have no meanings as such; they get meaning by the way they are used by individuals. Language is a means not "of *symbolizing references*" . . . but "for the *promotion of purposes*" (p. 16).

The pragmatic element and closeness to the later writings of Wittgenstein are clearly indicated.

Instead of the well-known relationship between word and object Ogden and Richards propose a triangular model (Fig. 36). In the sign-user occurs a

---

[5] Note the link between this view and the earlier discussion of the question of the truth-function of language.

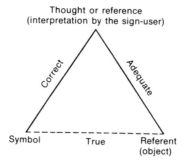

Thought or reference
(interpretation by the sign-user)

Correct

Adequate

Symbol   True   Referent
                              (object)

Fig. 36. Schema of the relationship between symbol, reference, and object. (Based, with slight modifications, on Ogden and Richards, 1952, p. 11)

process (interpretation) which is what is normally understood by meaning. The authors describe the nature of this process as follows: ". . . the peculiarity of interpretation (is) that when a context has affected us in the past the recurrence of merely a part of the context will cause us to react in the way in which we reacted before. A sign is always a stimulus similar to some part of an original stimulus and sufficient to call up the engram formed by that stimulus" (p. 53).

These sentences reveal the intermediate position taken by Ogden and Richards between the older view—meaning as connection with images or engrams—and the newer conception, according to which what goes on in the language-user is a third constituent (besides sign and referent) in the meaning relationship.

Moreover, for the further development of psycholinguistics it has been important that Ogden and Richards have interpreted the two dyads (word—language-user, and language-user—object signified) as a cause-effect or stimulus-response relationship. This goes back to Peirce who, as early as 1878, had written that in order to understand the meaning of a sentence all one had to do was to observe what habits it evoked.

By treating "meaning" as "stimulus" and "response" it becomes accessible to that type of psychological enquiry which seeks information not through introspection but through observable behavior. At the same time, meaning, understood as well-practiced connection between stimulus and response, or as "habit," places it into the area of the psychology of learning. But even for a philosopher, such as Telegdi, meaning is a generalization, accepted by society, which "manifests itself through action and through the use of the word, which implicitly expresses the rule governing this action" (1961, p. 210; cf. p. 277).

Morris, basing himself partly on Peirce and partly on Ogden and Richards, tried to bring logical positivism and pragmatism together. In this way he hoped to do justice to the logical, biological, and empirical aspects of the symbolic process and at the same time to confine himself to statements which are controlled by rules of operation and which express verifiable predictions (1938, 1946). In his *Foundations of the Theory of Signs* (1938) he attempts to produce a three-dimensional schema of "semiotic" (i.e., the science of signs) which integrates "a logico-empirical linguistic analysis with a basic pragmatic conception" (Apel, 1965). This schema will now be briefly described.

A necessary presupposition for the existence of signs is the goal-directed behavior of the sign-user. The essence of the sign does not lie in an abstract or ideational sphere; it lies in the fact that it is interwoven in a tissue which covers more than language, viz, the goal-oriented behavior of the sign-user.

This close connection between sign and action is also seen by Wittgenstein. For Bloomfield, speech events are embedded in practical events. In Russian psychology (e.g., Vigotsky), too, it is emphasized that the beginnings of infant speech lie in the activities of the infant.

A sign establishes relations in three dimensions: (1) the "syntactical" dimension relates signs to one another; (2) the "semantical" dimension relates signs to the objects to which the signs are applicable; and (3) the "pragmatical" dimension relates signs to human beings who use them.

Whereas Bühler holds that a sign can be analyzed as signal with regard to the receiver and as symptom with regard to the source, Morris saw the pragmatic dimension not as one of several others but as fundamental to the function of the sign. "It is precisely the interpersonal meaning of signs of a language system—however much its treatment in semantics may abstract from the concrete situation of language-use—which cannot be grasped without presupposing an act of interpreting situations as part of behavioral activity" (Apel, 1963, p. 30). Conversely, the use of signs is the major feature which distinguishes human from nonhuman behavior. Signs are the most powerful bonds humans have forged as well as the most useful instruments for the liberation of the individual and for the creation of societies.

A practical application of these arguments, developed by Morris, is found in Korzybski's and Hayakawa's General Semantics.

Apel has rightly pointed out that it is just this pragmatic element in Morris' procedure which leads to a humanistic integration and realization of linguistic structure. "Syntactical inter-relationships among signs and semantic relationships of signs to facts make sense as indicators of substantive truth only because they act as mediators in human behavioral settings" (1959a, p. 176).

This search for the "indicators of substantive truth" in language is not carried out without difficulties. The conviction that one needs only to consider syntax, semantics, *and* pragmatics is no longer reassuring. In the philosophy of language the question becomes more and more urgent whether the language of philosophy, which is used to think about language, itself must become subject to examination.

We might ask, for example, whether the fact that the English language has the noun "the meaning," misleads us all too easily to view the meaning of a sentence or word itself in terms of an object to be assigned to a word. Does this not create problems for the Platonic notion and for Weisgerber's "mediating spheres" of meaning? Instead of searching for the meaning of a word, we should think about ways of *explaining* what a word means. This is the starting point of the philosophical considerations of the later Wittgenstein, to which we now turn. If one wants to explain to someone what a "game" is, one does not enumerate all games in the hope that the listener will recognize in some mysterious way what all of them have in common. This approach is part of the old paradigm of mediating information, from Locke to Katz and Fodor. Instead, "One gives examples and intends them to be taken in a particular way—I do not, however, mean by this that he is supposed to see in those examples that common thing which I—for some reason—was unable to express; but that he is now to employ those examples in a particular way" (Wittgenstein, 1958, § 71). Thus the listener must share the intent for something which the speaker is trying to accomplish by means of his vocal utterance.

This orientation toward something, which becomes apparent in the act of meaning, was emphasized particularly by Husserl. Man always "means" something; even prior to the verbal expression, he always relates it to something. One can call something an "object signified" (das Bezeichnete) only after separating subject and object. As we speak we "always carry out an act of meaningful intent which merges with words and, so to speak, breathes life into them" (Husserl, 1929, p. 20).

The fact that in this formulation intentionality, i.e., a mentalistic act *par excellence,* is central, can hardly have appealed to a behavioristically oriented psychology which, with its mechanistic concepts, is certainly less sophisticated but epistemologically more consistent. In psychology such a formulation of intentionality is found in the writings of Brunswik, whose importance, along with that of his teacher Bühler, has only recently become apparent to psycholinguistics. Here we should mention Stenzel's fascinating formulation: "The breath of meaning defines the sentence" (1958, p. 53).

Aside from this channeled intentionality, an integration of language and action is a decisive factor for Wittgenstein. One can only explain the meaning of words or sentences by examining "the whole of language and the actions into which it is interwoven" (Wittgenstein, 1958, p. 7). All of this he calls the *language game.* "Only someone who already knows how to do something with it can significantly ask a name." In other words, linguistic elements can have meaning only against the available backdrop of the meaningful.[6] Meaning evolves from the interrelationship of people who live together.

[6] This is further expanded by Hörmann, 1976.

This notion has far-reaching consequences for psycholinguistics. It offers new approaches for the genetic-biologic requirements as well as for the acquisition of language.

One can elucidate this interweaving of verbal and nonverbal acts by trying to identify types of language games. This is what Searle (1969) has done. He calls them speech-acts, describing, for example, speech-acts of warning, of command, of promise, etc. Part of each speech-act is a network of verbal and nonverbal presuppositions and assumed consequences which, consciously or unconsciously, must be present in the speaker before he can generate the appropriate speech-act. Thus someone who makes a promise must at this point in time feel that he is ready and able to carry out what he has promised in due time. But the speaker must also make certain assumptions about the awareness of the listener. Part of a promise is, for example, that the listener prefers that the promise be kept rather than broken, otherwise it it is not a promise but a threat.

This network of presuppositions, of possible and anticipated consequences, goes far beyond the behaviorist's S-R formulation with its view that meaning is a verbal act embedded in nonverbal behaviors (Bloomfield). This leads to a conception of meaning which goes beyond speech itself. The meaning of a verbal expression becomes clear only after it is embedded in the totality of the speech-act. For example, the sentence, "Can you open the window?" while syntactically formulated as a question, is most often used in a requesting speech-act. So it is through the speech-act that an expression takes on its meaning.[7]

Let us look back from the vantage point of these philosophical reflections to the relationship between linguistics and psycholinguistics. What becomes clearly apparent here is the need for a relative weighting of every syntax-centered grammar, for example, the orthodox generative transformational grammar. If the listener is to understand a sentence in the sense that it is intended by the speaker, the listener must possess more than the so-called competence, i.e., knowledge of the rules for generating grammatically correct sentences. A native speaker interprets the statement, "Can you open the window?" as a request, although his *grammatical* competence tells him that the surface structure of this sentence has undergone a question transformation.

It is possible to attempt to solve this problem by introducing a super-competence. What Hymes (1972) describes as communicative competence or what Habermas (1971) calls universal competence, is supposed to ensure that, if need be, a sentence can be correctly analyzed by applying more than the usual grammatical rules.

Nevertheless, the introduction of additional competences does not really

---

[7] This last formulation leads us beyond Searle. For him, speech-act and sentence remain always vaguely reducible one to the other.

solve the problem. There is no final authority that decides whether or not, in a particular case, one of these supercompetencies is to be activated. What determines whether the statement, "Can you open the window?" is to be comprehended according to the syntactic competence (as a question), or according to a higher competence (as a request)? Applying psycholinguistic consideration to the solution of these difficulties, it becomes clear that the "level" at which a certain expression takes on meaning in a particular case is in no way determined only by the content and the form of the expression. Meaning and understanding are acts for which the range of significance is determined by the intention of the speaker and the listener. Viewed in this way, meaning is not a correlate of the sign or the association of sign and object signified. On the contrary, it is a process by which the speaker steers the listener's conscious awareness in order to assure that the latter understands what he means. For these acts to succeed it is necessary that the listener assume that the speaker's expression must make sense. Operating under this assumption, the listener will analyze the speaker's expression according to constantly changing procedural rules until it makes sense to him. That is the reason why the "smiling meadow" is not rejected as nonsense because of its semantic anomaly, but is continually analyzed until it satisfies the criterion of making sense. One could say that an expression of this kind is guided along the path of this criterion until it lands on the metaphoric plane. Thus making sense is the predetermined goal toward which the expression is analyzed. Sense is to be achieved or maintained under all circumstances. This is reflected in the concept of "sense constancy" introduced by Hörmann (1976).

As can be seen, the search for the philosophical bases and consequences of the process and the concept of *meaning* leads beyond a narrow definition of language. If we want to talk about *the* language which people actually speak, then we have to include nonverbal aspects like the situation, the intention of the speaker and the listener, and also the basic human tendency to make the world intelligible.

CHAPTER 8

Sign and Object Signified: Classical Theories of the Development of Meaning

Association through conditioning—Skinner's *Verbal Behavior*—Chomsky's critique of it—Meaning as a response—Meaning as disposition—MacKay's and Deese's contribution to it—Bloomfield's model—Mediational theories of meaning—Osgood and the Semantic Differential—Bilingualism and semantic satiation—A cognitive model of meaning.

In a previous chapter we talked about meaning as a connection, and regarded an association (as manifested in an experiment) as an indicator of the presence of such a connection. With the help of associations, we have tried to describe the network of connections within which a word is placed according to its meaning. Many of the assumptions that we had taken for granted became apparent only when we examined them within the context of the philosophy of language.

Now we are reminded that the concept of association can be used in a somewhat different sense, i.e., to designate the *occurrence* of such a connection. If we now turn to studies which focus on the process or the "mechanism" of this formation of associations let us remember, on the one hand, what we have said about the philosophical currents for and against behaviorism. On the other hand, we must also recognize that the approach to which we now turn attempts not only to explain how meaning evolves, but also to say something about the development of signs, and generally speculates on the evolution or the acquisition of language. We must consider these rather comprehensive claims in our evaluation of the achievements and inadequacies of the conditioning theories of meaning.

It is a well-known fact that associationism played a dominant role in psychology during the first half of this century. This was made possible by the fact that its supporters were able to demonstrate with relative ease the efficacy of this theoretical approach. By means of a conditioning process, Pavlov's dog came to associate the conditioned stimulus (CS, bell) with the unconditioned stimulus (UCS, food in the mouth) so that later the CS elicited the response (CR, secretion of saliva), which was originally elicited only by the UCS. For Pavlov, the factor which produces the association is the temporal contiguity of CS and UCS. For Thorndike, and later for Hull, the factor producing the association was the reinforcement or reward which follows the CS. Skinner emphasizes almost exclusively the sequence of response and reinforcement. Accordingly, in Pavlov's model the primary interest focuses on the association of the CS and UCS. In the Thorndike-Hull model it is the reinforcement or strengthening of the association between S and R. Finally, for Skinner, it is the reinforcement which increases the probability of the occurrence of the response.

As we have seen, behavioristic psychology views association through conditioning as the basis for, or even identical with, the process of sign formation. A sign becomes a sign, i.e., becomes invested with meaning, by being associated with the signified object. In orthodox behaviorism, this approach leads inevitably and rapidly to a total negation of the concept of meaning. Why talk about the "mentalistic" concept of meaning, which is difficult to conceptualize operationally, when one can talk about behavior and associations between S and R? In the following an outline of this orthodox behavioristic line of thought is presented not in the least because, in recent years, it has been discredited more than it deserves and in a manner which dumps the baby with the bath.

It starts with Watson himself, for whom the problem of meaning is "a pure abstraction." Humphrey (1951) admittedly views as a problem the question of how it is possible that a cluster of sounds emitted by A can evoke a certain reaction in individual B, but he regards the process as a learning problem, and in his view this learning problem should not be further complicated by giving it another name, i.e., "meaning."

The tempting simplicity of orthodox behaviorism and of an approach from learning theory can be witnessed nowhere more clearly than in Skinner's *Verbal Behavior* (1957). In the first place, the importance of this work lies in the fact that Skinner has attempted to design a psychology of language which, in view of the difficulties presented by the concept of meaning, dispenses with "meaning" altogether. The fixation on this notion, it can be argued, has led to stagnation in psycholinguistics. It is therefore justifiable to assume that a rejection of all mentalistic notions could lead to rapid advances in this area just as much as in other areas of psychology.

Skinner's approach is, secondly, of significance because his learning theory (in his view no "theory" at all), which naturally also permeates his psychology of language, has become widely known as a basis for programmed learning and for behavior therapy.

In his entire book Skinner avoids terms such as "language," or even "language behavior," or "linguistic behavior," because they suggest the notion of a linguistic "community," hence of something supraindividual, approaching Saussure's *langue*. Language for Skinner is no entity; he recognizes only behavior, and verbal behavior as a particular form of behavior.

His aim is—as Tikhomirov (1959) expressed it—to show in what respect verbal behavior and other forms of behavior are alike.[1]

Skinner intends to present a functional analysis of verbal behavior; the variables determining verbal behavior are to be identified and their interaction to be described. The mode of description must be objective; as far as possible operational definitions are to be used, hence such terms as "stimulus," "response" or "reinforcement" are employed. This functional analysis has achieved its object if, in this way, the verbal behavior of a speaker can be predicted on the basis of other observable behavioral or situational elements. The correct prediction, hence the control, of this behavior is the criterion of success of such an analysis. The search for variables determining verbal behavior is concentrated upon actual stimuli and earlier reinforcement, whereas the inherent structure of the language or structural elements within the speaker play no part in this analysis because they cannot be equated with behavior.

Although Skinner endeavors to analyze verbal behavior in terms of the same determinants as other forms of behavior, he discusses in detail why it is justifiable to treat verbal behavior separately from other forms of behavior. Behavior normally changes the environment of the behaving individual by means of mechanical operations. When I pick up a glass of water, it comes closer to me. Someone who is afraid of a dog and runs away increases the distance between himself and the dog. If someone slays the dog, the latter changes from a living creature into one that is dead.

Verbal behavior is different. If I don't go to the water tap but request a glass of water, such verbal behavior does not affect the environment directly, but indirectly through the intervention of another person. If I eventually receive a glass of water, this result is no longer directly or mechanically dependent upon my own physical action, i.e., the production of sounds.

Verbal behavior, therefore, is distinguished from other forms of behavior by achieving its object through the intervention or, as Skinner puts it, the "mediation" of other persons.

At least in principle it is only through the listener that verbal behavior attains its goal. This approach permits combining the speaker's and the listener's behavior into what Skinner calls a speech episode. In this episode there is nothing *beyond* the sum of the behaviors of the two participating individuals.

Let us remember that such interactions between speaker and listener are found also in the newer approaches of communication theories, such as in Searle, but in that case the encompassing unit is actually a structure which is *more* than just the sum of the individual behaviors.

---

[1] It will be remembered that in the introductory chapter of our book we were concerned with showing in what way linguistic behavior is different from other forms of behavior.

In order to be able to recognize the full weight of Skinner's last proposition, let us contrast it with the following: "Language is the thought-forming instrument. Intellectual activity—entirely mental, completely inward, proceeding, one might say, without a trace—manifests itself in the sounds of speech and thus can be perceived by the senses" (Humboldt, 1949 edition, pp. 52 f.). Humboldt's view represents in every word the extreme opposite to Skinner's behaviorism. In Humboldt's view, language has an existence transcending the concrete act of speech; it has power over the human being.

Skinner vehemently opposes this view. He argues that previously it was customary to "explain" verbal behavior as an expression of ideas; but are ideas more than words? A speaker does not utter ideas, images, or thoughts—these are purely subjective notions; what he utters are nothing more than words. Skinner's procedure is consistent. He rejects not only such notions as "idea" or "image," but also "meaning" and "information."

> Strictly speaking, this is one of Skinner's inconsistencies, because in a way the speaker does not utter words either, but at best sounds. That these sounds are perceived as words (and therefore have meaning), is already a mentalistic act which ought to be unacceptable to the behaviorist.

Let us now look again at another of Skinner's propositions: verbal behavior is behavior reinforced by the mediation of other persons. Thus, greatest importance is attributed to the element of *learning*. Human speech—in contrast to other forms of communication in the animal world—is learned; hence its acquisition and maintenance must follow the general laws of learning.

Laws of learning determine why, in a given situation, these and no other verbal utterances occur. Skinner (who does not claim to have a theory of learning) regards laws of learning as descriptive accounts of the events and of the conditions under which these events occur. This description is what he calls a functional analysis which, in his case, is inevitably made in terms of stimulus-response aspects of the present situation and earlier reinforcements.

According to Skinner, one can distinguish two major classes of responses: those which are elicited by certain a priori determinable stimuli (elicited responses) and those which are apparently produced spontaneously (emitted responses or operants). Particularly in the case of the latter, which are of particular interest to Skinner, one can change the probability of their occurrence through particular reinforcement. They can also be brought under the control of a particular stimulus by making the reinforcement dependent on the prior appearance of that stimulus. (For example, the pecking of a pigeon is brought under the control of a light, so that pecking for food occurs *only* if the light was previously presented.) Applied to language this means that if a chair is designated as "red," this response must be under the control of a particular stimulus attribute, namely the redness of the chair.

Skinner finds these different types of responses reflected in the types of verbal behavior. Thus, a "mand" is a verbal operant response which is reinforced by certain consequences. Mands are therefore commands, wishes, and threats. A command is a command because it is obeyed; and a wish becomes a wish because it is fulfilled.

A "tact" occurs whenever a certain response is evoked by a certain object or by particular qualities of that object. If mands are determined by the consequences, tacts are defined by the stimulus.

While, traditionally, the occurrence of an utterance was explained by referring to its "meaning," Skinner accounts for the occurrence of a word ("pencil") by asking what the stimulus situation must be like to elicit the response "pencil" in the speaker.

That a particular stimulus evokes a particular response is the result of a conditioning process. Whether the response is "emitted" or "elicited" it has become attached to a stimulus in a predictable manner because of the reinforcement of the S-R sequence. What acts as reinforcement? Broadly speaking, praise, approval, confirmation, success all act as reinforcement.

Thus we reach a group of empirical studies which—in addition to numerous investigations by Skinner's students on simple learning tasks—offer the most important evidence for the heuristic value of Skinner's interpretation for an analysis of verbal behavior. These studies can be summarized under the title of "conditioning of verbal behavior."

> In order to understand what is meant by that, the following situation should be imagined. Two persons are engaged in conversation. One of them has the intention of bringing a certain aspect of the verbal behavior of the other under his control by increasing the frequency of occurrence of this feature. For example, let us assume he wants to cause the other person to include in his talk expressions of opinions such as "I mean," "D'you see," "I believe," or "I feel," we can achieve this by reinforcing each appearance of such a phrase, by an expression of approval such as "mmm-hmm," "right," or "yes."

It is today beyond any doubt that it is possible to bring verbal behavior under control by means of such external direction of the learning mechanism and in this way to exercise a determining influence upon it. The verbal response can be attached to a certain verbal stimulus, and since the response is dependent upon the verbal stimulus, it is therefore also possible, given a knowledge of the stimulus qualities of the situation as a whole, to predict the verbal response.

But Skinner's claim that verbal behavior is always and in every situation under the control of the stimulus overstretches the applicability of this theoretical construct. The claim has had fateful consequences for the entire theory as has been clearly demonstrated by Chomsky (1959). Chomsky's critique deserves to be reported in detail as a corrective to the claim of orthodox behaviorism in psycholinguistics.

When verbal behavior is conditioned it is possible (just as in a Skinner-box experiment) to define the stimulus independently, e.g., the "mmm-hmm" of the experimenter, or the light signal in the Skinner-box. This stimulus is linked with a response by means of a well-known regular relationship; a response is what is evoked by a stimulus in accordance with a precise rule. If I talk about my friend Jack and therefore use a proper noun, this is, according to Skinner, "a response under the control of a person or thing." What does it mean in this context to say "under the control of"? The presence of a stimulus should increase the frequency of occurrence of the response. But we are likely to talk about friend Jack more frequently in his absence. Let us illustrate the point we are making by another example. Someone sees a red chair and says "red." According to Skinner, this verbal response is under the control of the stimulus aspect of the color red. If that same person says "chair," this response is made under the control of the stimulus aspect of the chair qualities. If, instead, he says, "Thank goodness, I'm tired of standing," the corresponding stimulus aspect is comfort-seeking or the like. It is quite clear that for every response the corresponding stimulus aspect is invented. The stimulus is inferred from the response and consequently has lost its objectivity which was so highly valued.

In Skinner's approach the essential dependent variable, i.e., the variable which is reinforced, is response-strength, defined as the probability of occurrence (and intensity) of a response. Skinner illustrates it by the following example: if we are shown a work of art and exclaim, "Beautiful!," the speed and intensity of our response are likely to influence the owner of the work of art. But if we take Skinner's definition of response-strength literally—and this is what we ought to do if we say that his experimental investigations on simple learning tasks have psycholinguistic implications—a person who is particularly impressed by the work of art would exclaim, "Beautiful!" in a loud voice and as often as possible.

Chomsky further selects the concept of reinforcement to show how Skinner attempts to give the psychological study of language the reputable aura of objectivity which notions such as "stimulus" or "response-strength" have acquired in the field of learning without at the same time ensuring that the concepts are used with the same rigor.

According to Skinner, reinforcement is the presentation of a certain stimulus in a temporal relationship either to another stimulus or to a response. The "mmm-hmm" of the experimenter acts as reinforcement because it follows immediately the response to be confirmed. If we examine the use of the concept of reinforcement in *Verbal Behavior*, it appears that a person talks to himself because this is "reinforcing" for him. A child imitates sounds it has heard because such imitation "reinforces." The speaker's verbal behavior is reinforced by the behavior of the listener—in short, a speaker says what he would like to say because it is "reinforcing" for him. The presence of reinforcement is inferred from the fact that verbal behavior occurs. This means that the concept of reinforcement has lost its meaning.[2]

The application of concepts taken from learning theory has led to difficulties here, because these concepts have lost their operational anchorage. The fact that Skinner uses the same terms in the psychology of language as in the psychology of learning creates "the illusion of a rigorous scientific theory with a very broad scope, although in fact the terms . . . may be mere homonyms . . ." "The magnitude of the failure of this attempt to account for verbal behavior serves as a kind of measure of the importance of the factors omitted from consideration, and an indication of how little is really known about this remarkably complex phenomenon" (Chomsky, 1959, pp. 30 and 28).

With regard to the problem of meaning, Skinner shared with many empirically oriented psychologists of that time a disinclination to appeal to states of consciousness and other subjective experiences. This was the starting point for his psycholinguistic *tour de force*. There was a feeling of being on safer ground if one spoke only in terms of behavior and explained the causation of such behavior according to the well-tried model of learning theory.

Fundamentally Skinner's approach belongs to the substitution theories of meaning. All of these start out from the fascinatingly simple assumption that the conditioned stimulus "word" serves as a substitute for the unconditioned stimulus "object" to evoke those responses which hitherto were evoked by the object.

This view gets into difficulties on two sides, even ignoring Skinner's overextension of certain concepts for which he was already criticized. On the one side, the reality of the object is being questioned and, on the other, the kind of response which was previously elicited by the US and which is now evoked by a CS.

What object is replaced by the word "justice" for example? What object is substituted by the word "or"? These examples show that, with the application of the substitution model, the sign or word is treated as a name, and thus the fact is overlooked that the entire vocabulary of a language cannot be fitted into this scheme. Admittedly, this accusation can be equally directed against linguistic philosophers with no behavioristic orientation: when Gadamer (1960) writes "language is the language of things," he is in trouble with such words as "or," "not," "if," and "against."

The difficulties which a view of *meaning as image or idea* had run into led, as a reaction, to the view of *meaning as response*. And within the framework of substitution theory, this was interpreted as a conditioned single response which, after a period of learning, was evoked by the CS (the sign) in exactly

---

[2] This is quite different from the use of the same concept in the work of Hull, Pavlov, Guthrie, or Thorndike where the definition of reinforcement has remained independent.

the same manner as it was previously evoked by the US (object or *desig-natum*). But which single response is evoked by the word "rain" in the same way as by the object rain itself? It is evident that there is no single or certain response either to the object rain or the word "rain." What follows the object or word depends to a large extent—although not exclusively—upon the situation in which they occur. From this results the difficulty that, as long as meaning is equated with the overt behavioral response to an object or sign, it becomes something quite unstable.

Moreover, which response is evoked if, for example, the reader of a novel encounters the word "rain"? No visible behavioral response at all is evoked. Yet, the behaviorist will hardly be inclined to say that in this case, therefore, the word has no meaning. Watson's stop-gap solution was the "implicit response," which was not observable in external behavior, but which would in the future be identified by means of special techniques of investigation, such as incipient movements of the speech apparatus, innervations and so forth.

It is now conceivable that one rejects the substitution aspect of the theory and yet conceives meaning as response to a sign. In that case it must be shown (Brown has emphatically drawn attention to this point) what the relationship is between the response to the object signified and the response to the sign.

This suggests the assumption of different but similar and interconnected responses—a Hullian habit-family hierarchy. This hierarchy can be brought into action by the sign as well as by the object signified. It then depends on the situation as to which response in fact occurs. Real rain will evoke responses that will lead to taking shelter, whereas the word "rain" is likely to be uttered before the actual event and leads to actions to avoid getting wet.

> It is clear that the search for the response evoked by the sign leads to the rejection of a rigidly dyadic scheme and to the addition of the situation—a pragmatic moment one might say—as a qualifying factor.

In this conception, represented above all by Morris, continuity between the object designated and the behavior evoked by the sign is established with the help of the argument that the sign does not evoke a single response but a *disposition to respond*. Additionally, the *situation* must be taken into account so that the disposition can manifest itself in actual behavior.

Thus, Morris in a very logical way comes to grips with one of the greatest difficulties presented by the theories of meaning as response. If meaning, as Bloomfield, for example, has it, consists in a sign being followed by a definite mode of behavior, how is it that the phrase, "It's raining," is at different times followed by taking a raincoat, or shutting a window, or running quickly, or sometimes even by nothing at all? Does this imply that, "It's raining," has various meanings? Morris' answer is that the uniform meaning of a word does not rest in behavior but in a disposition to behave, evoked by the word. The sign (or word) is a preparatory-stimulus which influences the behavior evoked by other stimuli. A preparatory-stimulus—Morris adopted this concept of Mowrer's—influences a response which the organism may make to another stimulus. Suppose a motorist asking the way is given the direction, "When you come to the white building, turn left." This sentence, although it does not immediately evoke a response, is a preparatory-stimulus (and therefore meaningful), because it influences the behavior of the driver which will be evoked by the sight of the white building.

In this way, Morris obtains a uniform correlate of meaning to which to relate the multiplicity of modes of behavior which follow signs without being fully determined by them. This also solves the great difficulty presented to theories of meaning as response by the act of reading because there is no visible response in behavior. "Whether a sign does or does not lead to overt behavior depends upon whether or not certain conditions of motivation and environment are fulfilled" (Morris, 1955 edition, p. 51).

While disposition as a carrier of meaning in Morris' theory can still be considered as a kind of response to a preparatory-stimulus (the sign), in Brown's theory the response notion has still further moved into the background. Brown writes: "When one comes to understand a linguistic form (i.e., a word or sentence) his nervous system is partially rewired (in the sense of changes in synaptic resistances or neurone growth process) so that one is disposed to behave appropriately with regard to that form. For the psychologist meaning is not any particular response. It is the disposition to behave in varying ways with regard to the form as the contingent circumstances are changed. The disposition has no substantial character other than the structure of the nervous system. . . . It is a response potential. A disposition is discovered by creating various contingencies and observing responses (1958a, p. 103).

This notion of the *modification of the disposition to behave,* which for Brown characterizes *meaning,* is found, interestingly enough, also at the center of what MacKay (1972) defines as *information.* Like Brown, MacKay cannot be accused of behaviorist leanings. Information, according to him, is that interaction between two organisms, A and B, through which A's signals affect the "central organization system" of B (that is his representation of events, knowledge, and judgment) in such a way that B's behavior is different from what it would have been without such influence. Thus information changes the *inner basis* for dealing with all that occurs in the world. It is important to recognize that these notions are far removed from behaviorism. They owe their existence, at least in part, to the futile search for *the* response associated with the sign.

This brings us close to Deese's (1969) notion of comprehension. On the one hand, orthodox behaviorism rejected outright the phenomenon and process of comprehension, while on the other hand, for the neobehaviorist, comprehension was at best an epiphenomenon of the (actually more important) response. However, to quote Deese, "understanding is the inward sign of the potential for reacting appropriately to what we see or hear" (p. 516). That caused the evaporation of the last remains of behavioristic theory which may still have lingered in "meaning as an association between sign and object signified." Becoming aware of adequate behavior possibilities is a phenomenal, "mentalistic" act closer to consciousness than to overt behavior. (This is discussed more extensively by Hörmann, 1976.) Let us still stay with the neobehavioristic approach and examine the development of another concept, namely mediation. It also originated from this approach and has gained importance both in psycholinguistics and in cognitive psychology.

Bloomfield, whose work has been influential, offers as a definition of meaning the situation in which the speaker utters the linguistic form and the response which it calls forth in the hearer (1933, p. 139). The behavior sequence in which linguistic behavior occurs normally begins with a practical event and leads via an act of speech to another practical event. Bloomfield gives this illustration: when Jill sees an apple, her speechless response can be represented as follows. The seeing of the apple (stimulus S) leads to grasping (response R). If this simple action is not possible (because, for example, the apple hangs too high), the sequence is as follows: Jill sees the apple (S) and says something (r) which causes Jack (s) to pick the apple (R); $S \rightarrow r \ldots s \rightarrow R$ is the model of a response mediated by speech. S and R are practical events; $r \ldots s$ is the speech act itself. The partial sequence $S \rightarrow r$ occurs in the speaker, and the partial sequence $s \rightarrow R$ in the hearer.

We now turn to a detailed examination of mediation because it represents the theoretical basis for numerous studies dealing with meaning, meaning acquisition, and change of meaning, published after about 1953.

In the preceding paragraphs we introduced what for the most part could be called "direct" conditioning, where a CS is associated with a UCS or an R. Only in the case of Skinner did we find the notion of mediation ("by means of another person").

A number of experiments in the psychology of learning, however, are known in which processes seem to be associated with one another which hitherto have not occurred together and to which the categories similar-dissimilar are not applicable either.

This connection can best be illustrated by the so-called Shipley example: tapping the cheek elicits eye blink as an unconditioned reflex. A weak light-flash is presented several times at the same time as the tap; as a consequence the flash elicits eye blink as a conditioned reflex.

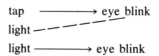

Next the tapping is paired with a pain stimulus to one finger which elicits the withdrawal of the finger. Once the connection

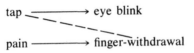

is well established the light-flash alone is offered to the subject, and although hitherto neither light and finger-withdrawal nor light and pain have occurred together, the light-flash elicits the withdrawal of the finger:

light ⟶ eye blink + finger-withdrawal

The explanation lies in the fact that in the second step of the described conditioning process the finger-withdrawal is 'hooked' onto the eyelid reaction evoked by tapping.

If we attempt to formulate this more precisely the finger-withdrawal does not become attached directly to the eyelid reaction but to the perception by the subject of his own response, in other words to the proprioceptive stimuli produced by the response. Since the light in the first phase of the conditioning experiment can elicit the eyelid reaction, in the second phase the light also evokes the finger-withdrawal mediated by the eye blink.

Thus a chain has been created by interposing a connecting link as mediator between light and finger-withdrawal, which hitherto have not occurred together; or, expressed in more general terms, if two elements A and B which have no connection with one another are each separately linked to C, they, in turn, become linked by way of C.

In the above example a connecting link is assumed as an explanation of the fact that a stimulus evokes a response with which it has hitherto not occurred. A second approach to this problem can be made by asking how it is that two different stimuli can evoke the same response. A preliminary answer is provided by numerous Russian investigations on the second-signal system. These investigations have been based on the following design. To begin with, a conditioned response to a particular stimulus-object is acquired. If the subject is subsequently presented with a word which designates this object this word also evokes the reaction. Thus, for example, the response "press lever" can be conditioned to a light signal. Once this conditioned response has been established, the word "light" alone can also evoke the response.

That this phenomenon is a case of generalization (i.e., a response hitherto evoked only by a particular stimulus is now also evoked by a second "similar" stimulus) can be further clarified by the experiments which, for example, Razran has undertaken to study the phenomenon of the so-called "semantic generalization." If, for instance, a saliva secretion response is conditioned to the word "style," the same response can be evoked, although more weakly, by the semantically similar "fashion." The less similar to the original stimulus-word the meanings of the words subsequently offered as stimuli are, the more reduced is the response. It is interesting to note, that in these cases semantic similarity is more influential than phonological similarity: generalization is surprisingly more marked for synonyms than for homophones. If in the given example "style" is not followed by "fashion" but by "stile," it evokes hardly any response.

What mediates between the first and the second stimulus, between "style" and "fashion"? Are both unconsciously brought in contact with a *genus proximum*? Whereas in the Shipley experiment the subject after the tap on the cheek is still blinking when he retracts his finger and therefore the blink as a mediating link is quite overt, in the case of semantic generalization the mediating link is entirely hidden.

The question of the origin and nature of these connecting links and the mechanism of mediation is today in the center of a great deal of psycholinguistic work. These studies will now be considered.

This construct can be traced back to Hull (1930) who argues that there are acts whose sole function it is to serve as stimuli for other acts. He calls them pure stimulus acts. Hull was aware of the significance of this argument: he describes these pure stimulus acts as the "organic basis of symbolism."

How should we imagine these pure stimulus acts? It may be illustrated by one of Osgood's examples (1953, pp. 400 f.), which—although not taken from psycholinguistics—explains the principle: the sequence of acts of tying a shoe lace. If we consider such a sequence in a five-year-old child who requires all his skill and attention to complete this task, it will be recognized that an initial situation describable in physical terms S_1, i.e. seeing the loose laces, is followed by the associated response R_1, grasping the laces with both hands. This response R_1 changes the situation for the child: hands and laces are seen in a new position S_2. This new stimulus S_2 must now be followed by the next response R_2, the movement of crossing and twisting the laces. This again changes the stimulus situation, so that we now have S_3 and so on (Fig. 37).

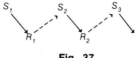

Fig. 37

How does this series of almost isolated stimuli and responses become the unitary sequence which an adult can execute without paying direct attention and even in darkness? The external stimuli which in the early stage in the child guide the action must lose their significance. Their role is taken over by proprioceptive stimuli. It is no longer necessary to see the laces; the feedback of hand movements is sufficient. All that is needed are the kinesthetic and sensory-motor input of the individual's own responses (Fig. 38).

$$S_1 \searrow$$
$$R_1 \ \text{---} \ S_{p_1} \longrightarrow R_2 \ \text{---} \ S_{p_2} \longrightarrow R_3 \ \text{---}$$

Fig. 38

Response R_1 is fed back and perceived as proprioceptive stimulus S_{p_1}. Each response has at the same time stimulus value, and this stimulus value is associated with the next response, so that the feedback of the completion of one response serves as the stimulus for eliciting the next response.

Lashley drew attention to the fact that the feedback of the individual's own action would require too much time to guide in this way very rapid sequences, e.g., piano playing. Consequently, Hebb has moved this organization from a combination between peripheral and central areas entirely into the central area. Hebb's phase sequence achieves the spatiotemporal organization here referred to. For our present purposes the following arguments are, however, more important than a detailed neurophysiological specification.

It was seen in the most diverse areas of psychology that it is essential to postulate, between the initial stimulus and the terminal response of an action chain, intermediate links which assume the role of mediator, i.e., which are to be understood as being at the same time response *and* stimulus. These mediation theories, which are widely recognized today, frequently appear remarkably close to linguistic processes, even where—e.g., in the psychology of thinking—they have been used outside the area of psycholinguistics proper.

On the basis of this general mediation theory, two constructs of interest to psycholinguists have been developed. They differ from each other in that in the first the nature of the link is specified as a *verbal* association, whereas in the other the mediating unit is an *emotional* link. Without going into the details and subtle distinctions of the argument, let us at this point attempt to understand the two basic models.

Bousfield assumes that repeated stimulation leads to the development of a representational sequence. Such a sequence (the order of presentation should be noted) consists of a representational response and a representational stimulus.

The representational response is a specially stable part of the total reaction system to a stimulus and is particularly conditionable. In the cases of interest to us here, the representational response is generally identical with a silent repetition of the heard stimulus-word. This implicit repetition of the heard word has in turn also the character of a stimulus (Fig. 39).

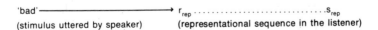

'bad'——————————→ r_{rep} .... s_{rep}
(stimulus uttered by speaker)   (representational sequence in the listener)

Fig. 39

The response part is r_{rep} and s_{rep} is the stimulus part of the representational sequence; s_{rep} is conditionable.

How can this model serve to explain the development of a meaningful response to a verbal stimulus? Bousfield illustrates it with the example of how the meaning of the word "evil" develops. How does a child learn what "evil" means?

> The developmental sequence begins when the small child hears the word 'bad' and at the same time is given a slap on his hand. This is interpreted as a conditioning process: the pain is the unconditioned stimulus US; it prompts also a representational response R_{rep}. The conditioned stimulus CS is the word "bad" uttered by the adult; it, too, is followed by a representational response r_{rep} whose proprioceptive stimulation is s_{rep}. As CS and US are almost simultaneous, s_{rep} is being conditioned so that in future s_{rep}, when the word 'bad' is heard, is capable of evoking the representational response to pain (Fig. 40). By running through this sequence several times a habit has been created which we call H_1.

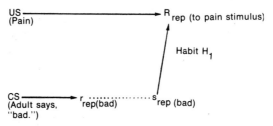

Fig. 40. The development of a meaningful response, first phase. (Based on Bousfield, in Cofer, 1961, p. 83)

At a later point in time the child hears the word "evil," which so far has been unknown to him, and, immediately after, the word "bad" with which he is already familiar. He might, for example, have asked his parents what "evil" means; or both words have been applied to him. The word "evil" here functions as CS which has its representational consequence. The word "bad" is the US which elicits the representational sequence belonging to "bad" as well as the habit H_1, acquired through earlier conditioning, so that the representational response to pain is evoked (Fig. 41).

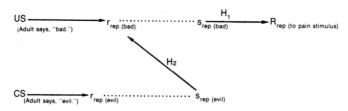

Fig. 41. The development of a meaningful response, second phase. (Based on Bousfield, in Cofer, 1961, p. 83)

If the child at a later stage hears "evil," we should expect that he should say "bad" either implicitly or, at least, think it associatively. Thus the habit H_2 is established by the new conditioning process.

Therefore, r_{rep} ("evil") evokes the entire representational sequence of "bad"; i.e., it leads as far as the R_{rep} (pain).

In Bousfield's model the representational response r_{rep} constitutes the mediating link between a relatively new stimulus and a response evoked earlier by another stimulus r_{rep} is a mediating response. Bousfield's interpretation is a mediation theory of the acquisition of meaning.

In the course of the use of language and as a result of such use, a certain equivalence of stimuli is created. Such acquired equivalence can also be regarded as the formation of classes of stimuli which is caused by the mediating function of the intermediate links.

Mediation theories also play an important role in explaining concept formation, a problem halfway between the psychology of language and cognition. Kaminski (1964) describes concept-forming mediation in an analogous manner to Bousfield's model.

How do we learn that apples and bananas are collectively referred to as "fruit," and cucumbers and cabbages as "vegetables"? How does a person who knows the names of the different sorts acquire the class concepts "fruit" and "vegetables"? The sight of apples is stimulus US_1, the sight of bananas US_2, that of cabbages US_3 and of cucumbers US_4. CS "fruit" is conditioned to US_1 (apples) and equally to US_2 (bananas). This means that the representational sequence following CS is the same for apples and bananas, and that the s_{rep} for apples and bananas are identical. The result is that—if one may use this expression—the total impression of apples (to which, besides US_1, $s_{rep\ fruit}$ also contributes) becomes somewhat more similar to the total impression of bananas ($US_2 + s_{rep\ fruit}$).

On the other hand, the CS "vegetable" with its representational sequence containing s_{rep} is conditioned to US_3 and US_4. This $s_{rep\ vegetable}$ brings cabbages and cucumbers closer to each other because it occurs with both of them. At the same time $s_{rep\ vegetable}$ is an additional means of distinguishing US_2 from US_4. Even if a particular banana might look very much like a cucumber, they will both be categorized differently, because US_2 evokes $s_{rep\ fruit}$ and US_4 the quite different $s_{rep\ vegetable}$.[3]

The conceptual aspect (i.e., the 'fruit-ness' and the 'vegetable-ness') is contained, in Bousfield's manner, in the communality of naming or the proprioception of naming. It is the connecting *verbal* link which creates the

[3] *Translator's note.* The reader may be interested to note that in the German text the author contrasts apples and pears as examples of fruit with tomatoes and cucumbers as examples of vegetables, and that the distinction between an apple that looks like a tomato or a tomato that looks like an apple is helped by the different verbal classification. In English this point would have been lost, because it is customary to classify tomatoes as fruit!

communalities and generalizations. To put it differently the *genus proximum,* in this view, is not a categorical entity on a higher level of abstraction, but a connecting link in the shape of a *word* which has been introduced by a process of conditioning.

To be sure, in recent times the rigid definition of the *word,* which was demanded by Bousfield's behavioristically based position, has largely been abandoned. The term "concept" is used without qualification, and without a commitment to any definition of the relationship between the concept and the word which signals it. The approach of Schank (1972) appears most promising, but we need not yet discuss it in detail.

Osgood's model to which we are now turning is different from Bousfield's in that it looks for a mediating connection in the emotional rather than in the verbal domain.

For Osgood—perhaps even more than for Bousfield—mediation is the central concept for grasping the psychological aspect of meaning. In his view the psychologist must concern himself, in a very large measure, with studying the mediating process which takes place in the organism during encoding and decoding. Osgood, too, conceives this mediating process as a covert response which serves as stimulus for what finally appears as the manifest response.

The introduction of this *emotional* factor, which so far has not been considered in the attempt to come to grips with the psychology of meaning, necessitates a brief digression.

Traditional theories of language (from Aristotle to Wundt) have tended to place in the foreground the rational or functional aspect of language. The expressive and emotional aspect was considered merely in connection with the evolution of speech from the prelinguistic state (e.g., Stevenson). Following the Scholastic distinction between various *modi significandi* and somewhat outside the main stream of historical development, a distinction was introduced between denotative and connotative meaning. "Denotative" is understood as the factual content of a concept. The denotative meaning of "moon," accordingly, would be "a heavenly body circling round the earth, partially illuminating the night of the planet earth by means of reflected sunlight." Denotation can, therefore, perhaps be equated with Bühler's symbol function. Connotative meaning refers to evocations which occur when the word "moon" is uttered or heard, e.g., night, cold, longing.

> The 'intellectualism' of most theories of language is further shown by the fact that semantic meaning is the approximate equivalent to denotation, whereas connotation has no such corresponding equivalent.

Stenzel sees a particularly close connection between emotion and meaning: " 'Fundamental meaning' often lies in the emotional stratum which maintains a certain tension between the conceptual parts. From the emotional stratum different meanings derive a more precise conceptual content.

But orienting impulse or emotive gesture is primary" (1934, p. 94). The experience of emotional set (the *Anmutungserlebnis* in the psychology of Lersch), the human tendency towards experiencing meaningfulness, and Ach's latent signifying disposition appear, in Stenzel's conception, as the meaning-substratum of words: the "incandescence of thought" has as its sole basis "the autonomy of affect" (Stenzel, p. 34).

We reach firmer ground and come closer to Osgood's model, which prompted us to digress, if we examine empirical investigations in the attempt to understand the role of emotive meaning. A consistent emotional set may establish similarity of meaning.

In these experiments an emotive and evaluative meaning dimension acts as mediating link which makes transfer possible. It is not, as in Bousfield, a covert *verbal* association. We are now ready to discuss Osgood's mediation model.

A stimulus S invariably and reliably evokes a particular behavior pattern R_T. A neutral stimulus $\boxed{S}$, the sign-to-be, is now repeatedly associated with this stimulus S. In this way the neutral stimulus $\boxed{S}$ is connected with a *part* of the total behavior pattern R_T; this part is designated as "mediating response" (Fig. 42).

At first sight this appears to be an orthodox conditioning process. But there is a decisive difference: the mediating response r_m, which follows sign $\boxed{S}$ as a representational mediating process, is not identical with R_T following the original stimulus S (the object or significate). r_m consists only of parts of R_T, in particular, of those parts which are most easily subject to conditioning (i.e., attachable to signs), require little effort and do not disturb ongoing processes of behavior of the organism. These are, above all, glandular and emotional components of R_T when elicited by S; hence, those parts which make R_T easily recognizable and readily distinguishable from other responses by the individual.

Osgood (in Bruner et al., 1957, p. 94) gives the following example: the object is a ball. S designates those stimulus characteristics of the object (its shape, its resilience, its weight and so on), which regularly lead to a particular behavior pattern R_T (eye movements, grasping, squeezing, bouncing, as well as the pleasurable associations of play-behavior). According to Osgood's hypothesis the easily conditionable part of this total response is conditioned as r_m to the sign $\boxed{S}$ for ball. This mediating link has also a stimulus aspect s_m which elicits the further behavior prompted by the sign.

This process can be called 'representational' because the response r_m

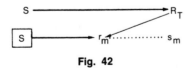

Fig. 42

following the sign $\boxed{s}$ is part of the behavior R_T which is elicited by the designate S. The process can also be called "mediating" because the proprioceptive stimulation s_m which originates in r_m can, in turn, be associated with the most varied instrumental acts R_x, one of which will manifest itself as most appropriate for the object designated and for the particular situation. The entire schema could be represented as in Fig. 43.

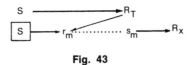

Fig. 43

Osgood, too, divides the total sequence between initial stimulus and terminal response into two parts. The associations between the sign $\boxed{s}$ and the mediator r_m he designates "decoding habits," while the associations between the mediator and the manifest instrumental response (i.e., $s_m - R_x$) are described as "encoding habits."

Osgood defines the meaning of signals, seen from the decoding end, as significance; from the encoding end, as intention.

In principle, Osgood's model is as behavioristic as Bousfield's. The difference between the two theories is the following. According to Bousfield's view the representational response to the heard verbal signal consists in a subvocal or voiced repetition of this word. Osgood rightly criticizes this conception, for a model of sign learning should also be equally valid for the infant at a prelinguistic stage when he is not yet capable of repeating a word. Bousfield's theory is basically a refined version of the old substitution theory, according to which a sign acquires its meaning by a process of conditioning which enables it to evoke those responses which originally were evoked only by the object signified. Osgood rightly raises the objection that even in classical conditioning the conditioned response is not identical with the unconditioned response; e.g., Pavlov's dog secretes saliva upon the bell-tone but he does not really feed. Therefore it is not a case of simple substitution.

Osgood's counter-argument now runs as follows. Signs do not become meaningful because they are linked with associated words, but—and this above all—because they are also connected with emotional and dispositional states. What a certain word means for a given individual, we learn not only through verbal associations which this word evokes in him but through his facial expressions, his gestures, his expressions of joy or of distress.

The most important function of the representational mediating process is, according to Osgood (1954), to provide mediation in generalization and transfer.

If we relate Osgood's model to Bloomfield,[4] we recognize that the representational process is in exactly that area in which Bloomfield places meaning. But whereas in Bloomfield's conception meaning is viewed as the connection between behavioral events before and after the speech event, in Osgood's view, meaning is to be looked for in the fractional *implicit* emotional and physiological responses which accompany the occurrence of a word.

The question now arises: are these conditioned phenomena associated with a sign as differentiated as the vocabulary of a language? According to Osgood, there could be no greater number of different meanings than the differentiations of mediating responses permit.

At this point Osgood has recently introduced an interesting extension of his model which provides a bridge to the concept of semantic features or characteristics. He claims that the mediating link $r_M - s_M$ (note that he now uses capital letters in the subscripts) itself consists of components which are now designated as r_m. A relatively small number of elementary r_m's which are independent of each other, can, by means of combining to form ever changing patterns, differentiate the meanings of a large number of $r_M - s_M$ links. Thus, for example, the mediating link r_{M_1} can consist of the components r_{m_a}, r_{m_b}, r_{m_f}, while the mediating link r_{M_2} can consist of the components r_{m_a}, r_{m_c}, r_{m_f}, r_{m_x}. Thus r_M is to be understood as a "simultaneous" bundle of distinctive features. Furthermore, there are fewer of these elementary distinctive features than there are mediating links r_M which differentiate concepts (or words).

Osgood takes up here that parsimonious approach to classification which at first had its greatest success in the field of phonetics. It also persuaded linguists like Katz and Fodor to postulate elementary semantic features. For Osgood, r_m's are such elementary semantic features.

In their historical origin Osgood's r_m's are linked with behavior (namely with an R_T), but this linkage applies only to the period during which they are first formed. The components of meaning are those which were originally responsible for *differences* in behavior. This notion, which in its final consequence also leads to Wittgenstein's point of view, asserts that it is not our disinterested *contemplation* of the world, but our motivated *acting* within it, which represents the basis of language.[5]

We should accept this approach even if we do not share Osgood's notion that a conditioning process is the basis for the formation of mediating links. It is not true that the entire Osgood model collapses if its foundation in

---

[4] "the *meaning* of a linguistic form (is) the situation in which the speaker utters it and the response which it calls forth in the hearer" (1933, p. 139).

[5] In contrast, Katz and Fodor have suggested that the semantic feature "leaps out" when a particular group of concepts is examined for their communality.

learning theory is shown to be in error. We can accept what is there and what is useful, even if we reject the manner in which it evolved.

The question about the efficiency of Osgood's model can be answered with a precision rarely possible in other cases, because Osgood has developed a technique for the measurement of meaning which we shall now consider. It was designated by him as "Semantic Differential."

If we ask someone to say what a word means, the answer naturally consists of a verbal output. This spontaneously produced output will vary considerably from subject to subject in quantity and subtlety. Consequently, the answers to the question of what a given word means are not easily comparable and therefore do not lend themselves readily to an exact empirical investigation of word meanings.

Osgood now draws the following conclusion: the subjects who are asked to give the meaning of a word should have at their disposal a standardized sample of verbal responses from which they can then make a selection. The number of such responses is not left to the subject; and the response possibilities offered must be representative of the dimensions along which meanings can be distinguished.

In practice, Osgood presents to the subject a series of bipolar, adjectival scales which refer to the word whose meaning is to be defined. The subject's task is to differentiate semantically the word in question, that is, to make judgments about it by allotting to it a position on each of the scales.

Figure 44 illustrates the procedure.

The subject sees "father" as rather sad, fairly soft, very slow and so forth.

In Osgood's view, the semantic differential represents a combination of controlled association and scaling procedures. The direction or, in more precise terms, the dimension of the associations is prescribed, but the subject is free to determine its strength.

Osgood aims at determining the functioning of the mediating processes which manifest their trends through these bipolar scales. As the number of such scales for a given word presented to the subject is determined by the experimenter, the question arises: how many dimensions are needed to differentiate the meaning of a word semantically in an adequate manner? Or, putting the question in another way: along how many independent dimensions can the mediating processes vary?

The answer to this question can be reached by the following consideration: anyone who classifies the word "sin" as "wicked," is also likely to regard it as "ugly" and not as "beautiful." If this happens with many words

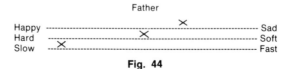

Fig. 44

and with a high measure of agreement among subjects, the scales *good—evil* and *beautiful—ugly* evidently measure the same dimension. Therefore, the intercorrelation of the different scales may give information as to the number of dimensions needed to order the mediating responses—or, putting it in more sophisticated terms, to define the dimensions of the semantic space.

To uncover these dimensions Osgood has carried out numerous factor analyses. These have shown that, for example, *good—bad, fair—unfair, beautiful—ugly,* and *sweet—sour* correlate highly with one another and can therefore be comprised in a single factor, labeled "Evaluation" by Osgood. The correlation of the scales *strong—weak, hard—soft, difficult—easy, masculine—feminine,* etc. yields a "Potency" factor; and the correlation of the scales *active—passive, fast—slow, excitable—calm, sharp—blunt* produces an "Activity" factor.

These then are *the* three factors or dimensions of the semantic space. It is true that more than three factors are found in most analyses, so that one cannot say with certainty that the semantic space has only three dimensions. However, evaluation, potency, and activity are three dimensions that are *always* found.

Every concept or every word scaled by the semantic differential is allotted a place along these three dimensions, dependent on what ratings for "good" or "strong" and so forth had been made.

As an example let us cite an investigation in which different groups of voters of different party affiliations before the 1952 American presidential election were studied by means of the semantic differential (see Fig. 45a and b). Among the concepts presented to them were the following: Stevenson (3), policy in China (4), Churchill (5), federal spending (6), Stalin (11), Truman (13), atom bomb (18) and McCarthy (19).

Figure 45a and b clearly shows how the "meaning" or in this case perhaps the "image" of different personalities varies from group to group.

As the example indicates there are numerous possibilities for the application of the semantic differential. Thus, it is possible, for example, to compare or correlate the profile, resulting from the ratings of a concept or word on the 20 scales (the number usually applied) of the semantic differential, with the profile of another concept on the same scales. It must be remembered that the rating of a concept on these adjective scales is regarded as an expression of the representational mediating process corresponding to the meaning of this word. Similarity of ratings between two words, accordingly, is an expression of the similarity of the mediating processes corresponding to these two words.

To illustrate this once more by a few examples: "red" is often called the color of love, i.e., "red" is vaguely felt to be semantically similar to "love." Hofstätter who calls the semantic differential "polarity–profile" (*Polaritäts–Profil*) has pursued the question whether what is called meaning here is identical with the meaning aspect expressed in the semantic differen-

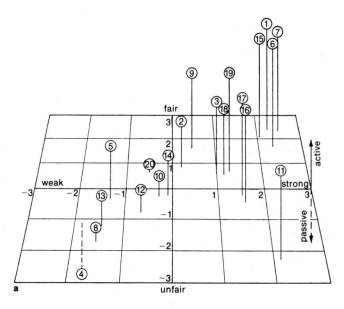

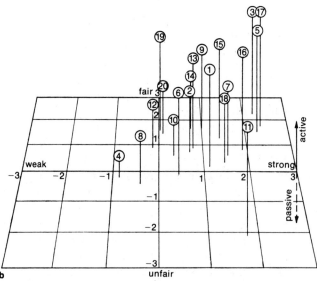

Fig. 45 a and b. Models of the semantic spaces for two groups of voters: **a** Taft voters, **b** Stevenson voters. The rated concepts are, for example: Taft (1), Stevenson (3), policy in China (4), Churchill (5), federal spending (6), Stalin (11), Truman (13), atom bomb (18), McCarthy (19), United Nations (20). The base of the projection indicates the position of ratings on the scales *fair–unfair* and *strong–weak*. The length of the projection corresponds to the ratings on the scale *active–passive*. (From Osgood, Suci, and Tannenbaum, 1957, pp. 114–115)

tial. If so, "red" and "love" should lead to similar profiles. Indeed, the correlation between the two profiles is 0.89. Thus the semantic differential offers a technique of giving a solid foundation to color symbolism—often the happy hunting-ground for speculation.

The introduction of the method of the semantic differential has, in turn, made possible a series of studies, the success of which can be viewed as confirmation for the heuristic fecundity of a conditioning theory of meaning.

Particularly relevant here are the studies of the modification of meaning which, for example, A. and C. Staats carried out extensively. The basic proposition from which these studies arise goes something like this: If meaning is viewed as a conditioned response, then it must be possible to associate the response elicited by a word which is heard or read $(r_M - s_M)$, with a stimulus which is simultaneously presented.

If a nonsense syllable is presented and immediately followed by a meaningful word, several repetitions of this process should make it possible to invest the nonsense syllable with the meaning of that word by a process of conditioning.

> There is of course a danger that the pairing leads to a direct association between the word and the nonsense syllable, i.e., that in future the nonsense syllable as stimulus will evoke a particular word as response. According to the Bousfield model, this process would be described as establishment of meaning. The two Staats, as adherents of Osgood, however, hold that in that case this would not be conditioning of meaning but conditioning of a word; and meaning, in Osgood's formulation, is not the same as the covert repetition of a word as a representational response. The two Staats, therefore, argue as follows: if the nonsense syllable is paired in close succession, not with a single word but with several words (with a similar meaning component), it is likely that the nonsense syllable will acquire this similar component of meaning without being strongly associated with any one particular word.

The semantic differential should lend itself particularly well to a demonstration of this "similarity of meaning" between the different words. The Staats' experiment in more than one respect offers the opportunity of reexamining the validity of Osgood's postulates.

In this experiment nonsense syllables are presented to the subjects visually. Immediately after the exposure of the nonsense syllable on the screen the experimenter utters a meaningful word. The nonsense syllables appear several times in random order and each time are paired with another word. Thus YOF is presented with "beauty," "win," "gift," "sweet," "smart," "rich," "friend," "happy," "pretty," etc., i.e., words with high loadings on a positive evaluative factor. For another group of subjects the same syllable YOF is paired with words of a high activity loading.

The subsequent ratings of the nonsense syllables on the semantic differential indeed indicate that they have acquired the meaning-tone of the words offered in the conditioning experiment.

This result could not have been predicted had the Bousfield model been applied because it would have led to the expectation that the different verbal responses conditioned to the nonsense syllable should cancel each other. Osgood's model, on the other hand, is ready to offer an explanation: the US "beauty" evokes a meaning (or mediating) response with an emotional or evaluative component which conditions the nonsense syllable. The US "win" elicits a differently composed meaning response, but it includes an evaluative emotional component which is similar to that of "beauty." As a result of the repeated linking with this common emotional meaning component, the nonsense syllable gradually acquires this meaning aspect, whereas the divergent components (i.e., those which distinguish "win" from "beauty") cancel each other.

In later experiments the Staats used the same method to modify the meaning of meaningful words, for example, the "meaning" of a nationality term—an experiment of interest from the point of view of social psychology. One reservation of importance to our subsequent discussions is suggested by the investigations by Cohen (1964) and Hare (1964). Both authors noted that the method employed by the Staats of conditioning emotional meaning leads to the expected results only when the subjects are sophisticated and are aware of the conditioning process. The question of the role of awareness of meaning, which is thus raised, will be more fully discussed at a later stage.

Whereas the experiments devised by the Staats had been based on the more immediate implications of a conditioning model of establishing meaning, another group of investigators has studied other, somewhat less obvious consequences: if meaning is something that can be conditioned to a sign, it should be possible also to study with similar means the phenomenon of extinction. This group of studies is generally summarized under the title of "verbal (or semantic) satiation." The basic hypothesis, as already mentioned, derives from conditioning theory: a constant repetition of a word alone without any possibility of reinforcement should lead to the extinction, or gradual loss, of meaning. Outside the framework of conditioning theories Titchener already, on the basis of introspection, reported similar experiences; they have been studied experimentally by Lambert and Jakobovits.

In these experiments selected words are first given ratings by the subjects on semantic differential scales. In the second phase of the experiment the subject pronounces the word repeatedly for 15 seconds and immediately makes his ratings once more on a semantic differential scale. Then he utters the word again for 15 seconds and subsequently makes his ratings on another scale and so forth. If the ratings before the satiation phase are compared with those after satiation, it is found that the ratings become more neutral and the meaning of the word loses color.

Lambert and Jakobovits explain these results entirely in Osgood's terms: meaning is a partial component of a total response. In the satiation phase this meaning response is evoked again and again, producing a reactive inhibition which temporarily reduces the availability of this response, i.e., weakens its meaning.

> Although Jakobovits and Lambert (1962a and b) were able to show (1) that satiation of a mediating link in a chain impairs learning of an association mediated by this link and (2) that satiation of a number prolongs the time needed for additions with this number, the whole problem appears more complicated than the original experiment led one to believe. For example, Yelen and Schulz obtained contrary results.

However artificial the satiation process may appear, the experiment demonstrates a phenomenon familiar from everyday life. The continuous use of a word without the reinforcement of an objective reference transforms the word into a meaningless hollow shell. To be sure, there are a number of unanswered questions (e.g., methodological ones) relating to this problem area (cf. Kasschau, 1969).

In its general formulation, conditioning theory of meaning also forms the basis for an attempt to elucidate another problem area, namely bilingualism. (We will later encounter other approaches to an understanding of this problem.) A bilingual is a person who expresses himself as efficiently and fluently in two languages as others usually express themselves in their native tongue. The learner of a second language ideally becomes bilingual. That is why the answer to the question, What mechanism underlies the linguistic behavior of bilinguals? is of fundamental interest even in cases where a second language is not mastered to the extent that it satisfies the suggested criterion. Genuine bilingualism generally occurs in children who grow up in a bilingual family, e.g., speak German to the mother and English to the father, or in situations where a child, through contact with a foreign nurse or servant, learns a second language from infancy. For example, British rule in India produced a considerable number of bilinguals in this way.

In the analysis of the psycholinguistic problem of bilingualism, Ervin and Osgood (1954) have introduced a fundamental distinction. If one starts from the assumption—as is commonly done in foreign language instruction in school—that the *same* object is referred to by two designations, a so-called "compound" system prevails. One representational mediating process $r_m - s_m$ corresponds to the sign stimuli in decoding (S_A from language A, and S_B from language B) and two verbal responses in encoding (R_A in language A and R_B in language B) (Fig. 46).

Such a compound system develops above all when, as in the school setting, a sign in language B is associated with a meaningful sign in language A. This system also develops in a child who lives in a parental home in which two languages are used indiscriminately, i.e., without separation of person and situation.

In the coordinate system, however, linguistic signs and responses in

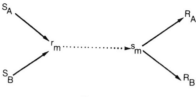

Fig. 46

language A are combined with one mediation process (r_{m1} . . . s_{m1}), whereas the signs and responses in language B are combined with a somewhat different representational mediating process (r_{m2} . . . s_{m2}). This is "typical" or "genuine" bilingualism which occurs when, for example, a child speaks language A with his parents and language B in school. Language A occurs in different situations from language B.

This theory of bilingualism leads to certain consequences which can be tested experimentally. The most important argument, perhaps, runs as follows: if in the case of bilingualism—to put it crudely—two words are available for each object, learning theory would lead us to expect negative transfer or mutual interference. This should be particularly so in the case of compound bilingualism, because here the same mediating processes lead to alternative verbal responses; the decision whether a response belonging to language A or language B should occur is determined by purely attitudinal or situational factors. Anyone who masters a second language knows quite well that often the second-language response dominates (i.e., suppresses the native-language response), if the second-language response has been evoked with greater frequency by the particular mediator.

According to Ervin and Osgood's theory, the ratings of equivalent words (e.g., "house"—"maison") on a semantic differential scale should produce more divergent results in the case of coordinate than of compound bilingualism, since in the compound system only one representational mediating process is present and since the semantic differential is supposed to tap particularly the mediating processes. Lambert, Havelka, and Crosby (1958) have empirically examined this hypothesis and found it confirmed.

Another attempt to test the distinction between the two types of bilingualism experimentally has been made by making use of the concept of semantic satiation. If in compound bilingualism (e.g., English/French) the word "house" is repeated several times, meaning impairment should also extend to "maison." In coordinate bilingualism "house" and "maison" have not the same but only similar mediating pathways, and therefore satiation in one should not lead to satiation in the other. Jakobovits and Lambert (1961) found in compound bilingualisn a confirmation of this hypothesis, but in the case of the coordinate systems they found, unexpectedly, a strengthening of meaning in one language if the equivalent word in the other was satiated.

In more recent studies we find indications that whether or not the two language systems operate independently and without disturbing interference depends on the nature of the task given to the subject. Kintsch (1970a) was able to show that, depending on the nature of the task, S was able to encode a word presented to him according to more language-specific or more general semantic features. However, between these two sets of features, there is a certain amount of overlap. The alternation between two languages is a process that requires time (MacNamara and Kushnir, 1970).

If it is the task, and thus the situation in which the speaker finds himself, which determines whether and to what extent the two language systems work independent of each other, then that, of course, means that this problem area can no longer be discussed exclusively in terms of psycholinguistic approaches. The problem of bilingualism becomes merged with that of diglossa which designates the use of different linguistic codes for different functions, like the use of a "high language" for official or ecclesiastical, and a "common language" for everyday purposes. Since this problem area is part of the domain of sociolinguistics we shall not explore it here.

Having pointed to the usefulness and limitations of a conditioning theory of meaning and the semantic differential let us now return to our starting point. What we have said should not deter us from a critique of this "technique of measuring meaning."

Carroll (1964a), in a most thoughtful and therefore serious criticism, has asked whether, in view of the necessarily limited number of scales and concepts rated with their help, it is at all possible to establish two or more independent dimensions of the semantic space.

> The presupposition for the claim that two dimensions can be considered as independent is that the points which are said to determine the dimensionality by their position must represent an adequate sample of this space. However, in Osgood's technique, the rated concepts are not a representative sample of the vocabulary of a language, nor are the scales employed a representative sample of all possible scales. If Osgood had not only used the red–green scale, for example, but also pink–turquoise, orange–pale green, strawberry red–moss green and had asked his subjects to rate the concepts cheek, grass, forest, tulip and glowing coals, his semantic space would have a fourth red–green dimension.

Another critic, Weinreich (1958), has represented the point of view of the lexicographer, i.e., of someone whose business it is to grasp the unique meaning of the individual word, whereas Osgood—in common, by the way, with nearly all other modern psycholinguists—is concerned with "meaning" as *similarity* of meaning, such as similarity between different words or similarity of mediating responses. In particular, Weinreich questions the results of Osgood's factor analyses, arguing that a too limited proportion of the total variance is accounted for by the extracted factors. This objection, however, is hardly apposite. An argument which would seem much more decisive to us would have been to question whether it is right to attempt to reduce the dimensions to the smallest number (the only condition under which factor analysis is the suitable method), or whether it would not have been better to find out the largest number of dimensions which could just about be distinguished in the semantic space.

> In the construction of tests, factor analysis is employed in order to operate with the most economic number of qualities needed to classify the responses of subjects; small differences between two variables are ignored and two slightly different variables are treated as equal.

Weinreich's critique culminates in the accusation that with Osgood's procedure the meaning of a word is related to "the infinity of *I's* and *today's*" (p. 350) and that the semantic differential grasps subjective and not objective meaning. But if we examine this objection more closely it turns out to be a compliment; for Osgood is primarily not a linguist but a psychologist, and as such interested in the interaction between language and language-user. Moreover, his concern with language-user and situation is entirely in keeping with the rejection, in the newer linguistic philosophy, of 'pure' semantics as a dyadic relationship between sign and object signified.

In more general terms, Osgood's procedure has been criticized for calling "meaning" what at best is only a partial aspect of the total meaning of a word, namely connotation. This objection is no doubt justified, and Osgood, taking note of it, has in fact modified his position. He has now come to speak of an "affective mediating system which is biologically determined and capable of some limited number of gross, bipolar discriminations. This is the system the semantic differential technique is assumed to tap primarily; I have referred to the aspect of meaning indexed as *connotative*" (1962b, p. 26).

Thus we come back again to the distinction between denotation and connotation. Carroll defines as denotative meaning "the properties or patterns of stimulation which are essential—that is, criterial—for the socially approved use in the speech community (1964a, p. 40).

Which are these properties? Is it really possible to view the meaning (and therefore also the choice) of words that are used in an expression as being dependent on the "properties of stimulation"? At that time, Carroll's notion still contained too much behaviorism to be acceptable to us. The determining "properties" for the use of a word depend on the communicative function which the particular word is supposed to have for the speaker and for the listener in the particular speech situation. In turn, this function does *not* permit a clear dividing line between denotation and connotation. If the linguist wants to demonstrate the existence of such demarcations with words like "moon" ("earth satellite" versus "cold, pale, lonely, longing . . .") then we should ask him where he would draw this line for words like "sad," "Jesus," and "love."

This lack of utility of the dichotomy of denotation/connotation may have been one of the reasons Osgood abandoned it himself. He did so after there had been impressive evidence for the fecundity of his approach. Across the world, numerous concepts from 20 different languages have been differentiated by means of the SD, and the resulting factor analysis showed everywhere the three factors, E, P, and A (1971). But after all that, Osgood again asks, what are the reasons for the universality of these semantic dimensions? His answer is that feelings and affects are basic dimensions of human life, as Wundt had already said. If we encounter something unknown we ask ourselves three questions:

Is it good or bad for me?
Compared to me, is it stronger or weaker?
Is its behavior active or passive?

The three dimensions E, P, and A correspond to these basic questions. They are universal because that is human nature. The universals of language reflect the universals of (affective) behavior and attitude toward the world.

Ertel (1967 and later) takes yet another step in this direction. In contrast to Osgood, his approach evolved from Gestalt psychology and therefore is actually beyond this chapter which is devoted to conditioning and mediational theories. For him the three basic dimensions are not related to content (affective or emotional) but are of a formal nature. Osgood starts with the association which, according to the findings of the SD, exists for example, between "father" and the adjective "round." In contrast, Ertel looks at the phenomenal relationship between "father" and "round" and finds that it is more true than the relationship between "father" and "square." Congruity or harmoniousness as a kind of relationship indicates a high phenomenal compatibility between the relational object and the self. According to Ertel, the affective quality of valence arises only from this formal relationship. Accordingly, the relational dominance of the judged object over the self stands behind the affective potency, while behind the affective dimension of activity we find the relational complexity of the connections.

Thus Ertel, in contrast to Osgood, views the basic dimensions which are threaded through our actions and our language, manifested not in affective but in formal relational structures of meaning.

There as here, we find that in addition to the cognitive factor, which was isolated by Deese's early word association studies and perhaps in Trier's concept of field, we need an emotional factor or even a relational one which would have to be located "below" the emotional one. Along with the cognitive map (Toman's concept) on which the meaning of a word is defined in terms of its relationship to other related or associated words, we apparently require an emotional map that contains the affective fields which lie between the word and the user of the language. (Perhaps this map also contains the "mountains of the heart" and the "homesteads of feeling" referred to by Rilke.)

A concluding evaluation of the conditioning theory and the related mediational theory of meaning leaves us somewhat dissatisfied, its undeniable successes notwithstanding. Above all, there are two reasons why we must take issue with these theories, although we are not in a position to offer a substitute which would have equal precision. What the learning theory model of conditioning predicts about the acquisition of meaning is incongruent with what has actually been observed in genetic and developmental psychology. Particularly critical is the following consideration: if meaning is acquired through a process of conditioning, then some form of reinforcement is required. Either, following Pavlov, this reinforcement can be found in the simultaneity of US and CS, or, following Thorndike and Hull, it can be seen in the fact that the response produces a pleasurable state for the organism. If this reinforcement is absent—and in many verbal situations there is no evidence of such reinforcement—this should necessarily lead to extinction or wiping out of meaning. Rapaport (1957) above all has raised this objection: a conditioning theory is unable to account for the stability of meaning.

The second argument is that the tenacious adherence to an S-R model of meaning (and the introduction of mediational theories is proof of just this tenacity) is explained, in the final analysis, in terms of a conviction that the cause of behavior (including verbal behavior) cannot be a steady state, but always is the change of such a state, i.e., an event. This point of view, which is related to the philosophical problem of free will, requires that every temporal gap between S and R be bridged by means of connecting or mediating links, all of which also have event characteristics.

But one of the identifying characteristics of language is that it permits, in a way, the extraction of a chain of events from the time span, storing them in form of a plan or a wish, and then releasing it back into the time span of behavior. This means that a theory of meaning must consider the factors which are always ignored by behavioristic and neobehavioristic approaches, namely those related to conscious awareness. Comprehension of a sentence does not necessarily change the behavior of the listener, but it changes, in any case the momentary content of his awareness (Hörmann, 1976). Accordingly, we have suggested (1967, in the first edition) that the meaning of a sound sequence should not be seen as lying in the fact that it is associated with other events. That such a link *exists* is not the decisive factor for the use of language; what is decisive is that we are aware of it. Meaning is not an association but knowledge of an association (which becomes actualized through the acts of meaning and understanding).

Admittedly this requires a more precise definition of the role of the concept of "knowing." What is meant here is a cognitive availability in the sense that relationships between experiences, acts, and sequences of acts can be reflected more or less consciously, and can become the basis on which acting and experiencing can be based intelligently. The conjunctive, disjunctive, and relational connections which link a particular word or phrase with other stored knowledge, enter into readiness.[6]

This awareness of connections, which becomes actualized in the process of understanding, is schematic in nature. Schema, a concept used by Bartlett, Piaget, and Church is, in a way, the principle according to which experiences and acts which belong together are organized. It retains common features of similar impressions. Perception functions by projecting schemata to the stimuli of the surrounding world. We are aware of the base line of a schema (and this awareness can have several levels) when we have comprehended or understood a *meaning*.

Our notion of "meaningful comprehension as awareness of connections" leads once more to Deese's definition of *understanding* as an "inner awareness of the fact that, if necessary, one could act adequately."

In order to clarify the problem of meaning it is necessary to take into consideration the *process of understanding* and the speaker's corresponding *process of meaning*. For this, the ability to learn and to form associations, which is seen as generating associations on a *tabula rasa,* is inadequate. On the contrary, it becomes necessary to take into consideration the biologic and anthropological equipment which man brings to the task of using language. The key to this central problem in psycholinguistics is not a concept of meaning which is tailored to the "language-in-itself" but a concept of meaning which corresponds to the cognitions and acts of the man who uses language.

[6] Bierwisch, in a critical discussion of the first edition of this book, pointed out the need for including some consideration of this.

CHAPTER 9

Imitation of Sound, Sound Symbolism, Expression

Imitation of sounds as the germ of human speech—Humboldt's dichotomy—Evolution of onomatopoeia—Traces of sound symbolism in linguistic behavior—"Maluma" and "takete"—Matching experiments in the mother tongue and an unknown second language—Concept of physiognomy—Werner's theory of symbol formation—Ertel's psychophonetics.

In the preceding chapter we extensively discussed the proposition that the connection between sign and object signified, i.e., meaning, is the result of conditioning. In principle, which meaning is conditioned to which sign is arbitrary. That would mean that the meaningful relationship between the sign and the object signified has an *arbitrary* nonessential component.

Questions can be raised about this from several perspectives. We have already touched upon this in discussing the philosophical bases of psycholinguistics. We asked, What is the basis for claiming that language is actually the true expression of the world as it is? Plato was cited and we referred to the controversy on the relationship between sign and object: does it originate in the nature of things (*physei*) or in human invention (*thesei*)? Starting from this debate we followed the "winner," Aristotle, and traced the anti-Platonic position down to the neobehavioristic psycholinguistics of our own day.

Today it is still possible to discover a refined version of the other, the *physei*, conception, which will be considered in the present chapter. The question is to what extent the meaning relationship between sign and object can contain an element of necessity or nonarbitrariness. We must occupy ourselves with "the belief, deeply rooted in our natural feeling for language, that meaning lies directly in the sounds of words; this belief is sustained by a peculiar feeling that it is self-evident,which certainly constitutes a very important experience in the mother tongue and in any other language of which we have a reasonable mastery" (Stenzel, 1934, p. 92).

This feeling of self-evidence and of an inevitable link between sign and object forms the basis of those phenomena which range from word magic—of interest to ethnologists—to the phenomena discovered by the General

Semanticists (Korzybski and Hayakawa). They are clearly illustrated, for example, by such remarks as: "Pigs are called pigs because they are so dirty."

A full discussion of the problems raised by the so-called sound (or phonetic) symbolism must be prefaced by a few remarks to show the deep rift which almost completely separates this complex of ideas from the prevailing view among present-day psycholinguists.

It may be regarded as certain that most linguists today (and most psycholinguists in their train) operate with the distinction between phoneme and morpheme. The phoneme is a unit of sound; the morpheme a unit of meaning. The meaningful morpheme is composed of phonemes which in themselves do not mean anything. Therefore there is a boundary between morpheme and phoneme: on one side of this boundary there is meaning; on the other there is not.

The existence of this boundary—and with it the phoneme-morpheme distinction—is called into question if meaning is already ascribed to the individual sound. In principle this applies even if the meaning value attributed to the sound is regarded as vague and purely suggestive.[1]

> Besides, the meaning value of the individual sound need not necessarily point to an object in the external world; it may well be an indication of a state of mind in the speaker. Bühler's distinction between symbol and symptom, of which one is reminded (cf. Chapter 2), may be phylogenetically and ontogenetically more advanced.

If even a single sound is meaningful, e.g., if, in all Indo-European languages right from the River Ganges to the Atlantic Ocean, the sound cluster "sta" designates the notion of standing and the sound cluster "plu" the notion of flowing (Curtius, 1858), we are led to the fascinating thought that the collection, comparison and analysis of such fundamental meanings may open up the possibility of reconstructing the original language of mankind (*lingua Adamica*). No lesser authority than Leibniz pursued this idea. In more recent times, Rimbaud, Rudolf Steiner, and Ernst Jünger, to name only a few, have speculated about the meaning content of speech sounds.

In Plato the idea of words following things guarantees that language can and does represent world. Leibniz finds the key to man's original language in the universals of sound symbolism which transcend national differences. Although Humboldt does not adhere to such views, he gave close attention to the relationship between speech sound and object. His exposition provides in a preliminary way the major division of this problem area.

"The advantages of language with regard to its sound system rest particu-

---

[1] Ertel (1969) is one of the few who draws a clear distinction between asemantic and semantic phonetic events and experiences. But he recognizes possibilities for sound symbolism in both areas.

larly in the relationship of this system to meaning . . . it seems certain that a connection between a sound and its meaning exists." Humboldt then distinguishes various possibilities:

(1)   "Direct imitation occurs whenever the sound produced by a resonant object is copied inasmuch as articulated sounds are capable of reproducing unarticulated ones. These signs can be likened to pictures" (1949 edition, p. 78).

"Since the copy in these cases always refers to unarticulated sounds, designation and articulation are, so to speak, in conflict with one another. This is why this kind of sign is little in evidence wherever there is a strong natural sense of language and gradually disappears in the advancing evolution of language" (p. 79).

This first possibility distinguished by Humboldt is the imitation of sounds, which today is generally known as onomatopoeia. In this case an original is copied.

(2)   The second possibility, sound symbolism, is different. Here the speech sound does not copy an original; it symbolizes it. To cite Humboldt once more, here we are not concerned with "a directly imitative sign but a sign which imitates a quality which the sign and the object have in common. This sign can be called symbolic. To designate objects it selects sounds which partly independently and partly in comparison with others produce an impression which to the ear is similar to that which the object makes upon the mind; thus *stehen* "stand," *stetig* "steady" and *starr* "stiff," "rigid" create the impression of firmness . . . *nicht* "not," *nagen* "gnaw," *Neid* "envy" create the impression of slicing or sharp cutting. In this way words pertaining to objects producing similar impressions have predominantly identical sounds, such as *wehen* "wave," "flutter," *Wind* "wind" and *Wolke* "cloud" in all of which the vacillating restless, and random movement— confusing to the senses—is expressed by the "w" which has solidified out of the naturally hollow and dark "u" sound.

"This kind of sign process which is based on the particular meaning of each individual letter and whole groups of letters has undoubtedly exercised a prevailing, perhaps even exclusive, influence on primitive word-formation. Its natural consequence has been a certain likeness of word-formation throughout all languages of mankind . . ." (p. 79)—a consequence which will engage our attention later.

Humboldt, however, concludes these reflections with the warning that this pursuit of language to its origins is "an altogether slippery path" (p. 80), because it is so hard to say which sound was the original one and what its original meaning was.

The term "sound symbolism," which so far in this chapter has been employed in a global fashion, represents a dimension ranging from onomatopoeia at one end to the freely chosen abstract sign at the other.

What varies along this unnamed dimension is closeness of connection between sign and object and the degree of cogency in the relationship, whether subjectively felt or objectively present.

> In linguistics it is quite common to talk in this connection about the "motivation" of a sign. Accordingly, a scream would be emotionally "motivated," whereas the use of representational words would be "unmotivated." "Motivated" in this context is almost equivalent to Bühler's "expressive"; "unmotivated" to his term "representational." This is a good illustration of an unfortunate use of psychological concepts, which is not uncommon in linguistics.

Let us now, following Humboldt's division, look at this whole problem from a psychological point of view and attempt to analyze the determinants or, perhaps more modestly, some contributing factors.

The origin of such words as "tinkle," "rattle," or "buzz" as an imitation of noises is immediately apparent; yet, they have been part of the language for a long time and have therefore been subject to the general historical development of all words so that the original relationship, "meaning as imitation of an object," is no longer quite so obvious. The question can therefore be asked whether the genesis of these words will reveal something about this connection. The German linguist Wissemann (1954) undertook a study of the creation of onomatopoeic words from noises. Various noises were presented to the subjects, who were not able to observe the manner in which the noise was produced; the instruction was to invent or select names for the noises.

Wissemann's experiments produced a large number of results, but an inadequate research design makes them hard to interpret. When subjects were asked why they gave preference to particular sounds in making up new words, it appeared that vowels served to represent the pitch and qualitative features of the noise. The /i/ sound is used to imitate a high-pitched, spiky noise, and /u/ for a low, dark noise. The evaluation of the words produced by subjects showed that the number of syllables in the word inventions was not proportional to the length of the noise; it reflected, rather, sections of the noise sequence. A noise with an abrupt beginning (e.g., when a tower of building blocks collapses) is described by a word beginning with a voiceless plosive (/p,t,k/). A gradually starting noise is generally given a word beginning with /s/ or /ts/.

According to Brown (1958a, p. 116), it follows that the initial sounds of onomatopoeic names copy the stimulus gradients of the noises they designate. At a closer inspection this will already reveal the limits of pure onomatopoeia. The details of the noise are not imitated; instead, a *formally* similar sound sequence is assigned to *formal* characteristics of the time extension of the noise sequence, e.g., its suddenness. In Cassirer's terminology (1953 edition) this case would be described as one of transition from mere "mimetic" to "analogical" expression; according to Humboldt it is the boundary area between the imitation of sounds and sound symbolism. If we look at this boundary from the other side, it will be even more clearly seen.

Gabelentz, in a book on linguistics which appeared in 1901, described the language of a child which contained a private word for "chair"—a feature which is not uncommon among children of a certain age. "Chair" was "lakeil"; a little doll's chair was "likil"; and the huge grandfather chair "lukul." Here the speech sound does not imitate a noise; it cannot be called onomatopoeia.

Another child calls a large bowl "mum," a plate "mem" and little stars "mim."

In the Ewe language of Africa most words have a high-tone and a low-tone form; the former describes small things, and the latter large ones (Kainz, II, p. 206). If a small specimen of a class of usually large objects is referred to, a word generally spoken in a low tone is uttered with a high tone. In another language the word "creep" is expressed by "džarar," creeping of a small animal by "džirir," and of a large one "džurur." In German "teeny-weeny" is expressed by "klitzeklein." In certain Sudanese languages high-tone words are used to express long distances or high speed, low-tone ones to express proximity or slowness. "And purely formal relations and oppositions can be expressed in this same way. A mere change in tone can transform the affirmative into the negative form of the verb" (Cassirer, 1953 edition, p. 194).

The development from sound imitation to phonetic symbolism becomes even clearer if we study another basic device of word formation, *reduplication*. Cassirer points out that reduplication first of all appears to have, as its purpose, the reproduction of certain objective characteristics of the referential object or process. Objects with the same feature occur several times or an event in time is composed of a sequence of equivalent phases; this is where "reduplication is most at home" (p. 195).

In these cases, therefore, there is something more than pure onomatopoeia; reduplication does not only occur to refer to repetitive noises, but to designate repetition in general.

This particular line of development can be pursued even further. "Repetition in general" becomes "plurality in general." In that case the repetitive element is not contained in the temporal succession of the *appearance* of the objects but in the *perception* of the objects. "Plurality in general" can further be analyzed conceptually into the expression of "collective" and "distributive" plurality. Some languages have a highly developed notion of such distributive plurality. The distinction is made between an act as a whole or an act which is composed of several individual acts. "If the latter is true and the act is either performed by several subjects or effected by the same subject in different segments of time, in separate stages, this distributive division is expressed by reduplication" (1953, p. 195).

The developmental trend which Cassirer's example here illustrates provides evidence for the importance of onomatopoeia and sound symbolism as components in the evolution of speech. The interest of a lawful relationship between word and thing does not lie in the fact that in everyday life we always imitate or symbolize things in a direct fashion, but in the observation—to paraphrase Bühler's words (1934, pp. 29 f.)—that, in the historical prelude to the matching of word and object, sound symbolism is likely to have played a role of which slight traces can, from time to time, be found even in our own speech.

We shall now address ourselves to those psychological experiments and theoretical approaches which are intended to explore how these less obvious determining factors operate.

The most impressive of these experiments is one described by Köhler (e.g., 1947).

Two nonsense line drawings as well as two nonsense words, "maluma" and "takete," are presented to the subject who is asked to decide which word matches which drawing (Fig. 47).

Looked at purely rationally, it is completely immaterial whether "maluma" is used for the round or the angular figure. If the designation is arbitrary, one would expect a random distribution of matchings, and approximately 50 percent of the subjects should assign "maluma" to the rounded figure and 50 percent to the angular design.

In fact the overwhelming majority of all subjects assign "maluma" to the round figure and "takete" to the angular one. This result has not only been found in Germany and USA (Holland and Wertheimer, 1964), but, for example, also in Tanganyika (Davis, 1961). It is as if there was a strange parallel or similarity between the visual and auditory shapes. Werner calls such similarities, transcending different sense modalities, "physiognomic" similarity; the theoretical conceptualization of this notion will be discussed in some detail below.

We need to examine this concept more fully before we turn to the methodology of the matching experiments.

Werner has developed a theory of symbol formation based on the concept of physiognomy, which introduced a new element into psycholinguistics.

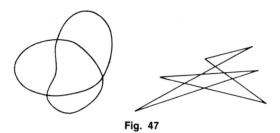

Fig. 47

This theory is a link between the problem areas of sound symbolism and developmental psycholinguistics.

In the primitive perception of animals, of children, and even of adults in a state of fatigue or illness, there is no categorical separation between the individual and the objects in the environment. But even at higher levels of evolution "at a stage where the object forms no longer an inseparable part of a psychophysically undifferentiated vital and total situation and is therefore distinct from the individual, we are still not simply in a sober world of objective facts; for objects are intimately interwoven with affective and motor activity" (Werner, 1953, p. 45). Things participate in the dynamic acts by which they are perceived; they also play a part in emotional and motor behavior. This is why they appear totally different to an animal, a child or a naive adult from the way they appear to an adult with a purely factual and rational orientation. "Things are not treated objectively, but physiognomically, i.e., as if they expressed an inner life and had a mind" (p. 45).

Thus, a landscape may be "cheerful," the contour of a mountain "threatening," a sloping pasture "melancholy" and a cup on its side "tired."

These assumptions supported by a wealth of examples from animal psychology, child psychology, and psychopathology are offered by Werner as presuppositions for symbol formation in general and, hence, also for sound symbolism.

If we relate Werner's approach to our earlier discussion, it will be particularly interesting to note how this approach brings language and expression closer to each other. This link has been stressed in psychopathology particularly by Goldstein, who, with reference to certain cases of motor aphasia, found that after the representational function of language had disappeared the expressive function of language alone had remained intact.

Werner, who believes that growth and decline of psychic functions move along identical paths, has made use of such findings to support his genetic theory. What constitutes a symbol is explained by Werner in terms of an account of its formation. His theory—developed fully in the work *Symbol Formation,* published jointly with Kaplan in 1963—is therefore a genetic one.

Objects are expressive. Physiognomic quality or dynamic properties are as inherent in objects or events of our perception as are their geometrical or technical features. The headlights of an automobile are not only round and brilliant; they also look like threatening eyes.

Identical dynamic-expressive features may be perceived in different objects or events. The contour of a rock or a musical passage may be equally "threatening." This transcendence of expressive qualities, as Werner and Kaplan have called this feature, does not only form the basis for analogies, metaphors and similes; but it is also the basis for seeing similarities in such fundamentally unrelated things as rounded shapes in a drawing and the word "maluma."

This interpretation is utterly unsatisfactory as an explanation. Whereas all earlier theories had attempted to answer *why* the same expressive qualities appear in parallel in different sense modalities, in other words, why it is that these qualities transcend *one* sense modality, Werner covers up this problem by asserting that this transcending of expressive qualities happens because expressive qualities possess transcendence.

Different factual processes can, according to Werner, be physiognomically similar; they may have the same expressive qualities. But an act of intentive and denotative reference must be applied to the factual process, i.e., an act of decision to interpret one similar objective process as a symbol for the other. Two hitherto equal objective processes are separated into a symbol carrier or vehicle (e.g., a sound pattern) and an object to which the symbol refers.

> This aspect of intentionality which is emphasized in this act may philosophically be referred back to Husserl and psychologically to Ach. In Ach's work the "latent, signifying set" plays an important role, but this set is a factor in a framework of thought which, in general, has a more associationist orientation. According to Ach the meaning-giving act is a process of fusion or "concrescence"; according to Werner it is a process of differentiation. Werner's view, therefore, comes closer to that of Merleau-Ponty than to Ach's.

Our account so far may easily have given too static a picture. The act of denotative reference is not projected upon two given independent objective states. Neither the symbol carrier nor the external object are finished products. (Without this proviso, Werner's thesis would come suspiciously close to associationism, which he rejects.) Latent expressive qualities in the symbol carrier and the object are first made apparent through the referential act, which is directed towards them. These are *"twin form-building processes, one directed towards the establishment of meaningful objects (referents), the other directed towards the articulation of patterns expressive of meaning (vehicles)"* (1963, p. 22). Werner names this directional, regulative, form-building process *dynamic schematization*. The semantic correspondence between sign and object has been established when the word, as well as the object, is rooted in similar or equal organismic states.[2]

Symbol formation is conceived here quite differently from the theories with an associationist orientation. It does not consist in the linking of two originally independent ready-made sets of data,[3] but in the gradual shaping and singling out of two factual processes from the common physiognomic fundament.

---

[2] This argument should be compared to Osgood's!

[3] Without such independence the possibility of postulates arbitrarily invented by man would not exist.

Two factual events take place: one leads to the formation of the symbol carrier or vehicle, and the other to the thing or referent. What is, literally, object of (or juxtaposed to) the word originates in the same act of creation in which the word is also created. This idea is again mindful of the great Humboldtian thought of language as *energeia* which transforms the world into the property of the mind. Stenzel speaks of "the primal phenomenon of the crystallization, from the buzzing confusion, of an object by means of the word. The word is so powerful that without it the object would not exist for the mind, but once the mind has a word it seems to be able to do with it what it likes . . . Mental activity which reaches awareness only through language helps to define more clearly the essential qualities of an object in all its manifestations . . ." "As a result (the word) now becomes an inherent part of the object and expresses it, and must henceforth be used to refer to it" (1934, p. 38).

An advantage of Werner's theory lies in the genetic priority it offers of the whole over the parts. The construction, implicit in the concept of association, of a comprehensive whole arrived at by a process of synthesis of separate elements has been questioned in various quarters. In the introduction to a work on the Kavi language of Java, Humboldt writes, "In fact, speech is not produced out of words which precede it; on the contrary words are produced out of the totality of speech" (1907, p. 72). Likewise, Bloomfield's approach (language develops out of speech events which are scattered within the total context of practical events) suggests an analytic direction. All signs in a speech event allude to an overriding total meaning (Merleau-Ponty). This also holds true for a Marxist theorist like Schaff, for whom the individual sign emerges only from the totality of verbal communication.

A second advantage of Werner's theory of symbol-formation in comparison with other theories on the same problem is that it offers the possibility of grasping psychologically the world-forming, rather than the world-reflecting, function of language. Thus, a link is created to another field of inquiry, i.e., "linguistic relativity," a field which we associate with the names of Humboldt, Cassirer, Sapir, and Whorf (cf. pp. 283 f.).

In view of the merits of this theory, the lack of clarity and other deficiencies of Werner's theory are all the more disturbing. The semantic correspondence between symbol and object, according to Werner, comes about "through the operation of schematizing, form-building activity which shapes the pattern on one hand and the referent on the other" (Werner and Kaplan, 1963, pp. 23–24). What is meant by "schematizing, form-building activity"? Let us attempt to clarify this statement with the help of an illustration given by Werner and Kaplan.

An individual is confronted by a configuration which has a "sitting tone" in Uexküll's sense; i.e., this configuration instigates in him a postural-affective state which is schematically organized as "something there to sit down on." This activity and this state cause the individual to apprehend the configuration as a "chair" rather than as a "table."

Werner now assumes that the same schematizing activity leads to the lexical item "chair" whenever a dynamic, intonationally molded sound /čɛr/ is articulated into a production whose expressive features parallel those contained in the percept "chair" (p. 25).

The present author must admit that this example, too, does not help him to find an answer to the question how it is that just the word "chair" comes to designate the object chair.

The merit of Werner's approach is threefold: it lies, first, in the suggestion of the importance of expressive and emotive processes in the genesis of word-object relations; second, he rightly draws attention to the fact that this relationship is rooted in the total state of the language user; and third, he recognizes the necessity of seeing the development of linguistic events not only synthetically, but also analytically.

The model of association—basically plain common sense—is certainly too simple to be able to account for the creation, stability and dynamic force of semantic relationships. But Werner's approach is too "physiognomic" to serve as an alternative theory.

Let us now return to the point at which we began our examination of Werner's theory, namely Köhler's juxtaposition of *maluma* and *takete* and the "matching" line-drawings. It was as intelligible as it was unsystematic.

One of the first psychological investigations going beyond anecdotal evidence for the existence of such sound-symbolic relationships was undertaken by Sapir (1929). More than 500 individuals were asked to imagine that the syllables "mal" and "mil" mean "table"; but one of the syllables refers to a large table, and the other to a small one. Which refers to the big one, which to the small one? Of all subjects 80 percent, i.e., a majority far greater than chance, agreed that "mal" fits better for the large table. Even more precise are the indications to be derived from an investigation by Bentley and Varon (1933): /a/ sounds are felt to be larger than /i/ sounds in the proportion 4:1, /i/ is three times as angular and twice as hard as /a/.

Accordingly one would expect that terms for large objects contain /a/ sounds rather than /i/ sounds. A corresponding systematic sampling of a dictionary (Newman, 1933), however, has not confirmed this expectation.

These arguments and investigations are all, implicitly or explicitly, based on the assumption that the causal relationship expressed by the term "sound symbolism" is naturally given. A general Gestalt principle of organization operates equally in things and in sounds, hence the "similarity" between thing and sound. The presence of such a Gestalt principle is a universal human characteristic and occurs in all humans alike. It is not the result of experience nor is it influenced to a varying degree by the acquisition of different languages.

On the basis of this argument the psychologists who have studied phonetic symbolism have always attributed considerable importance to the proof of *universality*, i.e., the universal spread and applicability of sound symbolism, as we shall see from the following studies.

Tsuru and Fries (1933) have undertaken a matching experiment in the manner of Köhler's "maluma" study; but instead of using nonsense material they operated with verbal data. This experiment has become the prototype of a whole series of studies. Lists of pairs of opposites in two different languages are prepared (e.g., big/small—groß/klein) and presented orally. Subjects who are speakers of only one of these languages are invited to match the corresponding words in the other language. Does an English speaker who has never heard or learned German identify "klein" as the translation of "small" or "big"? If correct choices exceed the 50 percent chance level, this would indicate a sound symbolism which is universal and therefore is not tied to a particular language.

According to Tsuru and Fries, English-speaking undergraduates who have never heard a word of Japanese can identify the meaning of Japanese words with a certainty exceeding chance.

Objections to such investigations have inevitably led, by a highly interesting process of elimination, to the exclusion of more and more possible sources of error. A first objection, expressed, for example, by Brown (1958a), was the following: authors operating with this type of study search for the words to be employed, having a full knowledge of both languages. Since in every language the number of phonemes is limited, it is possible that by pure chance similar phoneme sequences occur in both languages in words with equal meaning. Unconsciously the experimenter selects from the usually available series of synonyms a word which structurally (i.e., in its phoneme sequence) resembles the corresponding word in the other language. This would lead the subject—equally guided by the idea of structural similarity, matching A with A—to assign words correctly with greater than chance probability; but sound symbolism has nothing to do with this.

Allport was the first to correct this weakness. Brown, Black, and Horowitz (1955) have followed. The experimenter selected only English words and asked scholars of the particular languages to translate these into Chinese, Czech, and Hindi. The results of the subsequent experiment correspond to the earlier studies: the matching of English and foreign words is successful.

Another objection is difficult to formulate but can best be explained with the help of the experiment which has led to it. Maltzman, Morrisett, and Brooks (1956) carried out an experiment on phonetic symbolism in the already familiar way: the matching of English-Japanese and English-Croatian succeeds with more than chance probability. The authors now argue: if it is really the result of a universal phonetic symbolism that enables us to guess the meaning of unknown words, it is of no consequence whether or not the subject knows one of the two languages. It should therefore be possible to match the words of two languages unknown to the experimental subjects. The test of this argument—American subjects match a Croatian and Japanese list of words—yields a result which is not above chance expectancy.

What does that mean? In Köhler's experiment the hitherto unknown nonsense words were matched with a nonsense drawing. It is argued that this was possible because of the isomorphism in auditory and visual organization. This, however, is apparently not operative in the experiment of Maltzman, Morrisett, and Brooks. The factor that accounts for the negative result in the matching between two foreign languages becomes somewhat clearer in a subsequent experiment by Brackbill and Little (1957). In contrast to many other investigations, the matching does not succeed if a Chinese word is juxtaposed with an English word and the subject has to decide whether it means the same as the English word or the opposite.

The difference in results has evidently something to do with the change in the method of investigation. What is possible when the first-language word pair is juxtaposed with the second-language word pair is no longer possible when the word pairs are in two foreign languages or when only a single word of the native language is to be matched with one in the foreign language. This leads to the conclusion that the native-language word pair offers hints for matching which, in the other cases, are either totally absent or are at least not present to a sufficient degree.

This argument is analyzed further in an excellent investigation by Brown and Nuttall (1959). It is known as a result of the experiments by Sapir and others that the vowels /o/ and /u/ appear physiognomically "bigger" than /i/ and /e/; the consonants /b/ and /d/ appear bigger than /p/ and /t/; and polysyllabic groups appear bigger than monosyllabic ones. If it is assumed that experimental subjects possess this knowledge, without obviously having consciously formulated it, the method of paired comparison between native and foreign language is the only one which enables the subjects to employ this "knowledge" for guessing the meanings of words in a foreign language. When the subject inspects the word pair in the mother tongue (e.g., tall–short), he knows that the lexical dimension is "size," and he can now make use of his knowledge according to which this dimension can be symbolized by vowel contrast or by the monosyllabic-polysyllabic contrast, and so forth. If the subject is asked to match word pairs from two unknown languages, he does not know what dimensions are offered. He is likely, therefore, to make use of phonetic similarities which in the two languages are not necessarily linked in an equivalent manner. A certain semantic dimension (e.g., size) can, as is already known from empirical investigations, be symbolized by several sounds and sound contrasts. And, vice versa, the same sound may, according to the context in which it occurs, have different meanings; a /p/ may in one instance symbolize smallness, in another speed or suddenness.

If the influence of phonetic symbolism is to be experimentally demonstrated, the possibilities of choice open to the subjects must be restricted. Wilde (1958), in a related study of matching terms of emotions with drawings representing these emotions, came to similar conclusions. If drawings in which one group of subjects have expressed certain emotions (anger, anxiety, etc.) are submitted to other subjects with the request to write down freely their impressions, "correct" interpretations are hardly ever made. On the other hand, if subjects are given a list of terms of emotions from which to select the nearest approximation to the one expressed in the design, nearly all the expressive drawings are correctly identified. Quite similar conclusions were later reached by Müller, a student of Wilde, in an investigation on the emotional expression of the speaking voice. These studies indicate the transition from sound symbolism to expression: the expectation is that somewhere the graphic or vocal expression of anger, grief, etc. turns into a symbol of anger or a symbol of grief. It is regrettable that Wilde was no longer able to explore more fully this borderland between the two fields.

Certain formal properties of the graphic or vocal expression normally evoke a particular impression in the receiver. Wilde had intended to base a psychology of art on these relationships. In the investigation by Müller speakers were invited to utter the alphabet with varying emotional expression, e.g., with sadness, anger, yearning. The tape recordings of these speech samples were then submitted to subjects who were asked to state which emotion had been represented in each instance. It was found that some of these emotions can be identified by listeners with a high degree of assurance, whereas others cannot. Of course, a speaker who is supposed to express sadness, anger and so forth in his speech tends to employ a strongly conventionalized form of utterance, because he is not really sad or angry. What he utters could be described in Bühler's terms as half-way between symptom and symbol.

One way of narrowing down the possibilities in the phonetic symbolism experiment is to offer to the subject a word pair in the mother tongue in order to enable him to recognize the dimension in question. Another possibility is to influence the subject's decision by offering him associations with meaningful objects: if it is known that the topic is "tables" correct matching is facilitated (Weiss, 1964b). Once the experimental subject is familiar with the dimension or topic he can make use of sound symbolism to make accurate localizations along the dimension or within the area in question.

Ertel and Dorst (1965), modifying this technique in an interesting manner, have found confirmation for expressive sound symbolism in 25 languages. They asked native speakers to make tape recordings of terms of emotions in the different languages. Judges who listened only to these tape recordings had to decide whether the sound sequences had a positive meaning valence (lovely, good, sweet, right, loving, pleasant, joyful, happy) or a negative valence (ugly, bad, bitter, sad); whether they meant strength or weakness, movement or rest. Therefore the subject had only to make a decision on the feeling tone (i.e., a dimension of Osgood's semantic space); and such matching succeeded in all languages with a probability of $p < 0.01$.

Thus, it has been possible in the course of the past decades to overcome various methodological objections to the experiments which had been carried out in the attempt to elucidate the problem of phonetic symbolism.

A further confirmation—different from the usual matching experiments—for the existence of a universal phonetic symbolism has been given by Osgood, who reported on experiments in which American and Japanese subjects were presented with nonsense syllables composed of sounds which appear in both languages as phonemes. These syllables were rated on the semantic differential. It was found that the various phonemes were rated almost equally by Americans and Japanese. For both groups, front consonants (e.g., /p/) are more pleasant than back consonants (e.g., /g/); high frequency sounds are associated with smallness and impotence (1962b).

Osgood's results suggest a universal sound symbolism. But it cannot be denied that, even today, there is no agreement whether the "physiognomic" expression inherent in a word in a foreign language is identical for members of different language groups, or whether the development of sound symbolism is not, perhaps, to some extent determined by elements of learning, therefore leading to the expectations of differences in sound symbolism.[4] Hence the question, What is phonetic symbolism and where does it come from? is still open.

Brown (1958a) has put forward an elegant theoretical solution: what is mysteriously named "physiognomic" (and we have already seen how confused this term is!) is a result and consequence of a simple act of learning. In everyday experience there is a correlation between certain physical attributes of objects and the noises produced by these objects. A large object, for example, is more likely to produce a deep sound than a small object when it is pushed or when it falls. This relationship between size and deep sounds can therefore be learned; equally, a connection between sharpness and high frequency and between roundness or bluntness and low frequency.

Such relationships are therefore neither "prehistoric" nor physiognomic, but simply learned. Of course whether this theory can account for all phenomena subsumed under "phonetic symbolism" appears questionable.[5]

The success with which Osgood has made use of the method of the semantic differential in the study of phonetic symbolism prompts reflections which are long overdue. Most inquiries on sound symbolism select the linguistic material to be presented to subjects somewhat arbitrarily from the everyday vocabulary. But it is not to be ruled out that sound symbolism has certain preferred fields of manifestation, i.e., words with which a language

---

[4] See the controversy between Taylor (1963) and Weiss (1964a).

[5] Speculation about the origin of sound symbolism relations will also have to account for the findings of Pečjak's experiments on synesthesia. He showed that even the blind demonstrate a significant relationship between particular emotions and color *words* (1965).

expresses emotions. Perhaps it is not denotation but connotation which is the main field of action of sound symbolism (which in that case had better not be described as a *symbolism* of sounds). Stevenson remarks that the tone of a word may be "physiologically fitted" for the expression of certain emotions; this fitness and conventional factors merge into a unified form.

Ertel's numerous experiments in psychophonetics evolved from studies like those cited above and from an extension of Osgood's thinking. These studies were summarized in 1969. As we pointed out before, Ertel does not attempt to conceptualize Osgood's dimensions of meaning in terms of their content dimension (i.e., affective/connative). Instead he views them more broadly as an expression and a consequence of very formal phenomenal relations the "universal qualities."[6]

For example, the degree of *congruity* between the object and the self determines the factor of valence found in the semantic differential, while the number of connections embodied in the object determines the factor of activity. According to Ertel, connection, congruity, and dominance are the relational forms which structure various spheres of human life. Because of this, they lead to those parallels and analogies that we encounter between linguistic signs and object signified, and that at first glance appear so peculiar.

To begin with, Ertel can show that consonants differ in terms of their sound quality with respect to the potency dimension, and covariant with that, also differ with respect to their activity dimension. Thus, plosive consonants have higher values than those that are nasal. In the case of vowels, those which are articulated in front are experienced as more arousing than those which are articulated further back.

In the case of meaningful words, the impression of congruence of sound and meaning depends on whether or not the individual making the judgment is familiar with the sound or word form as conveyor of meaning. A person conversant with a language frequently has the *feeling* that the sound form is a "fitting" symbolization of a word. In spite of methodologically refined studies, Ertel still obtained similar findings, even with subjects not conversant in the particular language. Words with "*potency* +" meaning contain more "potency +" consonants, words with activity meaning are more likely to contain "activating" consonants.

This indicates to Ertel that, in the context of natural language development, the features of *universal quality* (that is, what he calls his congruency, etc., factors) of the phonetic process once had importance for the formation of words.

By positing the universal qualities as the fundamental formal relations, Ertel is able to generate extremely interesting hypotheses and studies that go far beyond the problem of sound symbolism that is the subject of our

---

[6] With this Ertel again picks up Köhler's concept of isomorphism which we discussed earlier.

discussion here. Let us, however, mention one important example. Ertel identifies fundamental similarities between, for example, affirmation and negation of sentences on the one hand, and the execution of certain hand movements on the other. For Ertel and Bloemer (1975) the affirmation of a simple sentence ("The sheep is small") combines two cognitive units, ("sheep" and "small"), while the negation ("The sheep is not small") separates them. If a subject is required to read and learn sentences of this kind and at the same time takes apart or puts together a paper square which was cut in half, he will learn significantly better if the sentence-dynamic and the action-dynamic are in correspondence (either both joined or both separated) than if there is no such correspondence.

Here Ertel goes far beyond the scope of simple sound symbolism. In a way he views the linguistic event as expression, but not at all in the sense that Bühler did, i.e., as the expression of the (emotional, connotative) inner state. For Ertel it is an expression or correlate of fundamentally cognitive, dynamic processes and relationships requiring the participation of the hearer's and listener's self.

This opens up the whole area of overlap between verbal and nonverbal events. We can orient ourselves here by using the thematic question which we raised earlier. Are there common structures that traverse both? But we can also look at it from the genetic point of view. How does something verbal develop out of something that is *not yet* verbal? What is the relationship between verbal and nonverbal communication?

Now of course the concept of communication becomes a problem once more. Is every expressive behavior which permits the listener or spectator to draw conclusions about the state or intentions of the sender, to be designated as communication? We are not going to explore this in detail, but refer to Wiener et al. (1972) and to Hörmann (1976).

Finally, let us look at another of the many important discoveries in this research area because we will need it later. Aside from the distribution of pauses (Goldman-Eisler), emphasis and prosody, above all, have been shown to be highly informative for the listener. Wakefield et al. (1974) showed that even a listener who is not conversant with the language to which he is listening can extract information from the text relating to the inherent linguistic organization of the utterance by just listening to the foreign language for about 20 minutes.

This discovery, like those concerning sound symbolism and those concerning the general validity of Ertel's relations, suggests that the similarity of articulation of verbal and nonverbal events can serve as an aid to understanding, and thus as a means for acquiring language. We will come back to this in Chapter 11.

CHAPTER 10

The Psychological Reality of Grammar

Limitations of Markov's model—The concept of grammaticality—Effects of syntactical structure on learning and retention—Temporal features of speech perception and speech production—The concept of the plan—Surface and deep structure viewed psychologically—Johnson's model of sentence-generating—Semantic factors of sentence structure—The semantic organization of memory—Paivio's dual coding hypothesis—Predicate/argument structures and their influence on sentence processing.

A wide gulf separates the subject matter of the present chapter from that of previous ones. We have considered at length the relationships that bind single speech events to other speech events. These "other speech events" may either precede the single event or be latent and simultaneous with it. The former relationships are probabilistic, the latter associative. Basically one kind can be transformed into the other.

The presentation of the consequences and mode of functioning of associative processes repeatedly led us to results which made it clear that there is an additional factor beyond the observed relationships. For example, the observation that most responses in the word-association experiment belong to the same word class (noun, verb, etc.) can, up to a point, be explained by a mediation model (see p. 162), but it is equally the consequence of a system which operates above the word level—this system is called grammar in linguistics.

The assumption that such a system does operate is further suggested by the argument (as pointed out by Lashley, 1951) that the combinations of word associations—and nothing else has so far been considered—are not sufficient to account for the structure of the largest linguistic pattern constituting a unit, i.e., the sentence. The order of words in a sentence cannot be accounted for in terms of associations which exist between the words in the sentence.

A similar relationship exists at a lower level between phoneme and word. As we utter a word, a sequence of specific movements of the vocal cords, tongue, and jaw occurs. The elements of this sequence have almost no associative interrelationships because, when we utter another phoneme or another word, the same tongue movement can be combined with a different positioning of the vocal cords and a different shape of the oral cavity. Therefore, the order of the elements of articulation cannot be derived from a directly associative combination of these elements; instead it seems, so to speak, to be imposed from above.

One might now be inclined to compensate for the inadequacy of the associationist model by employing a Markov model.

> When language is considered as a Markov process, we adopt—as is already familiar—the point of view that speech event A (phoneme, letter or word) at the producer or the receiver end is dependent upon which events (A-1, A-2, A-3 . . .) have preceded it.

As was seen previously this approach has been particularly useful in explaining a great deal in the area of speech perception; for, as we receive a single speech event, the only additional aid at our disposal is what we have already received. Starting from what we have just heard, we have to draw probabilistic inferences as to what speech event will follow.

However, even the Markov model, which like the associationist mode of explanation is a finite-state model, has its inadequacies. Miller (1962a) himself points to three limitations of the model: an incredible number of decisions would have to be made in a very short time; our subjective experience at best permits us to make only a few, albeit relatively far-reaching decisions, while the sentence is being processed; it would be impossible to correct an erroneous decision in the course of further processing, but, in fact, this is possible.

Let us turn now to empirical findings which challenge the fecundity of a Markov model, and thereby gradually develop what might be called the "psychological reality" of grammer.

The investigation by Miller and Selfridge on the connection between order of approximation and retention of linguistic material showed, it will be remembered, that the curve of retention after the fifth approximation no longer rises. This result was confirmed by a whole series of subsequent studies. Only combinations up to six words play a part in retention (and also, incidentally, in guessing omitted words, according to Deese, in Cofer, 1961a).

In certain studies, however, a surprising observation was made: at the seventh, eighth, or tenth order of approximation not only does the curve not rise any more, but it declines again. This observation was made the subject of an investigation by Coleman (1963) in which he attempted to answer the question, Do the transitional probabilities with which we operate when the order of approximation is raised constitute, in fact, a uniform factor?

His conjecture was that another factor should be separated from this one, one that is *not* probabilistic in character, i.e., a factor of grammaticality (or grammaticalness).

This concept takes us (it cannot be emphasized enough) out of the realm of a probabilistic-associationist perspective to a fundamentally different point of view which is dominated by *generative grammar*. Earlier we have sketched the salient features of this theory which was developed by Chomsky. Grammaticality, which is now the object of Coleman's search, is a key concept of generative grammar inasmuch as this theory attempts to conceptualize, by means of a rational model, the intuitive ability of the competent speaker/listener to distinguish between well-formed and not-well-formed sentences.

While the probabilistic-associationistic approach can at best describe the nature of a particular sequence of linguistic units, generative grammar, by the use of the concept of *grammaticality* attempts to recognize the demand of all grammars for the production of grammatically correct sentences, generated in a particular way.

Coleman's study (1963) stands paradigmatically at the beginning of this chapter, because it addresses the question of whether this primarily linguistic concept of grammaticality also has a *psychological reality* inasmuch as the effectiveness of this linguistic factor may be demonstrated by means of psychological data.

This "search for the psychological reality of grammar" represents the major thrust of psycholinguistic research between 1963 and 1972. During this time there evolved the (reductionistic) practice of using the concepts "psychology of language" and "psycholinguistics" interchangeably. The origins of this development within the history of science are discussed elsewhere (Hörmann, 1974, 1976).

All of these efforts were aimed at the goal of showing "in action" the competence of the speaker which had been described by the linguists. Miller[1] outlined the position of psycholinguistics as follows: A description of the rules which are applied in the use of a language is not identical with the description of the psychological mechanisms which are involved in the use of these rules; it is the task of the psycholinguist to design performance models for the language user, but the exact specification of what the language user uses must be supplied by the linguist (1965).

> Only recently has this come under attack. Is it possible for the linguist, who describes language-in-itself, to offer an exact description of the speaker/listener's speech processes which are in the domain of psychology (cf. Wettler, 1974; Schlesinger, 1967; Hörmann, 1972)?

Coleman attempts to investigate the psychological reality (or usefulness) of a very comprehensive linguistic concept, namely that of grammaticality. Later we will introduce attempts to analyze more specific linguistic concepts

---

[1] The psychology of language is indebted to Miller not only for his introduction of the probabilistic approach (1951a), but also for introducing the syntax-centered approach (1962b, 1965) which contradicts the former.

in this light as well. We begin with Coleman because his research can also show us the limited psychological value of a Markov model, while at the same time demonstrating the fecundity of applying grammatic-syntactic concepts to these limits.

Coleman submitted to a group of 12 linguists, who were not familiar with "order of approximation," sequences of varying degrees of approximation and invited them to rank the sequences according to the degree of grammaticalness.

It was found that the degree of grammaticalness did not rise beyond the fifth order of approximation. In other words, approximations of a higher order do not offer a higher degree of agreement between subject and verb, or between verb and object. On the contrary, one gains the impression that to make up a sixth-order approximation more unusual constructions are used than, for example, to make up a second-order approximation. The procedure for making up these approximations should be remembered (p. 101): at the sixth order a person is given six words and is asked to add a suitable seventh. In order to find a continuation for "humble because they have no electricity," one must no doubt think of something more unusual than if one searched for a continuation of "humble because."

Herrmann (1962) undertook syntactical investigations on the immediate recall of strings of words and equally came to the conclusion "that the exclusive concern with the expectancy structure basically does not offer an adequate psychological explanation for the immediate recall of verbal strings. Besides factual content, i.e., the semantic meaning, and the motivational context of the words to be remembered, the grammatical regulation of the sentences is always a factor to be taken into account.

Although grammaticalness—like order of approximation—is independent of meaningfulness in the semantic sense (cf. Chomsky, 1961, p. 231) grammaticalness is not to be equated with order of approximation. According to Coleman's investigations it appears that, for example, the amount of material retained on the lower levels of approximation is in keeping with the degree of approximation (and at this stage still rises with the degree of grammaticality), but after a certain point has been reached, the score of retention is more in keeping with grammaticality, which no longer increases, and less with the order of approximation, which continues to rise. In other words, the retention score, too, does not improve any more.

For the next step one must try to clearly differentiate the influence of the various factors, i.e., grammaticality, transitional probability, and association or meaning. Epstein's investigations (1961, 1962) concerning the effects of the so-called empty syntactic structure on the psychological processing of sentences address themselves to this task. We shall now examine these.

In order to isolate syntactical structure as a variable, Epstein produced categories of materials consisting each of two sentences (Table 11). The sentences in category 1 are nonsense-syllables mixed with two function

Table 11.   Learning materials.

Category	Sentence
1*	(1) A haky deebs reciled the dison tofently um flutest pav.
	(2) The glers un cligs wur vasing un seping a rad moovly.
2	(1) deebs haky the um flutest reciled pav a tofently dison
	(2) cligs seping a wur rad un moovly glers the un vasing
3*	(1) Wavy books worked singing clouds to empty slow lamps.
	(2) Helping walls met eating trees from noisy poor lines.
4	(1) worked clouds slow empty to wavy singing books lamps
	(2) noisy trees walls from lines helping eating poor met

* It should be noted that the "sentences" in categories 1 and 3 begin with a capital and end with a period.
From Epstein, 1962, p. 122.

words "a" and "the." Additionally, the grammatical tags "ed," "s," "ing," "ly," and "est" are appended to the nonsense-syllables. In this way sentences are made up which are nonsense but still have a certain measure of grammaticalness in Chomsky's sense.

Category 2 contains the same words but in randon order.

In these two categories 1 and 2 there is neither meaning in the usual sense (i.e., with object reference) nor are there statistical dependencies in the form of transitional probability because the "words" in these sentences have never been met before by the subjects and consequently cannot have been encountered in this particular order. The difference between categories 1 and 2 is purely the presence of the empty syntactical structure in 1.

Categories 3 and 4 consist of sentences with meaningful words, composed as patterns making up nonsense "sentences." Transitional probabilities should be extremely slight. In category 3 words are arranged in such a way that a syntactical structure is produced, whereas in category 4 the same words appear in random order.

The subject's task is to learn these sentences. The results are presented in Table 12.

Table 12.   Results (both sentences combined for each category).

Measure of learning	Category 1		Category 2		Category 3		Category 4	
	M	SD	M	SD	M	SD	M	SD
Trials to criterion	7.29	2.87	8.87	3.37	2.62	1.12	3.78	1.87
Errors to criterion	23.95	9.89	35.54	9.48	4.75	2.72	10.00	3.74

M = mean; SD = standard deviation.
Based on Epstein, 1962, p. 122.

If one compares the number of repetitions needed to learn categories 1 and 2, it will be seen that at work here is a sequential factor (1 and 2 are distinguished *only* by the order of words) which can have nothing to do with transitional probabilities or associations, for neither can be present since the subject has met them here for the first time. Meaningful words are learned more rapidly than nonsense words (compare 1 and 3), but even in the nonsense combination of meaningful words we can see the influence of an empty but syntactically correct sequential structure.

Characteristically, Epstein's findings apply only as long as the subject can read the sentences as units, as would normally occur when they are in a book. If the same sentences are presented in the form of a serial learning experiment, i.e., a word every two seconds, the influence of the syntactical structure is no longer present. All one finds is the usual serial position effect in the learning of nonsense-syllable lists.

What conclusions can we draw from these results of Epstein's investigations and similar results obtained by Miller and Isard (1963) and Marks and Miller (1964)? Syntactical structure operates as a comprehensive whole, characterized, for example, by a definite speed of occurrence.

In contrast, probabilistic and associative determinants are always attributes of a single unit, e.g., an individual word. For example, Noble describes how many associative relationships a single word possesses; the order of approximation tells us how many preceding words have to be taken into account in the choice of a single word.

The next step in the analysis of what can here be called comprehensive structure consists of investigations by Glanzer (1962). Here, too, the distinction made by Epstein, between function words (articles, prepositions, conjunctions, etc.) and content words, which have a correlate in reality, plays an important role. Function words are few in number, but they have existed in the language for a long time; they form the "skeleton" of the language. Content words are a huge open class; new words are added every day and old ones are discarded; they are the 'meat' of the language. Function words are always frequent, content words less so.

Glanzer now raises the question whether this linguistic distinction has a psychological correlate. To answer this question, he devised a learning experiment in which nouns, verbs, prepositions and conjunctions were associated with nonsense syllables (e.g., food—YIG, church—NIV, think—HUC, grow—FEP, of—TAH, with—SEB, and—KEX, if—NED). It was found that the association of a noun and a nonsense syllable was learned more rapidly than the association between a preposition or conjunction and a nonsense syllable.

It was fortunate that Glanzer was not satisfied with this first confirmation of his hypothesis, for he attempted to find a more convincing explanation. Function words, he argued, can only be regarded as separate words in a restricted sense; perhaps they are only complete if they appear in a context within which they can function as "function words." Content words, on the other hand, ought to be less affected by isolation. To express it differently: in the case of content words the addition of a context should therefore have less influence upon ease of learning. To put this argument to the test, Glanzer asked his subjects to learn the following:

> YIG—food—SEB
> MEF—think—JAT
> TAH—of—ZUM
> WOJ—and—KEX

The order of learnability is indeed changed now. Whereas previously nouns were learned fastest, and prepositions or conjunctions slowest, the order is now reversed. Similar results were obtained by Rosenberg and Baker (1964, in Rosenberg, 1965). Glanzer draws the conclusion that isolated function words are psychologically incomplete as units.

If this argument is taken further, it can be said, following Glanzer (p. 313): an utterance consists of a series of signals or units: some of these units are single words, but some of them are sets of words. Content words, in this sense, are one-word units, whereas multiword signals contain a function word embedded in them.

This result immediately reveals a fundamental difference between psycholinguistics on the one hand and nearly all other branches of psychology on the other. Whereas in general psychology or in personality research the psychologist often has an almost completely free hand in what he wants to choose as a unit of investigation, the student of psycholinguistics must find out empirically what the language user in fact uses as a functional unit and base his psychological investigation upon it.

Glanzer's study and the inquiries previously reported are almost at the end of a line which begins with Skinner who tried to explain verbal events without ever leaving the plane of behavior. But a verbal event is structured in a lawful manner. It might be said that this structure has an independent existence; in any case, it can become the object of scientific investigation.

One such attempt to grasp these determining structures operates with the concept of transitional probabilities, the Markov model. Transitional probabilities are relations between units which are always on a particular level, e.g., between phonemes, or between letters, or between words. As we can now see and as, for example, Carroll has repeatedly pointed out, these units are again organized into a more comprehensive whole; this organization is such that it cannot be reduced to transitional probabilities. What matters is not only which word follows another in a sequence, but also which function a particular word fulfills in this sequence. Grammar creates relations within a sequence which do not coincide with probabilistic relations.

If, for example, we operate in the framework of a Markov model of language at word level, each word is considered a unit which is linked to the following unit, and the one after, etc., by certain transitional probabilities. We now recognize that a word is sometimes the psychologically relevant unit and can therefore be considered as the base line for transitional probabilities. But, at other times, the single word does not constitute a psychologically relevant unit; it must be combined with other words. It is quite thinkable that the simple sentence, "There are men and women," should not be considered as a Markov chain consisting of five units; instead it should be represented as in Fig. 48.

"Men" and "women" on the one hand are complete units; on the other the "and" between them becomes a complete unit only if it is preceded and followed by a content word. This indicates that in the analysis of linguistic events it is necessary to operate with units on more than one level.

If the linear probability model lays emphasis on the conception of sending and receiving as a process of selection in which transitional probabilities determine which event is chosen as the next one, the importance of this selection process is not diminished as a result of the above considerations. Sending and receiving messages are indeed selective processes, but the question now is, What determines the time sequence of the command to select? It is by no means always a simple matter of preceding speech events determining subsequent events.

Looked at from the angle of the perception of speech, the view that the speech event is structured on several hierarchical levels has received valuable confirmation. Ladefoged (1959) assumes that the receiver, too, even if he had been specially asked to pay attention to these segments, would have difficulties in grasping the speech event at each single moment of hearing as if it were composed of small segments. In one experiment, the word "dot" was superimposed upon a spoken sentence. Subjects were asked to indicate the exact place in the sentence at which the superimposed word had begun. In many cases "dot" was located by the subject two or three words ahead of the place where it had actually occurred. This observation led Ladefoged to the conclusion that the processing of ongoing contextual information has different temporal features than the processing of isolated stimuli; ongoing speech events result in complex time patterns which have to be grasped as a whole. ". . . items of speech such as syllables, words, phrases, and even some sentences, have a perceptual unity; and any theory which attempts to explain the perception of speech in terms of the sequential identification of smaller segments is likely to be unsatisfactory" (1959, p. 402).

At this point we have the choice of moving in one of two interesting

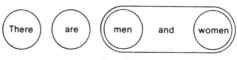

Fig. 48

directions. Along with Garrett, Bever, and others, we could examine more closely the structure of these components (phrases) which in terms of their size fall between the word and the sentence. For this purpose one could advantageously use the conception of levels first introduced by generative grammarians to distinguish, among other factors, between the deep and surface structure. This we will discuss later.

For the moment, let us glance back to the theories that view speech perception as an analysis-by-synthesis process and to the notion of lexical units.

It will be remembered that "dictionary units" were postulated because the process of recognition in the hearer was seen as an act of comparison. The fragments of the percept are complemented in accordance with the most fitting pattern of the inner repertoire; or to put it differently: what is perceived coincides with an already existing pattern. The difficulty of this conception of the process of speech perception lies in the assumption that the input must be compared in a fraction of time with an infinite number of such patterns.

As we know, one restriction of this infinite number is provided by transitional probabilities. In spite of that, it is hard to imagine that a huge number of dictionary units and a vast number of sentences can be stored as patterns.

To solve this problem, Halle and Stevens (1962) have advanced the hypothesis that these internal patterns against which the input is matched might be created only at the moment of receiving the message in accordance with the same rules of a generative grammar which the hearer would follow if he himself were the speaker.

The comprehension of the input, according to this view, begins with guesswork or a hypothesis. On the basis of this hypothesis the hearer generates an internal pattern of comparison to which to relate the input. Discrepancies in this comparison lead to the creation of a second pattern for comparison, matching better with the input. As soon as the match is judged to be satisfactory, the message is accepted or "recognized," which does not mean that it is necessarily "correct."

In the theory of Halle and Stevens the comparison of the input with a repertoire of possible patterns plays a role, but these possible patterns are not all stored singly, they are created at the moment of perception according to the rules of generative grammar.

Liberman's motor theory offers a parallel in that the hearer's production is decisive for the perception of what he hears. But, different from Liberman (hence circumventing the objections to his theory), what is produced by the hearer does not in Halle and Stevens' theory consist of an actual, if only covert, articulation. The hearer need not articulate what he hears; what he does is to activate the program which could generate the sentence which enters as input.

This Halle-Stevens approach was one of the first analysis-by-synthesis models. It was followed by many similar theories particularly in the field of visual perception.

Time markers in speech (as was clearly seen in Epstein's study) serve as indicators of the underlying structure of an utterance. As one would expect, the study of time features in the *production* of utterances will reveal this with particular clarity. Such studies were made by Goldman-Eisler (1968) in the form of detailed analyses of pauses in speech sequences.

Goldman-Eisler used as a measure for pauses—always in spontaneous speech—the proportion of the length of the pauses to the number of words in the utterance. It was found that pauses take up approximately 40 to 50 percent of the total time of utterances. Pausing regulates nine-tenths of the speed of speech, while the rate of articulation itself is remarkably constant. This can be explained by the fact that the articulatory performance constitutes the real "art" of speech, whereas pauses represent that part of the total event in which "verbal planning and selection" occur and in which, therefore, information is created. Pauses are related to the information content of subsequent words; fluency of speech is related to redundancy. The information content in these studies was measured in terms of transitional probabilities. In this context it became also apparent that the linear Markov model cannot be satisfactory: the relationship between information content and length of pauses became significant only when the transitional probabilities were estimated both in the reverse as well as the forward direction. The speed of an utterance, therefore, is determined by the probability structure of subsequent as well as preceding speech. That means that, at least as far as the production of speech is concerned, there must be a plan which, in the moment of event A takes into account not only the preceding events (A−1), (A−2), etc. but also future events (A+1), (A+2), etc.; this view will later be considered in detail.

Moreover, Goldman-Eisler was able to prove that a subject who has to fill blanks in a text as he reads it can complete this task successfully only if he makes the same pauses as the speaker who originally produced the particular sentence. This suggests the importance of time factors in the selection processes which are basic to the speech event (cf. Lashley). If a speaker describes the significance of an event, pauses are more than twice as long as when he gives a description of the event itself. During the repetition of previously narrated sentences, pauses are reduced. This is to say that length of pauses apparently is not only related to the information content of the utterance itself, but also to the creative activity of the speaker. Goldman-Eisler draws the conclusion that pausing indicates that, in the course of speech, information is being generated and an act of verbal planning is taking place.

The important influence of temporal factors on the articulation of linguistic utterances is not only shown by the importance of pauses; intonation also plays an important role. Here particular mention should be made of the studies by Martin (1972).

A first approximation of a model to represent the multilevel structure tentatively suggests two levels of encoding. The first of these might be labeled lexical, while the second might be designated syntactical, structural, or grammatical. A closer examination, however, shows that such a two-level model proves to be inadequate as an explanatory model for the empirical results that have been cited, as well as for many which were not cited. For example, the data reported by Glanzer require a more differentiated schema. The inadequacies of such a two-level model become even more apparent when we employ it to analyze the sentence, "He killed the man with the axe."

While the lexical meaning of the words is clear, the meaning of the sentence containing them is ambiguous. (The axe can be the murder weapon or serve as part of the description of the man who was killed.) Analyzing this sentence in order to understand it, we must proceed according to the rules of a grammar which tell us which lexical units (words) are to be combined in what order and with what other units of varying dimensions (phrases). That, precisely, is the goal of generative grammar, which after all is a grammar of phrase-structure with an added transformational component.

With the identification of the (linguistic) notion of the rules of phrase-structure, we not only return to the realm of generative grammar, but we also reach the point of origin for the long-standing, cooperative efforts between generative linguistics and psycholinguistics. Miller, Galanter, and Pribram (1960) developed the notion of the "plan" as a psychological analogue to the linguistic concept of rules of phrase-structure. Psycholinguistics, following the approach of generative linguistics, has more or less tacitly assumed that "rule" and "plan" are two aspects of the same thing.

We now turn to a more detailed examination of the plan concept. Of course, the problem of how to conceptualize the orderly sequence of behavior, i.e., the temporal *and* hierarchical integration of cognitive and behavioral units of varying dimensions, was well known to psychology prior to the introduction of generative linguistics.

A very clear but quite inadequate answer to this problem was the reflex chain theory. This theory, which originated in the early part of the century and was to a very large measure adopted by Watson in the development of his psychology of "behaviorism," assumes that the occurrence of each single reflex serves as the stimulus for eliciting the next reflex. The kinesthetic and auditory sensations which the articulation of a speech sound produces evokes the articulation of the next speech sound.

Toward the end of the 1920s, Lashley's investigations showed conclusively that this theory is unable to account for the temporal arrangement of behavior. Thus rats, for example, which have learned to run a maze are able to run the maze faultlessly, even if, as a result of surgical extirpation, they are forced to activate different muscle groups in quite different temporal patterns in order to reach their objective. Later, Lashley was also able to demonstrate, at the hand of linguistic examples, that a linear model is inadequate and that comprehensive integrating structures must be assumed. Here, then, is a first link to the notion of *plan*.

The second approach, following the reflex chain theory, was the Würzburg School, operating with the concept of "determining tendency," as it was evolved by Külpe and later by Ach. The arrangement of a sentence, for example, constitutes a mental set (*Bewusstseinslage*) in which the temporal sequence is not yet recognizable as such. Pick, for example, has drawn attention to the processes which occur in translating from one language into another with a different sentence structure. Suppose an English-speaking reader reads a German sentence and expresses it in a free English translation. As he moves from German to English, the German sentence must, in a certain way, be taken out of the time dimension and after that put back into it as an English sentence but in a different serial order. A speaker of several languages—at an international conference, for example—can express the same thought in different languages and in doing so change several times from one word order to a totally different one. This again suggests that the preconceived organization of thought does not necessarily contain a temporal organization.

Related to this point are the reflections of the Russian psychologists Leontiev and, particularly, Luria (1968), who was able to observe a deficit of just this ability of temporal ordering in patients with so-called dynamic aphasia. Wundt viewed the sentence as a transformation of a simultaneous representational whole (*Gesamtvorstellung*) into a successive sequence of words.

How complicated the factors involved may be was shown by Lashley with reference to the phenomena which psychoanalysis has studied as "slips" of the tongue and pen, etc.

Suppose a typist writing the word "manner" accidentally fails to double the middle "n" and writes "maner"; she crosses it out and at her second attempt writes "maaner." This means that the command to double the letter was carried out, but the instruction evidently had not included a sufficiently precise indication of serial order.[2]

Lashley (1960, p. 515), too, is finally led to postulate hierarchically organized levels: the order of articulatory movement as a word is uttered, the order of words in a sentence, the order of sentences in a paragraph, the order of paragraphs in a discourse.

---

[2] In Hull's psychology of learning this would be described as an anticipatory goal response; it is interesting to note here the fragmentation of a complex response.

We thus already approach a more differentiated conception: the order of words in a sentence is not on a single level, but is itself in turn the result of a hierarchy of factors.

In order to explain speech generation as well as speech perception, it becomes necessary to assume that there are control points which also provide a view of the future. Not only does the speaker know what he has just said, but he also knows what he is about to say, even if the latter takes place at a totally different level of consciousness. He develops his sentence according to a plan which anticipates future events. The listener applies the schema of a plan to the arriving sentence, in order to recognize the structure inherent in that sentence. The concept of plan may thus help us to overcome the weaknesses of a purely probabilistic-associationistic model of linguistic events.

A plan is to the organism what a program is to the computer. This modern analogy must not lead us to overlook the fact that what Miller, Galanter, and Pribram understand as "plan" is exactly the same as what Allesch described 25 years earlier as *Impulsfigur* ("dynamic pattern" or "directive configuration"). The *Impulsfigur* is a plan compressed into the formula of a program or a list of instructions.

The probability structure we discussed previously is a sequential structure on a single level. The assumption of a hierarchical plan as the organizing principle of the speech event takes into account the viewpoint that the speech event is simultaneously organized on several levels. It is important to recognize the distinction between a sequential and a sequential-hierarchical structure.

When a sentence is uttered, a motor plan must exist which regulates the sequence of articulating speech movements. Behind or above the motor plan, however, there must be a process which generates or selects the motor plan. In other words, above the level of the motor plan, other plans influence or direct the motor plan. Miller, Galanter, and Pribram refer to these collectively as the "grammar plan." It is made up of the hierarchy of general grammatical rules which come into play in sentence formation in the particular language. Chomsky's influence is evident here.

The grammar plan tests the sentence quality of the preliminary motor plan, or, in Chomsky's terms, the grammaticalness of the motor plan, and having tested it, passes it, as it were, as fit for articulation. For the notion of "feedback" distinctly suggested here, Miller, Galanter, and Pribram postulate a special functional unit which tests, modifies, re-tests and executes. They refer to it as the TOTE unit (test-operate-test-exit).

A TOTE unit has a certain affinity with the concept of the reflex arc—with the important distinction, however, that the TOTE not only carries impulses, i.e., energy, but also information or control.

In the view of the authors a complex plan, e.g., the grammar plan of a sentence, consists again of a hierarchy of such behavioral TOTE units; and the feedback mechanism which—as already mentioned—is also one of the features of this model serves to recognize and correct deviations from a standard.

This feedback mechanism cannot be of a purely sensory nature. From investigations on delayed speech feedback, it is known that sensory feedback plays an important part in the auditory control of the speaker's own productions. But the plan with whose help the grammaticality of a sentence to be uttered is tested is of a different order: it cannot merely consist of a sensory feedback device, because the corrections must be made *before* the utterance takes place. It is clear that, in the area of the *production* of speech, problems present themselves which are much more difficult to investigate than the problems which occur in the *perception* of speech.

Armed with the psychological concept of the plan, let us now return to the generative grammar which, after all, was the impetus for Miller's approach. The question is, Can one show the operation of a plan in the concrete case of verbal behavior, by showing that this behavior is articulated by means of those units which are used by generative linguistics to analyze the sentence? Again this question is one which relates to the "psychological reality" of this grammar as we discussed above.

We indicated earlier that Chomsky's grammar describes the sentence as consisting of phrases; nominal phrase, NP, and verb phrase, VP, hierarchically form the highest components of the sentence. Now we must ask, Are these linguistic units psychological units as well?

Fodor and Bever (1965) presented their subjects with sentences which, at one point, contained a click (shown here as an x); for example:

That he was happy was evident from the way he smiled.

            x   x   x   x   x
            1   2   3   4   5

(Each subject was given the sentence with only *one* click.)

If the subject is then instructed to indicate at which point in the sentence the click occurred, he is able to do so correctly only if it occurred at point 3, i.e., the point of maximal phrase separation. Clicks presented prior to or after that point (1, 2, 4, or 5) are subjectively moved by the listener to the phrase boundary. Thus we see that the phrase, defined linguistically, is a psychological unit as well. After all, psychological units are characterized to some extent by the fact that they resist partition.

Of course, one could voice the suspicion that the listener is made aware of the phrase structure and its boundary not so much through his linguistic knowledge (his "competence") but, on a much simpler level, through an acoustical signal, namely the pause between "happy" and "was." (That would still leave us with the problem why the pause would be placed at that particular point.) This suspicion was allayed by Garrett, Bever, and Fodor (1966) by means of a most convincing argument.

Compare sentences like these:

As a result of their invention's *influence the company was given an award.*

and

The chairman whose methods still *influence the company was given an award.*

If subjects are now asked to indicate where they hear the longest pause, they will place it between "influence" and "the" in the first, and between "company" and "was" in the second sentence. That means that the perceived pause corresponds to the articulation of the primary components of the respective sentences.

Now the tapes were cut and the second parts of the sentences—beginning with "influence"—were interchanged. These patched tapes were then used in a further click experiment. As Fodor and Bever had found earlier, here too the click was localized in the first sentence between "influence" and "the," and in the second sentence between "company" and "was."

These findings show that the beginning of the sentence determines the comprehension of its linguistic structure, i.e., its perception, even in the case where the perceptual (acoustical) signals are totally absent. We can conclude then that speech perception always incorporates a projective factor.

These studies have shown that, for the speaker/listener, sentences have a structure which is not identical to that which might be designated as their manifest stimulus structure, e.g., a possible structuring by means of pauses. In addition to its physical structure, the stimulus also has a linguistic structure which is determined by the totality of the sentence. The latter is often of greater importance to the perception of the sentence. As was indicated by the last mentioned experiment, the structural articulation is not determined by the actual conditions recorded on the tape. Instead we find that the listener's conceptualization of the linguistic structure of the total sentence is formed by extrapolating from the preceding components of the sentence. This indicates that the linguistic stimulus is, to a large extent, determined by the available knowledge activated by the physical stimulus, and then used to process it.

These diverse "structures" which we have contrasted here are to some extent the same as those which generative linguistics attempts to account for by the dichotomy of surface and deep structure. Is the deep structure of a linguistic utterance not as important as the surface structure for its processing?

Let us look at an experiment examining this question. Blumenthal (1967) instructed his subjects to learn sentences like these:

Gloves were made by tailors.

Gloves were made by hand.

Both of these sentences have quite similar surface structures but different deep structures. If the subject learns many such sentences and is then given the grammatical subject (gloves) as a cue to recall one finds no difference in the effectiveness of this cue for the two sentences. However, if the logical subject (tailors) or the adverb (hands) is given as a cue, the logical subject will be far more effective.

This shows that, at least under certain conditions, the deep structure is more "effective" than the surface structure of a sentence. The processing (in memory) is influenced more strongly by factors related to the deep than to the surface structure.

That, of course, leads immediately to the important question of how the listener arrives at the deep structure of the sentence when the surface structure is all that is available to him. After all, he hears only the word-sounds which are by definition the output of the surface structure with the addition of their phonological interpretation. In the case of the sentences above, how does the listener recognize that the word following "by" is in one case the logical subject, i.e., the actor of the act described, and in the other case the nature of that act?

Orthodox generative linguists cannot answer this question. Their model does not permit reference to the obvious factor of word meaning. For them, meaning is something secondary which cannot play a role in determining the syntactical sentence structure. But if one avoids prescriptions of this kind, the question raised above can be answered as follows: Apparently the listener must have some knowledge concerning the content, i.e., the meaning, of the relevant word in order to evaluate and place it properly (i.e., as logical object or as adverb). He must know that "tailor" refers to a living person capable of volitional acts while "hand" refers to a dependent instrumental appendage of such a person.

However, if the comprehension of the syntactic structure of a sentence requires such knowledge, it would appear that within the deep structure a clear separation of syntax and semantics is impossible.

Recently, this awareness has led to the development of the so-called generative semantics, represented by Fillmore, Lakoff, and Chafe, among others. In contrast to the orthodox generative grammarians, these investigators no longer view the dynamic relationship between phrases and elements as purely syntactic, and therefore independent of the meaning of a particular word. We will return to this conceptualization and its influence on psycholinguistics at a later point.

The concept of deep structure viewed as more than purely syntactical emerges as a useful construct for the development of psychological theory.

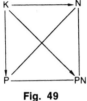

Fig. 49

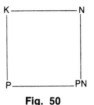

Fig. 50

Its value arises, in no small measure, from the way it suggests modification of the traditional view in the direction of greater precision.

The same is not true for the concept of transformation. It will be recalled that in generative linguistics rules of transformation form the second part of syntax. (The rules of phrase-structure, discussed above, form the first part.)

What is the psychological effectiveness of such rules? In an inquiry by McKean, Slobin, and Miller reported in Miller (1962b) the subjects were given a list of simple structure sentences ("kernel sentences")[3] which they were asked to transform in accordance with definite instructions: kernel sentences (K) were to be transformed into negative (N), passive (P), and passive-negative (PN) sentences. If these four sentence types were psychologically independent of each other, the transformation of K into P would require approximately the same time as from K into N or K into PN. According to Chomsky's transformational theory, a somewhat different result is to be expected: the six relationships, represented in the accompanying diagram (Fig. 49), can be reduced to a single pair of transformations: one transformation for the affirmative-negative aspect and one for the active-passive aspect. If Chomsky's hypothesis has psychological relevance, it follows that two steps are needed to transform K into PN, i.e., first, a transformation into the negative and, second, a transformation into the passive, or vice versa. Moreover, the transformation from N to P should require two steps: first into affirmative-active (K), then into affirmative-passive (P), or first into negative-passive and from there into affirmative-passive (P). Therefore, in place of the schema depicted in Fig. 49, the pattern according to Fig. 50 is to be expected, if the conception of transformation in Chomsky's sense is to be employed.

Transformations—so argued Miller and his collaborators—require time. Can one deduce from the different times required by the subjects for these transformations how many steps are involved?

---

[3] According to the generative grammar of that day, kernel sentences consist, so to speak, of the "least transformed" sentences. Today the standard theory holds that *all* sentences undergo such transformation on their way from deep to surface structure. Aside from these required transformations, however, there are also optional ones, as in the case of question, negation, and passive form, which may occur in addition to those which are mandatory. The nature of the experimental evidence presented here is not affected by these changes in the theory of linguistics.

Table 13. Mean numbers of sentences matched correctly by the experimental group (with transformations) and by the control group (without transformations). This figure is used to estimate the average transformation time per sentence.

Test condition	Mean number of sentences correct		Time for average subjects (secs.)		Estimated transformation times (secs.)
	Experimental group	Control group	Experimental group	Control group	
K : N	7.5	8.7	8.0	6.9	1.1
P : PN	5.5	6.4	10.5	9.3	1.2
K : P	8.1	10.1	7.4	5.9	1.5
PN : N	6.7	8.5	8.9	7.1	1.8
K : PN	6.9	10.0	8.7	6.0	2.7
N : P	5.6	8.4	10.7	7.2	3.5

Based on Miller, 1962b, p. 759.

Without going into detail (the experiments included some complicated comparisons with the control group), the inspection of the final column (Table 13) suggests the following conclusion: transformations into the negative require the least time. Transformations into the passive and from the passive require more time. However, times recorded are very much higher for those transformations which, according to the model developed above, involve two transformational steps (K:PN and N:P).

Further information on the processes involved in transformations of this order have resulted from an investigation by another of Miller's students, Mehler (reported by Miller, 1962b), who presented to his subjects sentences such as the following:

The typist has copied the paper. (kernel sentence)
The student hasn't written the essay. (N)
The photograph has been made by the boy. (P)
Has the train hit the car? (query: Q)
Hasn't the girl worn the jewel? (negative query: NQ)
The passenger hasn't been carried by the airplane. (PN), etc.

The order of the sentences was changed after each presentation. Subjects noted what they had remembered. An error analysis is offered in Fig. 51.

As is to be expected in a learning experiment, omissions decline from series to series. Other errors, such as intrusions of strange words or mixing up of two sentences, remain approximately constant. But the mass of errors is syntactical in character. Although the subject remembers the semantic content of the sentence, he changes its syntactic form so that a passive sentence, for example, appears as an active one.

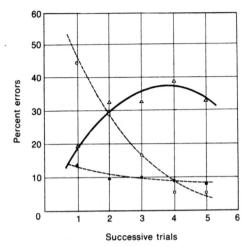

Fig. 51. Course of different error curves. $\triangle$: syntactic errors; $\bigcirc$: omissions; ● : other errors. (Based on Mehler, from Miller, 1962b, p. 760)

In order to explain these last findings Miller introduces an interesting psychological theory of retention. He assumes that the subject remembers each sentence as a kernel sentence plus an annotation of its syntactical form. For example, the sentence, "Didn't the girl wear her jewels?" is stored as, "The girl wore her jewels" plus the annotation "negative question form." We could say that the annotation represents a transformation command. Because kernel sentence and annotation can be forgotten independently after the experiment, it appears that they were also stored independently in memory.

But, we may ask, does this articulation, which characterizes our perception and retention, really take place according to the divisions described above? Let us take the sentence, "The train was not reached by the traveler in time." According to Miller and Mehler one would have to store first the semantic components "train-traveler-reached," and second the syntactic transformation command "passive/negative." However, among the reproductions of this sentence one will find, with high probability, the sentence, "The traveler did not reach the train in time," the active rather than the passive form and not, "The train was reached by the traveler in time," the passive/affirmative form.

That would indicate that the separation of "content" and "syntactical transformation" transpires in a manner different from that proposed by Chomsky and later Miller. It is far more likely that the general effect of affirmation or negation is part of the retained "content," than that it is an integral part of the transformation.

From here we could proceed in either of two directions. The first points to the fact that one possible reproduction of the original sentence could be, "The traveler missed the train." Apparently neither the semantic nor the syntactical "information" is stored in the listener's memory verbatim. More likely he retains information which enables him to construct, in his own words, that which the speaker intended, rather than repeat verbatim the sentence that he has heard. This approach takes us far afield from the problem area of the "psychological reality of grammar."

A second point of view, which does not take us quite so far afield, focuses on the concept of negation. Without documentation, we indicated above that, in our view, negation is not a transformation, it is not a syntactic but rather a semantic variable which in turn affects the syntactic form in which sentences are remembered. In one study (Hörmann, 1971) we presented subjects with sentences containing negative and affirmative forms. We then tested for retention. It was shown that sentences in which the predicate is negated ("The dog did not steal the bone.") are more likely to be remembered correctly than those in which a living being, carrying out the act, is being negated. ("It was not the dog who stole the bone.") The less precise the listener remembers the position of the negation, the more his reproduction will shift toward a generalized, unspecific negation of the predicate (Engelkamp, Merdian, and Hörmann, 1972; and Engelkamp and Hörmann, 1974).

It can now be seen that the relevant studies by Miller have, on the one hand, pointed to the probable psychological effect of transformation, but on the other hand they have raised the question about the extent to which the concept and process of transformation participates in the processing of the sentence. Up to now it has not been made sufficiently clear which aspects of a sentence are determined at the level of the rules of phrase structure, which at the level of transformation, and which are determined by purely semantic factors.

This ambiguity about the combined effects of the transformational components and the other grammatical units can be shown in yet another example taken from everyday communication. Carroll has already pointed out the fact that a speaker who uses the interrogative sentence, "Isn't it stuffy in here?" instead of the simple affirmative statement, "It's stuffy in here," applies a significant transformation, but psychologically in fact says the same thing. Furthermore, the question, "Can you open the window?" is not a question but a request, although it has undergone the question-transformation.

How does the reader know that in this case he is simply to ignore the question-transformation and take it to be a request? This problem takes us to the limits of what can be achieved by grammar-centered psycholinguistics; in fact it takes us beyond that limit. This approach breaks down at the point where another factor encroaches upon grammar and supercedes it, i.e., where the grammatical-syntactical determinants of understanding are secondary to its communicative determinants. The utilization of grammar must be part of a framework encompassing the speaker and the listener prior to the linguistic utterance and harmonizing their anticipation of possible acts and their mental sets.

Wittgenstein, in his philosophy of language, and Austin and Searle, in their theory of the speech act, both attempt to address part of this problem (see Chap. 7).

Up to now we have introduced models which examine individual grammatical-syntactical concepts in terms of their "psychological reality." The closest and probably most productive integration of the linguistic concept of structure and the psychological concept of plan is presented by the sentence processing theory of N.F. Johnson (1965).

Here the starting point is Miller's concept of "chunk." As we mentioned before, Miller was able to show that the capacity of short-term memory, which must play a part in the comprehension of a sentence, is limited by the number of the stored units. It was also shown, however, that the size of these units called chunks is variable, subject to change in the process of encoding or recoding. By recoding the material for purposes of storage it can be transformed into a more compact and therefore more parsimonious form. In principle it is always possible to combine units which have already been chunked into yet larger units, i.e., units of a higher level. At the point of recall these compressed units can then be decoded, i.e., translated into ordinary "long hand."

This description, originally applied to the memory process, which runs from a higher level of encoding "down" to the concrete indivisible units, is seen by Johnson as analogous to the processing of a sentence, which according to him proceeds simultaneously from "top to bottom" and from "left to right."

The first step in the process of generating sentence Σ, viewed as a unit, is to decode it into subject S and predicate P. The subject S is then further decoded into article T plus modified noun MN, etc. In this version of a tree diagram the nodes indicate encoding units and the lines decoding operations. It can be seen which words are determined or "dominated" by a certain encoding unit. When a terminal response has taken place, i.e., a word has been pronounced, the broken line indicates the next step in the sequence. Johnson, therefore, sees the production of a sentence as a series of decoding steps in which high order encoding units are reduced to units of a lower order. It is as if the speaker decoded his own products in the downward direction. In this process each coding unit is reduced to one or several subunits. While the first subunit continues to be decoded the others are stored in the immediate memory (Fig. 52).

Σ is divided into S + P. P is stored in the immediate memory while S is further decoded into T + MN. While T leads to the terminal response, i.e., the

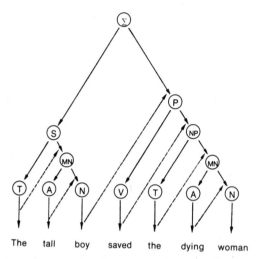

Fig. 52. Tree diagram of sentence generation showing decoding processes. (Based on Johnson, from Rosenberg, 1965, p. 54)

utterance of the word "the," MN remains stored in the immediate memory. As soon as "the" has been pronounced, the last stored unit, MN, is taken out of the store and decoded into A + N. N is stored until A has led to the pronunciation of the word "tall." Once N has also been led to the end response, the only unit stored in the immediate memory, P, is in turn decoded into V + NP and so forth.

The higher the level of the unit, the more operations are needed to decode downwards to the word level, but the greater the number of steps, the greater the susceptibility to error. Using this plausible analog, Johnson is now able to test his model experimentally. If the speaker first articulates the utterances into relatively large units, then he would make fewer errors *within* such units than if he took the more distant path between units. According to this notion, errors, i.e., the omission or substitution of a wrong word following a correct one, should occur less frequently *within* than *between* units.

To test this hypothesis, Johnson had his subjects learn sentences of the following kind: "The tall boy saved the dying woman."

Errors of the kind we have described are possible at six points, i.e., at each transition from one word to the next. According to the hypothesis they should occur, above all, at transition point 3, which lies between the two largest or earliest units into which the sentence is divided.

In a tree diagram it is possible to rank the nodes, at which the division into constituents occurs, according to height: e.g., the node between "the" and "tall boy" lies higher than the node between "tall" and "boy." The rank order arrived at in this way correlates significantly with the frequency of errors. The profile of error frequency reflects the sequence of the constituent analysis (Fig. 53).

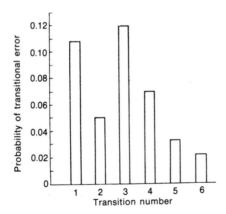

Fig. 53. Pattern of transitional error probabilities obtained when subjects learn the sentence, "The tall boy saved the dying woman." (Based on Johnson, from Rosenberg, 1965, p. 49)

A differently constructed sentence (Fig. 54) correspondingly produces a similar error pattern (Fig. 55).

According to Johnson's model a linguistic utterance is analyzed from "top to bottom" (i.e., according to a hierarchical structure), as well as from "left to right" (i.e., according to a sequential structure). Only the final coding process leads to the concrete words. The preceding coding processes and states (shown in the model as lying above) are recodifications which produce units of varying sizes at various levels (phrases, etc.) and are retained for ready recall.[4]

The influence of Miller, Galanter, and Pribram's concept of "plan," with its sequence control according to the TOTE principle, is clearly recognizable in this model. Undoubtedly Johnson's model represented, in its time, the most optimal integration of linguistic or, more precisely, generative grammatical and psychological theory. It was precisely this optimal integration that was lost when it became apparent to both linguistics and psychology that a conceptualization of language based (almost) exclusively on grammatically perfect form was inadequate. The speaker/listener's intent is not only to generate grammatically correct sentences, in line with Chomsky's ideal native speaker, but his utterance is also intended to achieve a purpose. This, however, requires that the semantic aspects, i.e., the meaning component, be included in the analysis of language and the communicative event.

In his interpretation of the above cited findings Johnson relies exclusively

---

[4] Levelt (in *Lingua* 1968, 20, p. 26) justifiably points out that the parallel processes of syntactical and psychological "generating" implicit in Johnson's model could also lead to the absurd conclusion that the speaker makes his decision about the *meaning* of what he wants to say at a very late point in the process. This criticism applies equally to Chomsky's model, on which Johnson's was based. For Chomsky, "semantic interpretation" is also a generating process which takes place after the syntactic structure.

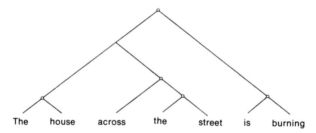

Fig. 54. Tree diagram of a sentence. (Based on Johnson, from Rosenberg, 1965, p. 48)

on syntactic factors. The "higher" the demarcation between two phrases or parts of phrases (in the generating schema), the higher is the probability that an error will occur at that point. The error profile reflects, so to speak, the speaker's structural "knowledge" of the particular sentence.

A large number of other experiments of different orientations, however, have shown that this syntax-centered explanatory model presents an incomplete picture of the factors involved in the processing of a sentence. This can be shown even in an experiment in the Johnson tradition.

Engelkamp (1973) presented subjects with sentences all of which had the same syntactic (phrase or deep) structure. Subjects were instructed to reproduce these sentences:

The soldier with the letter worked on the sculpture.

The soldier with the weapon worked on the sculpture.

The soldier with the chisel worked on the sculpture.

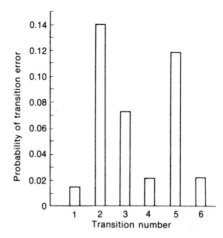

Fig. 55. Pattern of transitional error probabilities obtained when subjects learn the sentence, "The house across the street is burning." (Based on Johnson, from Rosenberg, 1965, p. 50)

Despite their identical syntactic construction these sentences produce quite different error profiles. The causes for these differences must be of a semantic nature, i.e., related to the content.[5]

In processing a sentence, the speaker/listener's awareness is apparently not limited to a recognition that its elements form a substantive phrase, or that they are classified as nouns, or that they function as the subject of the sentence. He "knows" something about their assigned meaning, and this knowledge plays a determining role in the processing of the sentence. How can this *semantic* knowledge be conceptualized in a theory?

This question takes us back to our earlier discussions of "meaning as association" viewed from a somewhat altered perspective. In Chapter 6 we introduced Katz and Fodor's model, which conceptualizes the meaning of a word as composed of *semantic features* and assumes that the user's lexicon is arranged according to dimensions which correspond to these features. The words "stone," "house," and "animal" all have the feature "physical object"; in other words, they are all localized on the "physical object" dimension. In addition, the word "animal" has the feature "living" which is not an attribute of the other words.

We also briefly discussed Clark's attempt to conceptualize the phenomena taking place in the association experiment in terms of a semantic feature theory. In line with his hypothesis about the types of processes occurring during the association experiment, Clark attempted to gain insight into the nature and sequence of linguistic units, i.e., the semantic features. At this point we face a very similar problem: We want to know something about the semantic relations within a verbal utterance by examining the processing of words and sentences in a way which will permit us to hypothesize what the speaker/listener "knows" about them.

The first study to which we turn asks quite directly what the language user knows about a "word," to be sure a word which, at the moment, he cannot recall. Brown and McNeill (1966), in a much-cited study, examined the tip-of-the-tongue phenomena. What happens to us, what do we "know" when, for example, we are trying to recall the name of the nautical instrument which is used to measure the height of stellar constellations? If we cannot think of the name, i.e., in the tip-of-the-tongue condition, we surely do not have an "empty" mental set. We know, for example, that the label that we seek has two syllables, with the emphasis on the second, and that it begins with "S." According to Brown and McNeill's interpretation of their findings, we already have some features of an intonational, orthographic, etc., nature with which we now begin the task of searching our vocabulary guided by the *semantic features*: "instrument," "nautical," "related to geometry." In the process we generate words like "compass," "protractor," "astrolabe," but as soon as we think of them we know that they are

---

[5] Engelkamp's interpretation of these findings will be discussed later.

wrong. We know it because we already have some of the features of the word we seek. If one presents several incorrect words to the subject at this stage, he can, without difficulty, rank them according to their similarity to the unknown target word. These rankings will correspond highly with the number of features that are shared by the correct and incorrect word.

Once the subject has reached the feature combination that corresponds to the target word, after repeated searches of his lexicon, he must yet succeed in "deciphering" the appropriate word that corresponds to this feature combination. This step, from the point of awareness of the proper feature combination to the appropriate word, remains rather obscure for Brown and McNeill. Presumably this is the same step that we take in the reverse direction when we understand a word.

This much is clear from the cited experiments: One can make the assumption that the memory representation of a word corresponds to an ordered list of semantic features, but the *use* of this list, i.e., moving from it to the word, is not an automatic association. Instead, it is an active process, with important contributions from a number of diverse factors.

There is an interesting economical aspect to the question about the classification system of the semantic features according to which words are registered in the "inner lexicon" of the speech user. What is the arrangement of this lexicon, this store of word meanings, permitting it to function as well as it does according to our experience and yet taking up a minimum of storage space? Is it really true that *every* bird (i.e., robin, sparrow, canary, starling) is assigned to the dimension "can fly"? Does the feature "can fly" appear next to every word that refers to a bird?

From this perspective Quillian (1967) and Collins and Quillian (1969, 1972) presented a very parsimonious and space-saving storage model.

To begin with, this model has three characteristics. First, it is hierarchically arranged, i.e., the relationship of lower and higher order concepts (dog/animal) plays an important role. Second, the semantic features that characterize a concept (a word) are in each case stored only along with the highest most inclusive concept applicable. Thus the feature "can fly" is stored only with "bird" but no longer with "robin" or "sparrow." On the other hand, "yellow" is stored with canary since it applies only to it. Third, operations with and within this lexicon that take place at only *one* level occur more rapidly than those that have to cross a number of levels. This characteristic is in a way the psychological consequence of the first two and thereby makes the model empirically testable.

Collins and Quillian have demonstrated the usefulness of this model empirically (Fig. 56). If subjects are instructed to examine the sentence "a canary can fly," they require more time to judge its truthfulness, than they require for judging the sentence "a canary is yellow," or "a bird can fly." Two of their findings, however, raise some question about the usefulness of this approach. According to Quillian's model, subjects should require less

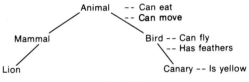

Fig. 56

time to process the sentence "the lion is a mammal" than for "the lion is an animal," because "mammal" stands between "lion" and "animal." In fact, exactly the opposite is the case.

To explain this requires the abrogation of an implicit assumption that has played a major role in feature theory from Katz and Fodor to Quillian, namely that the hierarchical structures, ordering the semantic features, are logical in nature. A system constructed according to a logical schema of *genus proximum* and *differentia specifica* appeared to be ideal for such a theory. After all, it would not be difficult to conceptualize the *differentia specifica* as an additional specifying feature that extracts a subcategory from the inclusive supracategory. But if our "inner lexicon" consists of a system of categories which are not, or at least not always, constructed according to a logical schema, then a description of the *arrangement* of these categories becomes a research task. In this connection we might mention a study by Henley (1969) who found that most people divide the animal kingdom according to the dimensions of size and ferocity. Another dimension encompasses farm animals (e.g., chicken *and* cow), while the elephant is in a class by itself. In light of these findings, it is not surprising that the cognitive path from "lion" to "animal" is shorter than that from "lion" to "mammal."

There is yet another critical consideration with more broad theoretical implications. Feature theories conceptualize semantic features as designating membership in particular categories. All words which share the feature "living" are equivalent *in this respect* and not distinguishable beyond that. *All* words marked by this feature are equal members of the category of words which may be combined with such verbs as "to die" or "to move." In the same way, *all* words belonging to the category "animal" are subject to the same rights and duties that arise from their membership in this category.

Is that a realistic assumption? Does speech function solely by regulating combinations of categories without differentiating further within these categories? We answered this question in the negative when we viewed categories to be exclusively syntactic in nature. This was, in fact, the reason for introducing the addition of semantic determinants to syntactic categories, as was shown in Johnson's studies. Are we making a similar error if we now conceptualize these determinants as well to be similarly defined in terms of features that apply equally to all single words belonging to that category? Are "eagle," "chicken," and "sparrow" identical members of the category "bird," because they all share the features "physical object," "alive," "animal," "can fly," "lay eggs"?

In a series of studies, Eleanor Rosch-Heider showed that this is not the case. For example, her studies in 1973 show that the language user does not view all of the words characterized by the feature "fruity" to be *equally* "fruity." An apple is far more "fruity" than say an olive or a fig. Malaria is more of an illness than rheumatism. Among all the colors that are unquestionably red, there are some which are more typically red than others. An eagle is more of a bird than a chicken.

Such findings cause us to abandon the view that semantic categories are simply compartments into which everything, characterized in terms of the features, fits equally well. It is more likely that semantic features form a focal center with a slowly blurring surround. The definition of a crime in the vocabulary of the layman is not characterized by a listing of common features shared by *all* crimes, but is instead centered around a definite configuration, "murder."

We could add here reflections about where to draw the line between a chair and a stool (Gipper, 1959). We are reminded that the philosopher Wittgenstein repeatedly asked his reader to define what a "game" is, and to differentiate it from a nongame (1960).

How are we to conceptualize the origin of such semantic centration? Is this focus in meaning innate? Can we demonstrate that the same tendency to form "prägnant" configurations, which were described by the Gestaltists in their studies of perception, apply equally to the study of meaning? This assumption would approximate that of Bierwisch (1967) who views the semantic focal points and structures as innate, functional forms of our "mental apparatus." According to this view, features such as "living," "round," "childlike," "uncomfortable" would be part of the human biologic equipment and not subject to more or less accidental learning during the acquisition of a specific language.

This, of course, takes us into the debate about the so-called language *universals*. Semantic features, according to the notions outlined above, are not peculiar to a particular language, but to language per se. Perhaps they are even universals standing above language and determining a person's linguistic and nonlinguistic notions of his world. We will have to return to this debate when we discuss the developmental aspects of language and also when we introduce the Whorfian hypothesis that language determines our perception of the world.

Now that we have discussed the notion of "meaning as focal prototype," and raised the question about possible universals which stand above language, we could take the next step. The question is, Do the semantic structures which the language user "knows" and with which he operates also contain nonverbal components? That brings to the fore a very old tradition in psycholinguistics which remained dormant during the decades of behaviorism's domination. We are speaking here of the notion that words and sentences correspond to images.

In Chapter 7 we introduced the futile attempt to capture the essence of meaning in terms of an association between the word and its relevant image. But even if this total reduction is impossible, imagery does play an important role in the language process. Paivio (1969 and later) particularly reported evidence of this nature. Paivio proceeds from the finding that words that designate something concrete are more easily perceived, understood, and retained than words that designate something abstract. He proposes a dual-coding hypothesis to account for this fact. Concrete linguistic material is stored according to a verbal-symbolic code *and* a nonverbal imagery code as well, but abstract material is processed only in the first mode. The "knowledge" that the speech user has of the word "house," for example, consists not only of the verbal-semantic features, "physical object," "inanimate," "made of stone," but also a pictorial image of "house." If, on the other hand, we are dealing with an abstract word (e.g., "justice" or "animal"), then no such images are available.

Parenthetically, it might be said that Paivio postulates that there are two different stores involved in the processing of verbal material. With this notion Paivio approaches an extensively studied area dealing with the nature of the process and the capacities of these different systems. This is not an appropriate place to enter into this discussion.

At first Paivio proposed his dual-coding hypothesis for the processing of (single) words. Reese (1970) added further precision by suggesting that it is not so much the fact that concrete words are more easily imaged that favors their processing over abstract material, but rather that the relevant image of this word links it with a comprehensive organization. That is shown particularly when the dual-coding hypothesis is applied to the processing and retention of sentences. Begg and Paivio (1970) found that the more difficulty a subject experienced in producing images for a sentence, the worse was its retention. There are a number of investigations that suggest that it is just this merging of smaller units into larger, integrated units that assists in the processing. Each verbal item that contributed to a unified image of this kind can be used to reactivate the total unit. A verbal item that includes images among its semantic features would, on the one hand, facilitate the formation of units (e.g., in a sentence), but, on the other hand, would also be more "accessible" within the "inner lexicon" because of its unifying and organizational characteristics.

There are also findings, however, that speak against such a theory of the effects of imagery. For example, sentences consisting of high imagery words are indeed more quickly verified than those consisting of low imagery, abstract words, but the time required is far below that which has generally been found for the formation of images (Jorganson and Kintsch, 1973). According to Holyoak (1974), it may not be so much the fact that there are two different stores, both of which process concrete sentences but only one of which processes abstract ones, but it may be that abstract sentences are generally "more complicated semantically" than those which are concrete.

With this we have reached a point that can no longer be subsumed under the heading of *semantic features*. Under this rubric we can still accept the notion of high or low imagery as a feature of a verbal item, we can even accept the notion that high imagery features facilitate unit formation, but the concept of complexity is no longer related to the characteristics or features of a single, verbal item (i.e., word or lexis) but to a more comprehensive structure.

This also implies, however, that with the introduction of the concept of semantic complexity (and all that it implies), we are moving away from the model that attempts to explain the dynamics of the sentence in terms of the rules of syntax and the features of words. As we begin our discussion of *semantic structure*,[6] let us return once again to a now familiar place, namely Johnson's findings and interpretations and their extension (or refutation or clarification) by Engelkamp.

Let us begin with a very vague formulation. A sentence consists of a dynamic, semantic structure that can be more or less complex. What type of structure can this be?

Fillmore (1968a) answers the question for linguistics. The predicate is the focal point of the sentence. Depending on its meaning, the predicate demands or facilitates certain supplementations, the arguments. For Fillmore and other representatives of generative semantics, the primary semantic structures of a sentence, which are the object of our search, are predicate and argument. These are *dynamic* structures, because an "agent" is only an agent at the bidding of and for that particular predicate. These are *deep* structures which can be transformed to surface structures in a number of ways. If the role of the agent is unoccupied, for example, it can be assumed by the instrument using a substantive in the nominative case, e.g., the knife cuts bread. If, in a particular sentence, the role of agent is occupied, the instrument for cutting has to be incorporated in the surface structure by means of "with," e.g., "Father is cutting the bread with a knife."

Engelkamp (1973) picks up on Fillmore's notions and attempts to use them in order to clarify the relationships that determine the psychological factors of sentence processing. He constructed three different types of sentences that we introduced earlier:

(K) The soldier with the letter worked on the sculpture.

(N) The soldier with the weapon worked on the sculpture.

(V) The soldier with the chisel worked on the sculpture.

---

[6] One could claim, of course, that we already dealt with semantic structures when we discussed "meaning as association." But here the term *dynamic* structures implies that one component demands the other.

These are distinguishable only by the phrase "with the . . . ." In the case of the sentence type (V), this phrase is an argument of the verb; in type (N), it is more an argument of the subject if one transforms "soldier" to "man with a weapon"; whereas in type (K), the phrase appears to be independent, i.e., it is conceived as neither belonging to the verb nor the subject.

A retention experiment in the Johnson tradition showed that sentences of type (K) are more difficult to remember than those of type (N) or (V). Engelkamp interprets his findings as follows: (K)-type sentences are more complicated because in addition to the structures that link "soldier" with "worked on the sculpture", there is an additional one (such as "soldier possesses letter") that must be stored. In contrast to this, the relevant phrase in the sentence type (V) is directly anchored to the predicate, and in the case of sentence type (N) somewhat less directly tied to the agent of the predicate.

Engelkamp presents additional data that confirm the assumption that semantic structures play a determining role in the (memory) processes of sentences. Subjects who are able to recall the predicate of a sentence are also likely to recall its noun, *if* it was an argument of the predicate. They are less likely to recall it if it cannot be conceptualized as an argument of the predicate.

In perception experiments, Hörmann and Lazarus (1976) obtained data pointing in the same direction. If "white noise" impedes the perception of a complex sentence, verb recognition encounters the greatest difficulty. Once the verb has been recognized, however, it is highly likely that the subject and object of the sentence will also be recognized. In contrast, recognition of the subject and object in no way increases the likelihood of recognizing the verb.

The analysis of a sentence apparently involves *dynamic* processes in which the predicate plays a central role. *One* of the determinants of these dynamic articulations are the predicate/argument structures, but they are by no means the only ones. For example, according to Bond and Gray (1973), it is likely that the listener articulates a sentence not only in terms of content (i.e., the syntactical and semantical relationships), but also in terms of the pattern of intonation with which it is spoken and the length of its phrases. Presumably we are dealing here with a complex interaction. The semantic structure determines what constitutes a phrase and what is to be stored jointly; conversely, the storage capacity also determines what can be conceived of as belonging together.

Kintsch's (1974) studies are based on a system similar to Engelkamp's. Here the basic structures are called *propositions,* i.e., aggregates of word concepts where one serves as a predicate while the other functions as an argument. Each argument is cast in a specific semantic role. The time required to read a particular text is determined by the number of such propositions, while the length of the text (i.e., the number of words) is relatively unimportant. In this task the reader finds it easier to process and store propositions consisting of familiar elements (word concepts) than those which introduce new concepts. Apparently, the new concept has to be coded first in such a way that it fits into the proposition.

Fortuitously we have now reached a totally different sphere, one which in traditional linguistics is separated from our previous topics by a deep moat. We have crossed the line between sentence and text. Let us remember that up to now the sentence has been the most important and most dominant unit. Generally this still holds for linguistics. The sentence is the playing field and domain of grammar. References pointing beyond the sentence we find in phenomena such as pronominality.

The issues that we discussed in this chapter were related to the semantic structures *of the sentence* as well. In order to determine the sphere of activity of these dynamic semantic structures, however, we now find it necessary to include the context beyond the sentence. For example, in order to determine the effect of the number of propositions on the speed with which a sentence or text is read, one must take into consideration whether the word concepts forming the proposition have previously occurred in the text, i.e., are part of the context. In other words, we are unable to investigate successfully the processes of applying specific (e.g., semantic) structures, without taking into consideration the speaker/listener's momentary set. The way in which a particular sentence is perceived and retained is not (only) a function of the sentence's deep structure, no matter how subtly its syntactic and semantic organization have been understood, but is a function of *all* factors that participate in the processing of the sentence. This, of course, includes factors related to context and, in a later part of our discussion, we will see that "context" must not be too narrowly defined.

Before we consider this point, let us turn to another problem, which at first glance may not be relevant here, namely the development and acquisition of speech. It is appropriate to do so here because we are going to be guided by the following reflections: Predicate-argument structures, which we introduced as dynamic centers of sentences (and maybe texts), *could be* part of the basic cognitive equipment that enables man to acquire his native language. Are agent and action, action and object, the intuitive forms enabling the human mental apparatus to gain systematic insight into his world? Do these basic structures of language reflect the schema with which we contemplate our world?

CHAPTER 11

The Developmental Psychology of Language Acquisition

The role of imitation—The language acquisition device (LAD)—Pivot-grammars—R. Brown's studies of Adam and Eve—The sensory-motor stage of intelligence—MacNamara's theory—The role of intention in language learning—Global behavior as the basis for language acquisition—The problem of the one-word sentence—The grammar of action—Strategies in language acquisition.

In the preceding chapters our discussion centered primarily on two broad concepts: *syntax* and *meaning*. These concepts were first introduced in terms of their linguistic conception, i.e., within the models responsible for their development and for which they had validity in the first place. We then attempted to "psychologize" the concepts, and where necessary their theoretical context, insofar as we wished to employ them for the prediction and explanation of empirically observable verbal behavior. Our approach was predominantly oriented toward general psychological principles. We spoke of *the* language user and we ignored individual differences.

Aside from this general psychological approach, there has always been another area of interest to the student of language, namely that of developmental psychology. The fact that we can observe in every child the ontogenetic development of language has consistently demanded that models of language and language use permit the inclusion of the phenomena and stages of language acquisition.

How does the child acquire his mother tongue? Surely the oldest answer given is, through *imitation*. But what does that mean?

First of all we have the fact that the verbal utterances of the child become more and more like those of the adult until, at age six or seven, they become almost indistinguishable. It is assumed that imitation is the cause of this increasing similarity, but this inference is by no means conclusive. If two people stop at the roadside, one after the other, we would likely assume that the cause is some environmental factor (e.g., traffic density) rather than imitation (Whitehurst and Vasta, 1975).

If imitation were the major factor in the acquisition of language, as is assumed by the layman, we would expect to find a high correlation between the frequency of occurrence of certain words or syntactic structures in adult language and the sequence of their acquisition by the child. That which occurs most frequently would have to be learned earlier, acquired through imitation, than that which occurs infrequently in adult language. In fact, this is not the case (Brown and Herrnstein, 1975, p. 480).

Those who postulate that imitation is the decisive factor in the acquisition of language often view language as an enormous collection of words and sentences that are slowly acquired by the child (through imitation of utterances of those around him), and which are then reproduced on more or less appropriate occasions. The increase in grammatically correct and semantically and pragmatically appropriate utterances, observed by the developmental psychologist, can then be attributed to either an increase in the ability to imitate, or to a particular learning process that leads to the gradual elimination of ungrammatical utterances.

We have to reflect on this last point, because the psychology of learning offers an alluring model of the "filtering" notion described above.

Classical learning theory has basically two possibilities of interpreting language acquisition: either, following Pavlov, the conditioning process can be said to produce a *stimulus* substitution so that the designated object is replaced by the sign, or, following Thorndike, conditioning leads to *response* substitution so that a less economical response is replaced by a verbal one.

Both conceptions have weaknesses that reveal themselves whenever the attempt is made to explain language acquisition as a conditioning process. The commonly applied concept of reinforcement is unable to account for the speed of acquisition or for the stability of meanings thus acquired.

The difficulties arising from the Pavlovian view have already been discussed in detail. We must now take a second look at Thorndike's view because its further development has led, in Hull's work, to the most sophisticated theory of learning and, in Skinner's work, to the most radical conception of verbal behavior.

According to Thorndike, the organism spontaneously produces many different modes of behavior. Among these occurs accidentally a certain mode of behavior that corresponds to the requirements of the stimulus-situation and therefore leads to a state that satisfies the organism. This satisfying state acts as a reinforcement of the immediately preceding mode of behavior, which then is more likely than before to occur again in the same stimulus situation. In Thorndike's view, trial and error leads to the selection of the mode of behavior which is followed by reinforcement. The organism must do something; and this act must be followed by reinforcement for an association to be formed between the S (situation) and the R (this mode of behavior), so that, in other words, learning takes place. Similarly, in Skinner's conception, a mode of behavior is learned if its execution is followed by reinforcement. It is singled out, by a process called "shaping," from among the mass of unnecessary and undesirable modes of behavior.

Now, even the psychology of learning recognizes a number of phenomena which indicate the possibility of learning without doing: latent learning explored by Tolman, latent extinction, learning with insight, and so forth.

Such phenomena are particularly common in language learning. The parents of a child do not wait for the chance appearance, among the random vocalizations, of a word or a word-like sound sequence and then reinforce it by a reward. Language learning is not based on the principle of trial and error. Nor are these vocalizations accidental preforms of words produced spontaneously by the child and then remolded by a gradual Skinnerian shaping-process. A child does not produce a vast number of random sound sequences, nor does it live in an environment constantly handing out differential rewards; consequently, the view of language acquisition as a selection process can hardly be justified. The model of a selective learning process in the sense of Thorndike or Skinner is too artificial to serve adequately as a model of language acquisition.

But there are further reasons why this model must be rejected. According to others who represent this view, the child learns those combinations of sounds with which he can control his environment (Brown and Dulaney, 1958; Brown, 1958a). But the child also learns elements or aspects of language (such as allophones) which have no sign function and which therefore do not, as these theories claim, have instrumental function. And, at least for the early stages of language acquisition, it is valid to say that the infant could manage without the instrument of language. He will be fed even if he does not speak and only screams, and therefore fails to utter any conventional signs.

The model of *language acquisition through selective reinforcement of utterances,* which goes back to Thorndike, and is upheld today above all by Skinner, must therefore be discarded for a variety of reasons.

That by no means settles the issue of "language learning through imitation." If selective reinforcement in a trial and error process can be eliminated, there still remains the possibility that a less precise learning by imitation is involved in the process. Indeed, some kind of imitation *must* come into play, because, after all, every child acquires the language that is spoken around him. Imitation is a most likely explanation for simple labeling. As late as 1964, Jenkins and Palermo described the beginning of the child's speech as "a form of imitation followed by a number of simple S-R connections between verbal labels and salient features of the environment to which they become attached. With the store of labels available, the child attaches words to other words in sequences, and the ordering or structuring begins" (p. 165).

That is surely oversimplified. It is perhaps possible to learn "book," "dog," or "cup" in this manner, but on no account can "beautiful," "or," or "why" be learned this way. We have already indicated this difficulty in Chapter 8. But even if we could employ this learning of labels by imitation for the acquisition of the entire vocabulary, we would still be left with the problem of whether imitation can serve as a useful explanation of the acquisition of grammar, i.e., the proper structuring and word-sequencing of sentences. Humans are able to use language *creatively,* i.e., they are able to produce and understand even those grammatically and semantically "correct" utterances that they have never before heard in this form. This fact is a potent argument against a much too naive notion of imitation as the sole factor in language acquisition.

There are a number of additional arguments against this position arising from empirical studies. It has been shown, for example, that the child relatively rarely imitates adult utterances spontaneously, once he has passed through the early stages of language acquisition. Lenneberg (1962) described a case of language pathology in a child who learned to understand speech, but due to organic damage, was unable to produce verbal utterances (and therefore imitate them). Finally, it is very difficult to induce a child to imitate (i.e., repeat) utterances that are grammatically more complex than is appropriate for the developmental stage of the particular child (cf. Whitehurst and Vasta, 1975).

We can summarize our discussion of the problem of "language acquisition by imitation" as follows: At best, imitation can be accepted as a partial explanation of language learning. We know of no "mechanism" in the psychology of learning (such as selective reinforcement) that could be responsible for the decrease in the child's incorrect and the increase in correct verbal utterances. This "failure" of the psychology of learning, as well as the creative nature of language, has led the proponents of generative linguistics to reject empirical explanations of language acquisition and caused them to espouse a nativist approach, to which we now turn our attention.

Let us recall that the competent speaker/listener has such knowledge as enables him to produce and understand *all* grammatical utterances that are possible in his language. He possesses a set of rules for generating sentences. Where did he get it? According to Chomsky and his followers, he can have acquired it only by abstracting, from the verbal utterances surrounding him as a child, those rules according to which the utterances were constructed. To do this, one must postulate some "apparatus" which, so to speak, produces the grammar from the perceived utterances. After all, the competent adult speaker/listener is in possession of this grammar. This "apparatus" is called Language Acquisition Device (LAD). (Related to the following discussion, see Levelt's (1975) excellent treatise.)

This conceptualization brought about a sweeping change in the interpretation of infantile speech. Until then, the child's language had been interpreted as an imperfect and incomplete adult language (because the child has not learned to imitate it sufficiently!). Now, along with the concept of the LAD, we find the notion that the child speaks *correctly, according to rules* at *every* level of language development, albeit not according to the rules of adult

grammar but rather according to his own, perhaps more or less idiosyncratic, infantile grammar. This is the beginning of developmental psycholinguistics' search for the nature of the rules of infantile utterances. We
shall return to this repeatedly.

If the LAD is an "apparatus" that produces grammar from perceived
linguistic utterances, then this apparatus must of necessity have an inner
structure of its own. This structure, which generates an English grammar
from English utterances and a Chinese grammar from Chinese utterances,
can itself not be learned, argue the advocates of generative linguistics. They
claim, first, that there is no known learning mechanism (see above) and,
second, that the cultural differences between linguistic communities are too
great to justify the assumption that these universal structures, represented
by the LAD, originate from analogous cultural factors.[1] Therefore, if this
structure is not acquired individually, it must be innate.

In this way, the notions about language acquisition come under the influence of a strong nativistic and, therefore, biologic orientation.[2] As a transition to the theoretical level to be examined now in detail, we cite G.A. Miller:
"It is difficult to imagine how children could acquire language so rapidly
from parents who understand it so poorly unless they were already tuned by
evolution to select just those aspects that are universally significant. There
is, in short, a large biological component that shapes our human languages"
(1965, p. 17).

Here maturation is contrasted with the learning aspect which had hitherto
been stressed. It is true that Carmichael (1964), in a comprehensive survey,
had already shown that the anatomical and physiological basis of the receptor and motor mechanisms of speech are ready to function at birth, but that
the actual functioning of these mechanisms was still dependent upon further
cerebral maturation after birth. Not until then, says Carmichael, does the
infant reach the state of "speech readiness" which is the precondition for
the acquisition of meaningful linguistic patterns.

This emphasis on the biologic and developmental aspect comes out particularly clearly in Miller's account of causative factors in language acquisition: "He learns the language because he is shaped by nature to pay attention to it, to notice and remember and use significant aspects of it" (1965, p.
20). The child is capable of abstracting, for example, grammatical structures
from the incoming flow of speech and to learn these because he pays
attention only to a restricted number of possibilities.

This restricted number of possibilities is a given for the LAD. In this
respect, the generative linguist can say, for example, that the conception of
the *sentence* as such is innate, or, putting it differently, that it represents a
linguistic universal applicable to *all* languages.

---

[1] This is a point of contention, as we will find later on.
[2] However, this biologic orientation is contrary to the view of the orthodox generativists who
propose that competence is unitary and either totally present or not present at all.

The process of selecting linguistically significant details from the flood of other events which in the past was supposed to find an explanation in differential reinforcement, is now looked upon as a biologically given fact which cannot be reduced any further.

In this connection we might remind ourselves of a pronouncement by Lenneberg, cited at the beginning of this book (p. 2), which stated that the capacity to acquire and use a human language does not depend on the fact that the organism is intelligent or has a large brain, but that it is a human organism (1964b).

From the atomistic and therefore associationist theories of language acquisition, we move into a more biologic and more holistic climate of opinion.

Impressive evidence for biologically based determinants of language can be found in the studies of Molfese (cf. Freeman, 1973). Here it was shown that infants, long before the verbal age, show a sensitivity for verbal stimuli in the left cerebral hemisphere and for nonverbal auditory stimuli in the right hemisphere.

In a way this could be neurolinguistic evidence for the existence of that which generative grammarians wish to include in the LAD concept.

The output of this apparatus, we have learned, is a grammar (by no means *the* grammar), which corresponds to the linguistic competence of the particular individual. This notion incorporates the hypothesis that every child at the various levels of this language development, conforms to a (his!) grammar. Therefore the task is to find to which grammar the particular child conforms when he generates his utterances. Braine most of all deserves credit for attempting to write a child grammar from this point of view. Based on very exact recordings of utterances of a child (in this case Steven, 23 months old) over several weeks, Braine gains insight into what does and what does not occur (Table 14).

Asking the question, "*What* can appear *where?*" (i.e., by establishing the "privilege of occurrence"), Braine, was able to define two word classes: "X-words" and "pivots." There are only a few pivots; they appear in various combinations, mostly however in position 1 (P_1); only "do" occurs in P_2. X-words are a large open category, comprising the entire remainder of the infant's vocabulary. If the classes of the sentence constituents are defined in this way, it is possible also to describe the syntax or arrangement in which these constituents occur. Steven's syntax has two rules:

$$P_1 + X$$
$$X + P_2$$

If this represents the grammar which at that point in time was the basis for Steven's utterances, it should be possible to use it to predict[3] which utter-

---

[3] Strictly speaking it is impossible to test an hypothesis related to the competence of a speaker by means of prediction from his performance (cf. Hörmann, 1976).

Table 14.   Verbal utterances of a 23-month-old child.

want baby	it ball	get ball	there ball	that box
want car	it bang	get Betty	there book	that Dennis
want do	it checker	get doll	there doggie	that doll
want get	it daddy		there doll	that Tommy
want glasses	it Dennis	see ball	there high	that truck
want head	it doggie	see doll	there momma	
want high	it doll	see record	there record	here bed
want horsie	it fall	see Stevie	there truck	here checker
want jeep	it horsie		there byebye car	here doll
want more	it Kathy	whoa cards	there daddy truck	here truck
want page	it Lucy	whoa jeep	there momma	
want pon	it record		truck	bunny do
want purse	it shock	more ball		daddy do
want ride	it truck	more book	beeppeep bang	momma do
want up			beeppeep car	(want do)
want byebye car				

Other utterances:

bunny do sleep	baby doll	find bear	eat breakfast	
Lucy do fun	Betty pon	pon baby	two checker	
want do pon	byebye car	pon Betty	Betty byebye car	
want drive car	Candy say	sleepy bed	Lucy shutup Lucy	shutup Lucy

Based on Braine, 1963b, p. 7.

ances Steven can and cannot produce. Presumably one would find "want candy" or "want truck" but not "baby want."

We see that such *pivot grammars* describe the *general* structure according to which the particular child forms his verbal utterances. Braine's explanation of the emergence of these general structures deviates from the LAD concept. His approach is based on learning theory and introduces the concept of "contextual generalization" which he defines as follows:

"When a subject, who has experienced sentences in which a segment (morpheme, word or phrase) occurs in a certain position and context, later tends to place this segment in the same position in other contexts, the context of the segment will be said to have generalized . . ." (1963a, p. 323).

Braine made children of different age levels learn miniature artificial languages. This procedure suggested that what is learned is the localization of a linguistic unit within a larger more comprehensive unit. Unit formation, it appears, occurs on different levels so that a hierarchy of units is formed. Within the sentence it is possible to isolate, as a first unit, the so-called primary phrase ("the book," "has thrown"); within the primary phrase the units generally consist of a noun or verb and one or several words from such form classes as articles, auxiliaries, etc.; the latter indicate the relational order of content words and facilitate the recognition, identification and learning of the primary phrase. They are designated as functors or pivot words.

The primary phrase consisting of a content word and one or two pivot words is a characteristic feature of speech development. It can be seen from Table 15 below that the grammar of the child in question could be expressed in the following generative rule: first take a pivot word (i.e., a word from class M), then add a word from the large class of content words N.

These two classes, M and N, which are here needed to describe the child's grammar, no longer occur in the language of the adult. Between the stage of language development described here and that of the adult, there is not only an increase in differentiation and complexity of the generative rules that come into operation, there is also a change of the functional classification of the vocabulary, to which we are now turning. The child, for example, must learn that "a" and "two" do not belong to the same class since "a" is followed by a singular and "two" by a plural. He must also learn that the word "more" is followed by a plural of some words ("more nuts") and the singular of others ("more coffee").

Table 16 taken from Brown and Bellugi, will show the stage of differentiation attained 16 weeks after the stage described above.

In the earlier two-word utterances, the article had appeared immediately before a noun as in other examples the demonstrative. At this stage in three-word utterances the article normally occupies the first position and other modifiers ("nice," "blue") are placed between the article and the

Table 15. Noun phrases in isolation and rule for generating noun phrases at Time 1.

A coat	More coffee
A celery[1]	More nut[1]
A Becky[1]	Two sock[1]
A hands[1]	Two shoes
The top	Two tinker-toy[1]
My Mommy	Big boot
That Adam	Poor man
My stool	Little top
That knee	Dirty knee

NP → M + N

M → a, big, dirty, little, more, my, poor, that, the two.
N → Adam, Becky, boot, coat, coffee, knee, man, Mommy, nut, sock, stool, tinker-toy, top, and, very many others.

[1] Ungrammatical for an adult.
Based on Brown and Bellugi, 1964, p. 145.

Table 16. Subdivision of the modifier class at Time 2.

Obtained	Not obtained
A. Privileges peculiar to articles	
A blue flower	Blue a flower
A nice nap	Nice a nap
A your car	Your a car
A my pencil	My a pencil
B. Privileges peculiar to demonstrative pronouns	
That my cup	My that cup
That a horse	A that horse
That a blue flower	A that blue flower
	Blue a that flower

Based on Brown and Bellugi, 1964, p. 147.

noun. If a demonstrative appears, it may be placed in front of the article. At Time 1 the generative rule M + N was sufficient; to describe what is happening now requires far more complicated rules:

Dem. + Art. + M + N or
Art. + M   + N   or
Dem. + M   + N   or
Art. + N
or generalized: (Dem.) + (Art.) + (M) + N.

And six months after Time 1 of the investigation, Adam had already subdivided his large class M into five different sub-classes.

After a precise analysis of these developmental phenomena one must surely admit that "contextual generalization" is not an adequate mechanism for making these differentiations. The gradual adaptation of the child grammar to the adult grammar itself proceeds according to rules that are not explained sufficiently by the nonspecific concept of LAD. Roger Brown, undoubtedly the leading researcher in the field of language development, resorts in his explanation to a particular form of imitation and role playing which takes place between mother and child.

His observations on Adam (27 months at the start of the study), Eva (18 months), and later also Sarah, produced the results shown in Table 17. The mother says something and the infant copies it. But what is this imitation like?

The order of words remains identical. This is by no means obvious; but in this way the order of words which applies to grammatical sentences, hence their comprehensibility, is guaranteed. Only short sentences are copied

Table 17. Some imitations produced by Adam and Eva.

Model utterance	Child's imitation
Tank car	Tank car
Wait a minute	Wait a minute
Daddy's brief case	Daddy brief case
Fraser will be unhappy	Fraser unhappy
He's going out	He go out
That's an old time train	Old time train
It's not the same dog as Pepper	Dog Pepper
No, you can't write on Mr. Cromer's shoe	Write Cromer shoe

Based on Brown and Bellugi, 1964, p. 136.

completely. If the sentences exceed a length of three or more morphemes the child omits words. The cause for these omissions cannot lie in the limitations of the child's vocabulary (the omitted words are known to him) nor do the limitations of his immediate memory account for them; for the child's spontaneously produced sentences are also only of this length. It is probable that a child can only plan utterances of a restricted length.

The limitations of his planning capacity compel the child, when he copies, to omit some of the words of the model. It becomes evident that these omissions are not accidental. Omissions include inflections, auxiliaries, articles, prepositions, and conjunctions. These words are comprehensively referred to by some linguists as "functors," because their grammatical function is more important than their semantic content. Among the words copied and not omitted by the child are nouns, verbs, and adjectives, i.e., words that are important not for their function in the sentence but for their content.

The child proceeds exactly like an adult composing a message in telegraphic style: words with a high information content are kept; those with a low information content are dropped.

We are not forced, however, to assume that the child undertakes an analysis in terms of information theory followed by a sifting process of what he has heard. His procedure is facilitated by a device that is much more obvious to the ear: the child can confine himself to copying the stressed words because they are the content words.

We shall return to the role of the *stressed* words when we discuss the concept of *strategy*, i.e., the child's strategies for the analysis of perceived utterances.

Returning to Brown's studies, we find again this first division of content and pivot words which we encountered in our discussion of Braine's pivot grammars. We see that even if the child repeats words, he follows the rules of his *own* grammar.

The recordings show that it is not only the child who copies the sentences spoken by the mother, but also the mother who copies sentences first uttered by the child (Table 18). It should, of course, be noted that while the majority of the child's imitations entail a *reduction* of the heard utterance, the mother *expands* the child's utterance; and more specifically, she again adds those functors which are absent in the child's speech. Such expansions on the part of the mother were found in approximately a third of the data collected by Brown and Bellugi.

The verbal interaction between mother and child consists largely of a cycle of reductions and expansions. The modifications made by the infant are perfectly predictable, so that a machine could be programmed to turn a mother's sentences into baby-talk; but the expansions which the mother adds when she repeats the child's utterances cannot be specified so well. In the above examples the child always produces a proper name plus a common noun. The mother turns these into quite a variety of sentences. Thus the child's "Eve lunch" is not expanded into "Eve's lunch" nor into "Eve will have lunch," but into "Eve is having lunch," because in this particular situation this expansion is more appropriate. Therefore the expansion encodes aspects which the child, instead of encoding, had left to the situation to express. The expansion on the part of the mother translates from the situational into the verbal the functional entity of a message which had relied less on specific verbal elements. The inserted functors give information about the time at which the action is set (e.g., in the past), whether it is completed, and what the relationship is between participants; e.g., "Throw daddy" will be interpreted more precisely as "Throw it to daddy." By expanding the child's sentences, the authors argue, the mother teaches more than just grammar; she teaches a world-view.

Could these expansions be a preferred control mechanism used by the adult to guide the child's language acquisition? Cazden, a student of Brown, pursued this possibility by means of an experiment in which one group of children were subject to an extensive "expansion" program, while a control group grew up without such a program. It was shown that the expansions

Table 18. Expansions of child speech produced by mother.

Child	Mother
Baby highchair	Baby is in the highchair
Mommy eggnog	Mommy had her eggnog
Eve lunch	Eve is having lunch
Mommy sandwich	Mommy'll have a sandwich
Sat wall	He sat on the wall
Throw Daddy	Throw it to Daddy
Pick glove	Pick the glove up

Based on Brown and Bellugi, 1964, p. 141.

carried out by adults on the utterances of the children had no influence on language development.

A more critical look at these expansions leads to the question whether the child in fact *means* that which the adult makes of his infantile utterances by means of expansion. Is there not a danger that the adult (and following him, the psychologist) attempts to overinterpret what the child says? We can ask this question differently: What linguistic knowledge and what intentions are involved in a child's utterance? What does a child really *mean* and what *does* he really *know* it he says "mommy sock" when he sees mother's socks on a chair, but also a few days later, when mother puts his socks on him. This is the problem area to which Brown addresses himself in his later studies.

In a few cases it is relatively simple to determine the level of a child's knowledge of linguistic rules. That is particularly true in those cases where the child overgeneralizes the rule, applying it to situations where they would not be applied by an adult. An error of this sort cannot be a desultory imitation (after all, the child has never heard the relevant form), but must originate in the child's "stock of rules."

If a child employs the plural correctly and says "dogs," it cannot be inferred whether he imitates a particular word (perhaps he has heard his parents say this word) or whether he has already mastered the plural rule and constructs plurals accordingly. But if the child says, "Two mans," the mistake indicates that he has begun to construct forms according to rules— even though in this instance the use of the rule was inappropriate. He is unlikely to have ever heard "mans," but constructs this word according to the rules applicable, for example, to "dogs."

Modifying this incidental observation into an experimental procedure, collaborators of Brown, in particular, have carried out systematic studies. One of these investigations, a study by Berko (1958), will be described.

A total of 50 children (one group of 4½-year-olds, another group of 5½-year-olds) were shown line drawings as illustrated in the accompanying figure (Fig. 57).

The rule of plural formation is studied in the following way. The investigator points to the first picture and says, "This is a wug. Now there is

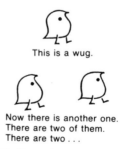

This is a wug.

Now there is another one.
There are two of them.
There are two . . .

Fig. 57 (From Berko, 1958, p. 154)

another one (second picture). There are two of them. There are two . . . . .''
If the child has mastered the rule he will complete the sentence and say "two
wugs". The mastery of the rule for the comparison of adjectives is tested
with another example. The child is shown a picture of a spotted dog, next to
it a dog with more spots, and next to him again a dog with many more spots.
The experimenter points to the first dog and says: "This dog has quirks on
him. This dog has more quirks on him. And this dog has even more quirks on
him. This dog is quirky. This dog is . . . And this dog is the . . . .'' If the
child employs the rule for the comparison of adjectives, he will insert
"quirkier" and "quirkiest."

Berko's investigation shows how these rules gradually appear during the
growth of the child; but there are considerable differences in difficulty of
different grammar rules. Unknown words are treated by children according
to the rules that are applied most frequently and have the smallest number of
exceptions.

Brown's search for the rules that the child actually employs in his utterances is, in fact, a search for the rules that determine the sequences of words
in a sentence or utterance, because the rule-like nature of language primarily
manifests itself in the word order. (At least this holds true for most of the
Indo-Germanic languages.) Thus Brown is primarily interested in the two-
word sentence.

The active verbal expressions of the child, however, begin with the *one-
word utterance*. In order to "understand" and theoretically interpret this
phenomenon, we must set aside Brown's query for the moment, because it
arose from the preoccupation with issues related to the child's knowledge of
grammar. Before we can even begin to speculate about this knowledge, we
must ask more globally, what is it that begins to surface here, what is the
situational context from which it arises, and how should one conceptualize
the transition from the preverbal to the verbal stage?

This takes us of necessity into a more biologic, more wholistic environment. We search not only (psycholinguistically) for the rules that apply to
verbal utterances, but now we ask (in terms of a psychology of language)
about the *function* required of that utterance in the given situation which
embraces the child and adult, the speaker and the listener.

A modern work on child language begins with the sentence, "A child is
born a speaker and born into a world of speakers" (Lewis, 1963). (a) The
infant utters sounds from the first days of his life; (b) he responds to the
human voice; (c) the mother responds to the child's voice; and, (d) she speaks
to him. These are the four fundaments on which later speech development is
based. If one of them is absent, the whole structure of later linguistic growth
is imperiled. From the very beginning, even before speech proper, constant
use of speech characterizes the child's environment. Long before the sound
utterances of the child have any definite meaning, they serve—though
imperfectly—the same goals as the skilled language use of the adult.

Therefore, it is false to think in terms of the child facing a world to be depicted and to be named by him; instead, one must think much more of a dynamic whole comprising the two poles: child and world.

A powerful interpretation of the infant's situation is to be found in Bloch's *Tübinger Introduction to Philosophy:*

"A self alive does not yet mean awareness of self—and least of all awareness of its activities. All the creature feels is hunger and want . . . All is centered around this non-aware self; yet it is not self-sufficient; . . . its wants make it dependent on the outside world; its own hunger takes it beyond itself. 'I want' is the first glimmer of awareness" (pp. 12 f.). The infant is inevitably a part of this dynamic unity. "Even to sense its own existence the creature must reach for something beyond" (p. 11).

The experience of this dynamic reality—and with it the experience of being part of it—can, according to Church, be characterized by three components: realism, phenomenalism, and dynamism. This is to be understood as follows. All events are equally real; as yet there is no distinction between doing and wishing, or between fear and pain. All events are accepted as they appear. The closer in time two events appear, the closer appears their "causal" relationship. The infant sees his world as endowed with energies which make him—through the phenomena of animism, anthropomorphism, and magicalism—subject and object of active processes.

Perception and action, looked at from "inside," are hardly different. Both involve, as Church says, total mobilization of the organism.

> Under the concept of "mobilization" Church subsumes what, on the stimulus side, is referred to as "attention" and, on the response side, as "set"; it is therefore a form of directed concentration upon an activity.

Similarly, Piaget starts from the principle of this primordial lack of differentiation between action and perception. According to him, the child, interacting with his environment during the so-called sensorimotor period, learns, through the interrelatedness of action and perception, that he can effect and cancel constantly changing centrations in relation to his environment. Yet the physical object remains constant. This object-constancy is a first knowledge about the world arising from the flow of sensorimotor acts. The independent existence of objects is a schema emerging as something that remains constant in time and space. It is not only the independence of objects which emerges as a constancy schema, however, but also specific acts and the self as initiator and sustainer of such acts. What emerges as a schema are specific roles in the dynamic relationship between act and actor, act and instrument, etc.

There is a direct connection between this Piagetian notion and Fillmore's view that the case and predicate/argument structures are the focal points of verbal utterances. These are central *linguistic* structures, their schemata determine the construction of our notion of the world. A study by Huttenlocher et al. clearly shows how the child's language comprehension is determined by this early differentiation between an active "agent" and a rather passive object serving as a goal of the action. Children were given toys with which to act out sentences like these:

The green car pushes the red car.

The green car is pushed by the red car.

One of the cars was fixed so that the other had to be placed in relation to it. It is much easier for the children to move the car which is the "agent" than the one which is the "object" in relation to the "fixed" agent. The all-embracing dynamic that organizes the child's perception and action is not the only one that must be considered in an explanation of language learning. As we have mentioned before, the child is faced with the dynamics of the total situation which is comprised of speaker and listener, action and sound.

Originally, action and sound are not distinguished in their meaningfulness. The question, therefore, is not how a primarily meaningless combination of sounds becomes meaningful (this has been the problem of all associationist theories of meaning); the question now is how, out of the flow of stimuli and modes of behavior, some which are collectively referred to as speech are singled out.

It appears, therefore, that the infant does not first learn to understand and use words; what happens is that in the total stream of behavior the verbal aspect becomes more and more clearly differentiated. Well before speech sounds have established unambiguous and socially binding relationships to other events, and therefore have acquired semantic meaning, they already have functional value in the totality of behavior.

From this point of view, we should once more consider a model previously discussed, Bloomfield's diagram of the speech event. The usual behavior sequence leads from stimulus (S) to response (R): S→R. Jill sees an apple (S), grasps and eats it (R). If this simple sequence meets an obstacle, e.g., the tree is too high for Jill to reach the apple, a change in the behavior sequence occurs. Jill sees the apple (S), says something (r) that causes Jack (s) to pick the apple and to give it to Jill (R): S→r . . . s→R. For Jill the direct action (R) is replaced by a verbal one (r); for Jack a direct stimulus (S) is replaced by a verbal one (s); in Jill's case it is a Thorndike response substitution; in Jack's it is a Pavlov stimulus substitution. The simple S→R sequence, the "speechless reaction," occurs within one person; it becomes a verbal reaction which links two persons with each other—a reaction which, as Bloomfield said, is "mediated by speech."

Bloomfield's mediation is an interpersonal event; it becomes—as we shall see later—through a process of internalization, an intrapersonal mediation in Vigotsky's sense as, for example, in Osgood's theory.

In Bloomfield's conception the speech act is the mediating link between two practical events. But from the point of view of our previous discussion, it is important to remember that the speech act does not link two separate practical events; on the contrary, in the "preverbal" stage these practical events were contiguous members of the dynamic structure of a behavioral unity.

The speech act does not link what previously had been apart. (This is the reason why the concept of association cannot be the main key to the speech event.) The speech act makes it possible to part what previously had been combined. Speech makes it possible to pull practical events apart.

> The relationship between practical events and speech events is repeated on a higher level in Weizsäcker's conception of the relationship between language and formula. "A formula makes sense only through the connection which has been established by words." "There is always a known area of shared knowledge within which comprehension is quite adequate enough to make it possible to use this common ground for an advance upon new fields" (1960, pp. 144 and 152).

The practical events can be seen to be distributed upon conduct in two directions: the speaker's and the listener's. The more these two forms of conduct are pulled apart, the more reliance must be placed on the speech act.

Speech bridges practical events and is crystallized out of the behavioral totality. This point of view can be related to the tendency to fall back on nonverbal behavior whenever verbal communication is inadequate. The scientist, for example, uses "operational" definitions; he reverts to operations or actions.

And, vice versa, the more clearly defined the business of practical events is, the less care need be taken of the verbal link. "Exactitude of the object . . . permits inexactitude of language" (Weizsäcker, 1959, p. 139). To summarize, we can say: language is the continuation of action with other means.

This proposition is to be further clarified by the following discussion. To begin with, Bloomfield's definition of meaning should be recalled. Meaning of a word is the situation in which a speaker utters it plus the response it calls forth in the hearer. We recognize now that this definition is to be interpreted as far less "primitive" and "associationist" than Bloomfield presumably had intended it to be understood. The word whose meaning is in question is, at first, no independent element to be regarded as distinct from the stimulus-response sequence of the situation and as labelling the sequence. The child, to begin with, does not understand what a word as such means, but he does understand what a person talking to him means (Church, 1961, p. 61).

With that we have reached what is probably the most acceptable, contemporary theory of language acquisition, that of MacNamara (1972). The child is able to understand what the (adult) speaker means because both are involved in the dynamics of the total situation. The child can then use this comprehension to determine the linguistic code used by the speaker in formulating the utterance. Putting it another way, because the young child already understands the speaker's intended meaning, he is able to infer the meaning of the utterance. Thus speech comprehension is older than speech production, but "understanding others" is even older yet.

From this perspective the philosophical and linguistic notion that the imperative is the basic form of verbal utterance becomes attractive to the psychologist.

Heidegger argues: "Calling is fundamentally not naming; it is the reverse; naming is a kind of calling in its original sense of 'calling hither' or 'summoning' " (1954, p. 151).

Wittgenstein regards the command call which the individual directs to his situational partner as the nucleus around which an emerging language-game becomes crystallized.

Similarly Höpp (1970) views the "Einerspruch" as the acoustical tool mobilizing the individual contributions for meaningful communication and work-sharing acts. We would go further than Höpp and assert that the imperative is not so much an intervention in the action of the addressee of the message than in his conscious awareness (cf. Hörmann, 1976).

This notion, that language acquisition arises from an awareness of the intentions of the speaker, is expressed most precisely by Schlesinger (1971a). According to him, the child perceives the total situation as a "structure of intention markers." The actual task of language acquisition, or more precisely of learning to use the language, consists of acquiring the rules that govern the transformation of these structures of intention into linguistic surface structures. The child is able to perceive these rules because the verbal utterances addressed to him by the adult are situation-specific and usually highly redundant. Because a child who is past the earliest development is able to grasp the dynamic structure of the situation, and because he is already able to classify object and agent in preverbal cognition, he can use this available knowledge to decipher the linguistic formulation of that situation.

In communicating with the child, the adult characteristically uses two speech forms which in this sense particularly facilitate understanding, namely question and command. While the normal conversation within the family typically contains 1 to 25 percent interrogative utterances, one finds up to 50 percent of such utterances addressed to the baby.

According to MacNamara and others, it is not so much the meaning of words that is learned by the child, but rather how to verbally label an already available meaning, concept, or idea.

One can also show this preverbal existence of the concept in the case of Washoe, the chimpanzee, who challenged many fond linguistic and philosophical convictions by acquiring and using some 200 signs of the

American Sign Language (Gardner, 1969). Washoe learned the sign for "open" originally related to a door. Immediately, without any further training, she was able to employ this sign not only with respect to other doors, but with respect to a cola bottle and to a briefcase which she suspected contained food. Apparently, even here the concept of "opening" is one that stands ready to be assigned a verbal sign.

That is not to say, by any means, that these notions or concepts are in fact innate. It also does not mean that they are always "attainable" to all persons in the same manner. Most importantly, nothing is said about whether or not in later stages of speech development, prior linguistic forms determine what concepts will be formed. We will say more about that in the next chapter. Let us now return to the main theme of our discourse.

Perceiving the origin of the sign in the dynamics of the total situation makes comprehensible why the philosophy of language had so little relevance to the psychology of language until Peirce and Morris had introduced a pragmatic element. Looked at in this light, language does not appear as the sum of basically separate parts; and further, the concept of association loses its explanatory power. To sum it up in Humboldt's terms, "Speech is not put together out of words that precede it; on the contrary, words are singled out from the totality of speech" (1907 edition, p. 72).

How very much the comprehension of utterances of early childhood is dependent upon the support of the total situation is indicated by Sherman's experiments. A number of subjects, mothers and nurses, were asked to state what caused an infant, lying behind a screen, to cry. The actual causes of the cries were varied: hunger or pain, etc. The observers were unable to distinguish between the cries and to identify their "meaning."

And looking at the problem from the other side, we cite a case to demonstrate how much the situation which surrounds and accompanies the speech event in the narrower sense is the carrier of meaning. Meumann asked his little son in German (his mother tongue), "Wo ist das Fenster?" and the child pointed in the right direction. He then asked him in French, "Où est la fenêtre?" Again the child pointed to the window; and equally so in response to the English question, "Where is the window?" Meumann went on and asked him in German, "Where is the door?" and the child again pointed to the window! The child did not react to the meaning of individual words but to the dynamic configuration of the total situation.

The close interaction between word and total situation becomes clearer through Luria's experiments (1959) on the directive function of speech. A child at the age of approximately 1;3 is shown a toy fish.[4]

The experimenter said, "Give me the fish"; the infant followed the instruction. Next, a toy cat was placed between the infant and the fish. The

---

[4] Translator's note. In this notation, the figure before the semi-colon indicates years and the figure after months, i.e., 1;3 reads "one year three months".

experimenter said, "Give me the fish." The infant reached toward the fish but, as his hand passed near the cat, seized the cat, and handed it to the experimenter. In a dynamically unambiguous situation the word can already perform its directive role. But as soon as there is a possibility of conflict in the dynamics of the situation, the child cannot yet resist the orientational pull of the situation. The forces determining the dynamics of the situation do not lie in the words on the one side and the stimulus configuration on the other, but partly also in the "mobilization" of the infant as determined by the immediately preceding modes of behavior. In another series of experiments, Luria placed before the child a tumbler and a cup. A coin was hidden under the cup; the child lifted the cup and picked up the coin. Having repeated this sequence four times, the experimenter placed the coin under the tumbler within sight of the child and asked again, "Find the coin." If the child is immediately allowed to pick up the coin, most subjects (aged 1;4 to 1;6) go straight for the tumbler. However, if a pause of 10 seconds is introduced between instruction and action, the motor habit, i.e., the old mobilization, is dominant: the child reaches for the cup.

In a third experiment, after the coin had regularly been placed under the tumbler, it was placed under the cup without the child seeing this. The experimenter said, "The coin is under the cup." The child, following the dynamics of the situation, reached for the tumbler. To put it in different terms: the word achieves an independent status only gradually and relatively late, and its dominance over the dynamics of the situation, comprising both child and situation, is an end phase.

To what extent reliance upon the total situation can delay the developmental differentiation of language can be illustrated by the speech development of twins. Twins, as siblings of the same age who may even be monozygotic, find themselves in similar situations. We recall what was said earlier (pp. 3 ff.) about the interaction between spontaneity and life space. If twins grow up together, they share common life experiences to such an extent, and patterns of behavior fit together so well, that additional verbal guidance is hardly necessary. The mutual understanding can still be carried entirely by the parallel structure of practical events. Correspondingly, language development of twins in comparison with only children is delayed (Davis, 1937; Forchhammer, 1939; and Zazzo, 1960). This delay can be even more marked in one of the twins if the other assumes the role of "ambassador," making contact with the environment (thereby normalizing his own speech development) and transmitting to the other twin the verbal signals of the external world in form of behavioral clues. Frequently the speech development in the latter partner, in comparison with speech development of his contemporaries, is seriously retarded.

Luria and Yudovich (1959) have thrown further light on the close interaction between speech and total situation in a detailed study on a pair of neglected twins. The vocalization of these children had meaning only in concrete-active situations. Verbalization was closely interwoven with the rest of the activities; sometimes the word functioned as grammatical object whereas the subject remained on the level of concrete activity. (This distribution between verbalization and activity has already been mentioned previously.) Luria, who called this use of language "synpraxic," meant more or less the same as what Bühler had previously called the "empractic" use of language.

The twins' verbal comprehension was confined equally to concrete situations. Since language here was not yet distinct from actions, the child was unable to arrive at generalizations and, consequently, at abstractions. Any ordering of concrete individual objects and events into classes, hence a "new principle of nervous activity" (1959, p. 91), was not yet possible. Corresponding to the primitive use of language, therefore, the organization of activity had still remained equally primitive at the level of direct action.

This raises the question of the influence of language on cognitive development, which Vigotsky has described in detail (English edition, 1962). Vigotsky treats the formation of the first meaningful words as analogous to the intellectual operations which Köhler's chimpanzees had to perform. "Words enter into the structure of things and acquire a certain functional meaning, in much the same way as the stick, (has meaning) to the chimpanzee" (p. 123). To be true, the analogy does not take us very far; thinking in relation to the use of tools can be related to the use of speech only in man, but not in any animal. According to Vigotsky, anthropoids have some speech components of a phonetic, emotional and social kind, but these components never form a language because the component of a specifically human intelligence is absent. If we wish to lay as much emphasis on the evolution of thought as Vigotsky has done, it is possible to detect, in the phylogeny of thought and speech, a prelinguistic phase of the development of thought and a preintellectual phase of the development of speech.

Crying, babbling, and perhaps even the early autistically acquired words, just as much as the social contact with persons in the environment, are the preintellectual roots of speech.

Up to a certain point in time, thought and speech develop separately; at this point they meet and thought becomes verbal and speech rational (Vigotsky, English edition, 1962, p. 44). We shall return later to the localization of this stage.

> We should note parenthetically that if the lines of thinking and speaking run independently of each other for long stretches, this has important negative implications for the Whorf thesis of linguistic relativity.

For the following ideas Vigotsky makes use of Piaget's notion of egocentric speech. According to Piaget, the child up to about the age of seven does not use speech with social intent; he uses it egocentrically because his thinking is still egocentric.

At this point we might recall Mowrer's autism theory, which also claims that the child's speech is "egocentric."

This theory undoubtedly lays too much stress on the intellectual component and too little on the social component of the total behavior. But more important for Vigotsky than the theory itself is one obvious observation, i.e., that the child frequently talks to himself. Why does he do it and on what occasions? Vigotsky's answer is: he always starts talking to himself when his activities meet obstacles. The combinations of thought needed to help him across a difficulty and the reorganizations of earlier experiences are made in the medium in which these experiences (in abstract and generalized form) are stored: in the medium of language.

Bloch (1963, p. 14) says, "Necessity is the father of thought." We may add: Necessity is the father of speech. The "naked self," which, according to Bloch, reaches for something beyond itself in order to become aware of its own existence, seizes what it can most easily manipulate: the fabric of sounds, language.

But in Vigotsky's theory such "speech for oneself" originates through differentiation of the originally social function of "speech for others." The so-called egocentric speech is "a phenomenon of the transition from interpsychic to intrapsychic functioning, i.e., from the social, collective activity of the child to his more individualized activity—a pattern of development common to all the higher psychological functions. Speech for oneself originates through differentiation from speech for others" (1962, p. 133). At the early stage of its development to inner speech, egocentric speech is still very much like the speech used for social, inter-individual communication. Gradually a tendency emerges towards abbreviating, and towards phonetic and syntactic "economy." Nevertheless, according to Vigotsky, the origin of inner language functioning as the vehicle of thought always remains clear; it derives from socialized external speech and, therefore, in the last resort, from the activities of man. Thus the sentence, "In the beginning was the Deed,"[5] even applies to speech development if one lays stress on the word "beginning."[6]

The connection between language and thought, which Vigotsky so convincingly describes, is not only an important topic in the language development of the child; it is also important at the "opposite" end, the pathological deficit and loss of speech. Neurologists assumed for a long time that definite anatomical centers within the central nervous system corresponded to the organization of speech so that the loss of such a center would entail the disturbance of a particular psychological element of speech. This view has

[5] Translator's note, i.e., Faust's reply to the Biblical "In the beginning was the Word" (Goethe, Faust, English translation, Part I, 1. 889).

[6] More than 100 years ago, Setchenov had already described thinking as a "reflex with an inhibited end."

been abandoned almost everywhere. Instead, the attempt is made to explain in phonetic and psychological terms the significance of the functional disturbances which appear in the different forms of aphasia.

> From this point of view it can easily be understood that the connection between thought and speech and the various possibilities of its disturbance play a large part in the discussion of aphasic pathologies. Thus, Goldstein, for example, has attempted to explain a certain group of these diseases as a disturbance of the capacity to categorize, i.e., as a disturbance of cognitive ability. The change in verbal behavior is the manifestation of a loss of Vigotsky's "inner speech."
>
> However, the way in which both Vigotsky and Goldstein operate with the concept of "inner speech" and the connection between thought and language reveals a difficulty which is inherent in such views. The diagnostician, in these cases, makes it necessarily his business to find out whether the capacity to categorize is impaired or whether "only" that act is affected which translates categorizing activities into speech. But in practice there is no possibility, as Teuber (1964) emphatically pointed out, to grasp thought processes and their results without reference to linguistic processes.
>
> To put it in more general terms, the problems of the relationship between thought and language are immeasurably confused (or may even have been created) by the circularity of the definition of language and thought as well as by the methods used to study these relationships.
>
> After this necessarily sketchy digression into the psychopathology of linguistic behavior, we now return to the main line of our argument.

In the beginning was the Deed. Necessity is the father of thought. Necessity is the father of speech. But soon speech detaches itself from the motor of need, for "the hunger of humans, unlike that of animals, is not easily satisfied. What he eats gives him a taste for more" (Bloch, p. 15). It is not necessity alone that stimulates speech; at an early stage questioning and wonder appear on the scene as well. Next to the cry, "I want to eat," another call is heard, first feebly, then stronger and stronger and more and more frequently: "I want to know."

We thus come to an aspect that most theories viewing the differentiation of speech from the totality of behavior have tended to neglect: in speech, consciousness plays a part that must not be underrated. When we discussed the concept of meaning, we drew attention to the necessity of taking this fact into account: meaning is knowledge of a relationship. The urge to know is directed towards language; the possession of knowledge requires language; the achievement of knowledge serves as reinforcement in learning language and meaning.

The next question is at what point of speech development does the role of consciousness become evident? In our view this point can be located with the help of Lewis' theory of language development.

Lewis (1951) distinguishes three stages of imitation. In the first, which comprises the period up to approximately the fourth month of life, the infant responds with vocalization to human sound utterances. Then follows a pause in vocalization or at least a marked reduction. A third stage around 8 or 9 months is characterized by increased vigor, frequency and accuracy (1963, pp. 23–24).

According to Lewis (1963) this revival of vocalization coincides with the observation that, at that time, the child is beginning to understand what is said to him.

Lewis offers an explanation of the second stage, i.e., of the period of marked decline of vocalization; he says that the child becomes more attentive to the circumstances in which the sound event occurs. The sounds—as it might be formulated—have become sufficiently detached from the total situation that the infant can perceive them as independent entities. This enables him to relate sounds to practical events—a fundamental feature of all language. Since the infant's attention span at this stage is, however, still very limited, he is unable to attend and vocalize at the same time.

Following Lewis, we assume that in this second stage a silent latency phase between the fourth and eighth month of life, a new consciousness factor becomes effective: the infant, so to speak, catches on to what is called language. It seems reasonable to speculate that it is at this point that the child grasps the relationship between what the speaker means and what he says, which is what MacNamara and Schlesinger are talking about.

> Stern (1914) expressed a similar view. It is between the ages of 1½ and 2 years that the child makes the most important discovery, i.e., that everything has a name. Perhaps Stern puts it somewhat too intellectually and therefore places it too late chronologically.

During Lewis' vocalization pause, a new psychic function emerges in a preparatory way, a function which decisively intervenes in the development of speech and of the human being generally: we call it the symbol function. Man has a biologically given tendency—hence a tendency not derived from experience—to make and use symbols. The principle of symbolism is, one might say, the key to the specifically human world.

The early vocalizations of the infant are always part of the total behavior of the infant. Their motivation is "orectic," as Lewis calls the mixture of affect and conative strivings which characterize the early period; striving and emotion are, so to speak, the devices by means of which the infant is inducted into the dynamics of the total situation. The dawning symbolic awareness, which makes speech out of these orectically motivated vocalizations, is a result of attention which briefly arrests the fleeting moment of the flow of events. Thus, certain events become detached from their context and are thrown into relief. This process initiates a trend whose characteristic development Langer noted (1963, pp. 116–117); i.e., genuine symbols have a dissociated character and are produced without practical motive.

If we assume that speech develops through a process of differentiation from the flow of behavior comprising two individuals, consciousness has the task of imposing "constancies" upon the flow of sounds and events. Man's symbolizing capacity is identical with his ability to discover constancies in the flow of events. The beginning of this most human of all capacities lies in the exclamation which William James expressed so aptly in the telling phrase: "Hallo—thingumbob again."

We must make it clear that there is more to this phenomenon than the crystallization of permanencies described by Piaget as well. Even an animal is capable of guiding behavior by making use of generalization from many similar situations. James' exclamation indicates, however, not only the process of detachment of common features in similar situations but, at the same time, it indicates the *awareness* of communality: the common features have become part of our knowledge, or the "beam" of cognition has picked them out.

The combination of sounds produced by the adult and heard by the infant is, to begin with, part of the total situation. The various situational aspects may change, the speakers may change, the orectic characteristics may change also—yet there is something that is not lost. Included among these permanencies and recurring features is a complex of sounds. The awareness of a relationship—transcending the here-and-now of every moment—between constancies in the sound combinations and constancies in the situation, in other words, the act of taking note of this relationship—however dim and ill-defined it may be—is at the root of the experience of verbal meaning.

There is a case on record in the psychological literature where this experience has been described with unusual insight. In this case it did not occur in an early phase of childhood, when it is no longer accessible to the adult's memory, but at a later stage. Helen Keller, who grew up blind and deaf, described it in her memoirs.

Helen Keller became deaf and blind when she was about 1½ years old. She grew up without speech, until, at the age of nearly seven, she had a teacher, Anne Sullivan. Miss Sullivan soon began to teach her the finger alphabet. The child liked the game without knowing of course that these were letters—she did not know anything of words or language. Eventually she was able to imitate letter sequences without grasping that they had a constant relationship to an object. Her teacher wrote: ". . . 'mug' and 'milk' had given Helen more trouble than all the rest. She confused the nouns with the verb 'drink' . . . (She) went through the pantomime of drinking whenever she spelled 'mug' or 'milk' . . . We went out to the pump-house, and I made Helen hold her mug under the spout while I pumped. As the cold water gushed forth, filling the mug, I spelled 'w-a-t-e-r' in Helen's free hand. The word coming so close upon the sensation of cold water rushing over her hand seemed to startle her. She dropped the mug and stood as one transfixed. A new light came into her face. She spelled 'water' several times. Then she dropped on the ground and asked for its name and pointed to the pump and the trellis, and suddenly turning round she asked for my name. I spelled 'Teacher' " (Keller, *The Story of My Life*, 1905, p. 316). And Helen Keller herself wrote, "I knew then that 'w-a-t-e-r' meant the wonderful cool something that was flowing over my hand. That living word awakened my soul, and gave it light, hope, joy, set it free! There were barriers still, it is true, but barriers that could in time be swept away."

"I left the well-house eager to learn. Everything had a name, and each name gave birth to a new thought. As we returned to the house every object which I touched seemed to quiver with life. That was because I saw everything with the strange, new sight that had come to me . . . I learned a great many new words that day . . . words that were to make the world blossom for me . . ." (*op. cit.*, pp. 23–24).

We therefore assume that meaning is the perception of a constancy. Viewed from this aspect, meaning has close similarity to what cognitive psychology calls " concept." Carroll, above all, has drawn attention to this close relationship: ". . . concepts are properties of organismic experience—more particularly, they are the abstracted and often cognitively structured classes of 'mental' experience learned by organisms in the course of their life histories . . . One necessary condition for the formation of a concept is that the individual must have a series of experiences that are in one or more respects similar; the constellation of 'respects' (references) in which they are similar constitutes the 'concept' that underlies them" (1964b, pp. 180f).

In Carroll's conception, the "experiencing of similarities" has still a rather passive character. We should like to view this process somewhat more actively. The similarities are not only and not always contained in the events from which the individual abstracts them, but they may equally, at least sometimes, originate in the individual and may be imposed by him upon the events. The notion of "abstracting" does not mean a passive subjection to impressions; it is a psychologically active process. There is a natural human trend to arrest the flow of events and to capture the ephemeral character of concrete events in images which man himself created. Cassirer comments upon this as follows: "Another indication that the creation of the various systems of sensuous symbols is indeed a pure activity of the mind (and not merely a passive reflection—*the author*) is that from the outset all these symbols lay claim to objective value. They go beyond the mere phenomena of the individual consciousness, claiming to confront them with something that is universally valid." This claim in itself "belongs to the essence and character of the particular cultural forms themselves . . . It is characteristic . . . that they do not clearly distinguish between the content of the "thing" and the content of the "sign" . . . the mere word or image contains a magic force through which the essence of the thing gives itself to us . . . For consciousness the sign is, as it were, the first stage and the first demonstration of objectivity, because through it the constant flux of the contents of consciousness is for the first time halted, because in it something enduring is determined and emphasized'' (Cassirer, *The Philosophy of Symbolic Forms*, I, 1953 ed., pp. 88–89).

The part the language-user plays in establishing order in the world will occupy us in greater detail later in the discussion of the Whorf hypothesis. But even before that a similar trend will be met in certain views expressed by Brown.

Nelson (1974) recently addressed herself to the problem of concept formation in children at the language acquisition stage. In agreement with Piaget, she views the object as emerging out of the interaction between the child and his environment. At first, ''ball'' is constituted as in Fig. 58.

$$
\text{Ball}_1 \left\{
\begin{array}{l}
\text{in the living room, in the hallway} \\
\text{mother throws, picks up, holds} \\
\text{I throw, pick up, hold} \\
\text{rolls, bounces} \\
\text{on the floor, under the table}
\end{array}
\right.
$$

Fig. 58

Thus ''ball'' emerges through the formation of a cognitive map consisting of dynamic relationships, relationships between what is now ''object'' on the one hand, and what on the other hand is the child himself, the mother, or certain loci and events. Within the variability of all these relationships the covariation, i.e., the ''common fate,'' clearly indicates what belongs with what. In the second situation, the following is integrated into the developing cognitive map (Fig. 59).

$$
\text{Ball}_2 \left\{
\begin{array}{l}
\text{on the playground} \\
\text{boy throws, catches} \\
\text{rolls, bounces} \\
\text{over the ground, under the fence}
\end{array}
\right.
$$

Fig. 59

We can see that through this interaction a number of ''agents'' become differentiated, eventually leading to a concept of agent per se. But, above all, it is important that $ball_2$ bounces, rolls, and is thrown like $ball_1$, and therefore permits the emergence of a concept ''ball.''

According to Nelson, concepts of this type have a *functional core* that is formed by the various relationships and acts that encompass the concept.

We do not only summarize a large number of different-looking quadrupeds as ''dogs'' but a variety of percepts, changing in time, as ''the landlord's dog, Prince.'' This aspect is of greatest importance because it demonstrates a link with other branches of psychology and therefore establishes the universality of the principle: even the individual object or thing in this sense is a *category*. We include a series of very different retinal images in the class "this table." The designation "this table" is not the verbal label of one particular retinal image but the correlate of a constellation of slightly varied, but similar, retinal images. In accordance with a profoundly human tendency, we project upon this constellation a unitary and unifying designation.

As the introductory chapters of this book have stressed again and again, this setting up of constancies is a fundamental psychological feature, a tendency which manifests itself in the psychology of perception as constancy of objects or as size constancy and reaches right into social psychology, where it accounts for such phenomena as prejudice and stereotyping.

Thus the child must also learn to recognize the *repetition of vocalizations* as identical. This means he must learn to ignore variations in intensity of the sounds which are caused, for example, by varying distances of the speaker, or by varying frequency spectra of different speakers. He must recognize that "dog" uttered in a low and deep voice is equivalent to "dog" uttered in a loud and high voice. He must learn—even on the acoustic side—what are "criterial attributes" in Brown's sense, i.e., attributes on which depends the decision whether a sound belongs to this or that category. He must learn to ignore "noisy attributes" which are irrelevant in subsuming a sound to a certain category (the intensity of a heard word is a "noisy" attribute in establishing meaning). The child must further learn to employ the criterial attributes, not only for word recognition, but also for word production (Brown, 1956 and later).

What attributes of the words and expressions used by the child does he *have* or *know*? With this question we have returned to Brown's basic question. He asked, "What semantic structures are represented in the verbal utterances of the child?" (1973). What does he mean by the single word "ball"? What does he mean by "mommy sock"? Brown wants to attack this question first at the level of the two-word utterance, because he feels that at this level, the order of the two words could provide a clue to these structures. Meanwhile we have seen that one cannot and should not approach this question at the two-word level. We even want to approach it *prior* to the evolvement of the one-word level. We must remain aware of the fact that temporally prior to the stage to be discussed, namely the stage of the earliest *verbal* utterances, there was another stage. In this stage the child understands the adult not only by grasping what he means but by employing the adult's linguistic utterances to clarify this meaning. But what is the story about speech *production*?

The child sits in his play-pen and whimpers. Mother arrives and sees that the ball has fallen outside, lifts it up, and hands it to the child. At the base of this "expression" of these whimpering sounds there presumably are emotional tendencies.

Since the child does not live by himself, but in a social environment which is receptive to signals, these sounds act instrumentally: mother comes and does whatever is needed. What she does *may* not be exactly what the child would have liked her to do, because the sound sequence produced by the infant does not as yet contain any information; the mother is simply likely to perform whatever the situation as a whole suggests.

This is to say that up to this point meaning is conveyed almost completely by the situation. The sound sequence produced as a result of orectic pressures is rather like a non-specific signal to do *something*. It does not yet point to an object (and is clearly not yet conventionalized), nor does it say what is happening or ought to happen with regard to this object nor does it express a hope or a fear.

If we refer once more to Bloomfield's model of the speech act as a link between two practical events (cf. p. 162) and remind ourselves that the speech act does not connect two unconnected events, but, on the contrary, permits the separation of two neighboring links in the chain of events, we can now raise the question whether this separation which is dependent upon the speech act can be related to the genesis of predication.

The next step which characterizes this development is the following situation: The baby sits in his play-pen and cannot reach the ball outside. He reaches towards the ball and whimpers. In one way this is entirely emotional, yet in another we see here the beginnings of predication. The gesture of the hand, as Brown (1958a, pp. 197–198) says, defines the function of whimpering. The coordination of gesture and sound means "Please, Mummy, give me the ball."

On the next level of development the infant no longer simply whimpers; he says "ball" or "want." For the first time a word is used here to bridge, in a specific way, the gap between two practical events (the infant seeing the ball outside and the mother giving the ball to the infant). We are faced here, for the first time, with a verbal event which can be described as a sentence— admittedly, a sentence in which either only the object (ball) or the predicate (want) is encoded in a socially binding fashion.

Such sentences are called *one-word sentences*. In this situation the single word "ball" means "Give me the ball"; in another situation the same word "ball" may mean "This is my ball" or "This is a lovely ball." The single word "want" in this situation means "I want the ball"; in another it might mean "I want something to eat."

> These one-word sentences or holophrastic words are discussed in detail in psychological writings. What Clara and William Stern wrote on this subject at the beginning of the century constitutes one of the classical texts in the literature of psychology.

But in each single case of such an expression we should not lose sight of Brown's concern. There is no need for a linguistically structured sentence, we could be dealing with just (unstructured) labeling! But psychologically even such labeling is not totally unstructured. Let us pursue this thought a little bit further.

The one-word sentence is the first instance of a sound combination or word establishing the link between two practical events. This also explains why the first infantile utterances in genuine language always relate to an immediate situation and not to the past or future: the contribution of the concrete situation is still an essential part of the meaning-carrying process. Likewise the receiver still needs to know the concrete situation to be able to decode the message. This, in effect, means that the one-word sentence is not a true sentence. The so-called one-word sentence "want" is more accurately a two-term sentence; it is already a kind of predication. The child utters the predicate that goes with a nonsymbolized, physically present object of the sentence, the ball lying outside the play-pen and pointed to by the child. He does not have to say "ball" because he can point to it.

And vice versa, he can confine himself to designate the ball by a word, while the predicate can be added by means of a gesture and the situation. Accordingly, Mowrer calls the one-word sentence "quasi-predication."

McNeill (1970) speaks more precisely of an *intrinsic predication* which emerges earlier in the development than the extrinsic. At this level the encoding capacity of the sign maker is not adequate to put the whole message into words; part of it must still be carried by the situation; or to put it differently, words still serve only to define more precisely the meaning of the total situation.

With that we have returned once more to MacNamara's theory of language acquisition. But in certain circumstances, e.g., under conditions of neglect, hurry or laziness, even the adult who has full command of the power of speech may regress to this stage of development. Messages are left incomplete because the receiver can complete them on the basis of previous experience or situational context.

An impressive confirmation of our thesis that the degree of elaboration of speech is inversely related to the degree of communicative support supplied by the situation is given by a relevant finding of Meier's linguistic statistics. Among the texts examined by Meier for sentence length, the dialogue in a film ("In Those Days" by H. Käutner) displays the highest frequency of extremely short sentences (Meier, 1964, p. 191). The sequence of visual events supports communication to such an extent that extreme shortness of sentences is possible.

But as soon as an utterance refers to something which is not here and now, constructions of more than one-word length are needed. The object which is not present cannot be referred to by a gesture; it must be "re-present-ed" by a word.

The preliminary schema of predication discussed so far must be further refined and differentiated.

The reason for this is that the child generates more than one word in sequence. That brings us to the two-word utterance which affords the opportunity for studying the nature of the structure of the word sequence.

We have returned to the pivot grammars, to Brown's notion from which we digressed some time back.

The above discussion has shown us that the rules that govern the sequencing of elements in the utterances of the child are laid down in a preverbal stage, during which the relationships between the child and his world are structured. Parts of this structure are then gradually transferred to the verbal level. What the child means is gradually translatable to what he can say.

This rule-like sequencing, which we first detect with certainty in two-word sentences, has not only a preverbal, semantic root but a syntactic one as well. The child already behaves according to rules in cases (1) which are not related to language or communication, and (2) where there is no need for it. The best evidence for this is reported by Patricia Greenfield *et al.* (1972). In this study, children, ages 11 to 36 months, play with nesting cups. First the experimenter presents to the child five cups of varying sizes and then stacks them according to a particular rule (strategy). Children are then permitted to play with the cups that have been separated again. It was found that the majority of children, in repeated trials, follow a certain strategy (but by no means the strategy demonstrated by the experimenter). The strategy used is independent of the order in which the cups were presented, but is typical for the child's age level.

This shows that in his nonverbal behavior the child also follows rules that are related to age and developmental stage. Furthermore, he follows rules even when this would "not be necessary." There is no reason why cups have to be stacked always in the same manner.

However, Greenfield's findings go beyond showing the structuring of sequences in nonverbal behavior. She is also able to demonstrate that these play strategies correspond in a *formal* way to various sentence forms which are produced by the child, months later of course. The developmental sequence is the same for both nonverbal and action verbal strategies. The "grammar of acts" (that is Bruner's term) becomes apparent in both the nonverbal and verbal acts. We can conclude that presyntactic structures are already an integral part of ordering the preverbal acts of the child.

From this vantage point let us once more return to MacNamara's theory of language acquisition. The study of Greenfield et al. has shown that the child's behavior is guided by rules even in the case where such rules are not necessary for reaching the goal. Because this is the case, the child can apply rules to the sound waves characterizing the communication of his fellow beings. Furthermore, he can apply rules to the relationship between the sound waves and the relevant situation; he can, as required by the theory, recognize the relationship between what the adult speaker means and what he says. For this purpose the child employs pat rules which Bever (1970) calls *strategies*. These would include:

comprehend as belonging together all which is not separated by pauses
attend that which is emphasized

attend to the sequence
combine the individual words according to their meaning in a manner
   which is most likely to make sense

Let us look at an example of the last-named strategy. In order to understand this sentence, *The man gives the dog a bone,* it is sufficient for the child to know the meaning of the words "man," "dog," and "bone." In the processes of understanding the child needs only to combine the words in a manner that makes the most sense in terms of the situation that is described. The man is more likely to give the bone to the dog than the other way round. The man is more likely an "agent" than the bone, the bone more likely the patient than the dog, etc. Thus, based on the meaning of the words and without recourse to syntactic instructions (subject in the nominative, object in the dative), the child constructs the informational content of the sentence which presumably corresponds to the meaning intended by the adult speaker.

A child who is able to grasp the essence of what is said by the speaker, however, without necessarily being able to analyze the verbal utterance in terms of its linguistic components, can now use this insight to examine the rules that govern the relationship between what is meant and what is said. If we know what is inscribed on the Rosetta stone we can decipher the unknown language. The child is able to recognize the rules inherent in the adult's verbal utterance because he knows the intended meaning conveyed by that utterance.

The tendency to act according to rules, on the one hand, and the situational cues and perceptual strategies, on the other, are all resources for the young child's acquisition of knowledge about rules, which he must employ later to ensure verbal comprehension as well where the intended meaning is not discernible from the dynamics of the situation.

We agree with Brown that one of the major dimensions of language development consists of "learning to express always and automatically certain things (agent, action, number and tense, and so on), even though these meanings may be in many particular contexts quite redundant" (1973, p. 245).

The child learns to use and operate with language because he attempts to apply rules even to situations where this is not required. He learns to use language by using it in the first instance even where he is not required to use it.

CHAPTER 12

Language Comprehension and Man's View of the World

Olson's cognitive theory of semantics—Situational determinants of meaning—Comprehension as constructive process—Levels of comprehension—Influence of language on the speaker's view of the world—Categories as guides to attention—Linguistic determinism and linguistic relativity—Whorf—Studies of color coding—Language universals—*General Semantics.*

At the end of Chapter 10 we observed that an adequate study of the use of linguistic structures requires the inclusion of the "speaker's state" in the equation. In the last chapter we learned that the "state of the language user"—in the case of the child and probably the adult as well—is determined to a large extent by the course of action in which he is involved, by the intentions which he wants to effect by means of language as either a speaker or a listener. We will now expand on these reflections.

MacNamara's theory of language acquisition assumes that the listener can grasp, at a preverbal level and admittedly imprecisely, the meaning of the speaker's utterance. How are we to conceptualize this integration of situational and specific linguistic factors?

A systematic answer to that question would require an extensive excursion into the domain of so-called nonverbal communication. This would include a far-reaching study of those theories of philosophy of language and anthropology that postulate that the origin of meaning is to be found in the verbal specification of the (social) act. This volume is not the place to do so. The reader is referred to Wiener et al. (1972) and to Mehrabian (1969) for a discussion of nonverbal communication, and to Wittgenstein (1960) and Höpp (1970) for the genesis of linguistic meaning.

We begin our own discussions relatively "late," with the individual who is already able to use speech. Here we find that a great deal of general information is conveyed by intonation and the placement of pauses. These are the factors that participate extensively in contrasting linguistic figures from the undifferentiated ground of the entire expression. These figures or elements must then be defined in terms of their relationships within the expression (e.g., as agent or object) by means of linguistic forms in the more narrow sense. Bolinger (1972) correctly pointed out that characteristics of intonation are more uniform among the various languages than any other linguistic phenomena. Thus a spoken verbal utterance is already articulated in a way that is relatively isomorphic to the intentions of the speaker (VanLancker, 1975). Verbalization consists at first of a specifying encoding of a *part* of this whole expressive act, the general dynamic of which was already apparent. Olson (1970) carried out a number of studies related to this. We shall now examine these.

A little paper star is hidden under a wooden block. A spectator is instructed to tell someone, who has just entered, under which block the star is hidden. The block, under which the star is hidden, remains the same for all trials, it is small, round, and white. Now, what does the speaker say when there is a second small, round, and black block next to the one under which the star is hidden? He says, "Below the white one." For the second trial a small, angular white block is placed next to the one with the star. The speaker now says, "Below the round one." In the third trial there are three blocks, a round black one, an angular black one, and an angular white one. Now the speaker says, "It is under the round, white one."

Olson interprets his findings as follows: By his utterance, the speaker distinguishes the intended reference object from other alternatives available in the situation. The utterance restructures the listener's perception of the situation. He is told to what he is to direct his attention. But he *can* be instructed in this way only because the speaker has verbally coded precisely that aspect of the situation which is required to "complete the task." The object does not determine the label, rather the speaker uses *various* words to designate one and the same object according to the particular intentional mode.

In the listener's *comprehension* of the verbal expression we find the same dynamics of meaning that guided the *selection* of the terms used by the speaker. This can be shown by two studies, one of which also analyzes the influence of the nonverbal situation on the processing, i.e., the comprehension, of the verbal utterance.

Hörmann and Terbuyken (1974) instructed subjects to rate, by means of the semantic differential, verbs appearing in short expressions ("I *beg* you," "I *trust* you").

A second group of subjects rated the same sentences which in this case did not appear in isolation but on a cartoon drawing indicating that they were spoken by characters that had been rated as ranging from very dominant (or very active) to less dominant (or less active). It was shown that the way in which the word is experienced depends to a large extent on who is saying what to whom. If a small, feeble character says to a large strong figure: "I *beg* you," this is perceived as much weaker than if the same words are spoken by the large to the small character.

Apparently, the features that are relevant to the particular perception of the word are determined only after its function in the communicative situation has become apparent.

What functions it must satisfy are determined not only by the total communicative situation, but even more so by the verbal context. It should be clear, however, that there is no fundamental difference between the determination by the verbal context and that arising from the situational context. For that reason we shall look at a second experiment.

The subject is presented with sentences like these:

The man tuned the piano.

The man lifted the piano.

The man shattered the piano.

The man photographed the piano.

It was found, for example, that the phrase "something heavy" facilitated the recall of the second sentence far more than did the phrase "something wooden"; just the opposite was true for the third sentence (Barclay et al. 1974).

Apparently we store in memory those features of a word which are relevant to the emergence of the meaning of the total expression.

If one reflects on findings like these, it becomes clear that the common sense notion of "understanding an utterance" must be revised. After all, it views "comprehension of an utterance" as a sort of combining of information contained in the single elements. The fact that the word "piano," however, also contains the information "heavy" becomes manifest only after it is combined with the verb "to lift."

These semantic scaling and memory experiments show that comprehending an utterance consists not so much of analyzing incoming information; it is, in fact, a process of constructing something new, involving the broader context and the total situation along with the immediate verbal input. This new construction determines to a large extent what is, and what can be extracted from these various sources.

We can see now that findings from two quite different subareas of psychology can be usefully applied to psycholinguistics. As a student of the psychology of memory, Bartlett (1932) identified two phases in the memory process, namely storage in terms of an adaptation to a schema and recall as a reconstruction, based not on specific memory traces, but on a general schema. In the psychology of perception (e.g., Arnheim, 1947) we find the notion that perception involves the application of idiosyncratic perceptual categories to the stimulus input. That a constructivist approach of this kind might be useful for psycholinguistics was demonstrated primarily by experiments on retention. Such studies showed repeatedly that it is not the literal text that is retained, but rather the propositions contained in a sentence, i.e., what is being asserted.

Sachs (1967) presented her subjects with short texts consisting of several sentences. Later they were presented with a single sentence and asked whether or not it had appeared in the previous text. The single sentence contained either a small semantic or syntactic alteration, or was identical to one of the sentences in the text. She found that small *syntactic* changes (e.g., a change from an active to a passive form) were no longer noticed if the distance between the two critical sentences was more than about 80 syllables. *Semantic* changes, on the other hand (e.g., changes from an agent to a patient role), were identified even when there were 160 syllables of intervening text. Flores d'Arcais (1974) points out that it is the primary semantic information contained in the original that is remembered, i.e., who did what to whom and under what conditions. But this information is not stored in sentence form and reproduced *verbatim* at the appropriate moment; rather the sentence recalled during the test phase is a new construction based on the stored abstract semantic information.

For this reconstruction, the listener not only calls upon his linguistic knowledge (i.e., his knowledge about the meaning of words and syntax) but also his general knowledge of the world. According to Bransford the process of comprehension generates a "semantic description" of the situation. He demonstrates this point by the following experiment.

First each subject is presented with either sentence (a) or sentence (b):

(a) Three turtles were resting next to a floating log, and a fish swam below them.

(b) Three turtles were resting on a floating log and a fish swam below them.

Both sentences have the same deep structure, but the "semantic situation" described is different in each case. Sentence (b) suggests that the fish is below the log as well. This is suggested not by any particular information tied to a specific word, but by the knowledge one has about the spatial relations in the world. Now the subject is presented with sentence (c):

(c) Three turtles were resting (on/next to) a floating log and a fish swam below it.

Bransford argues that if the subject stores the exact linguistic form of the first sentence he should be able to notice the change both with respect to (a) and (b). But if what is recalled is a semantic description of the situation based on reconstructions of either sentence (a) or (b), then sentence (c) would be identified as nonequivalent only by those who first heard sentence (a). In fact, that is the case. A person who hears sentence (b) formulates a "semantic description" based on his knowledge of the world that is indistinguishable from that represented by sentence (c), although the latter differs somewhat in its linguistic form.

Thus this "semantic description" is something that is relatively uniform. What determines the components used for its construction, which are extracted from the verbal input, and what determines the specificity or generality of the information extracted? This question connects the psycholinguistic issue of comprehension with the issue of retention and recall in general psychology. Providing the connection between these two approaches is the concept of *coding*. Therefore it is necessary for us to examine briefly the general psychological models of information processing.

Such models are generally conceptualized as flow charts on which a number of stores are connected in sequence. There usually is an iconic (or echoic) store with relatively short retention, followed by a short-term store that permits recoding (i.e., transformation into an other format) and which is able to retain its content long enough to facilitate silent rehearsal. Connecting this short-term store with the long-term memory, one usually finds a channel with limited flow capacity, but this is not of concern to us here. (For a detailed description, see Norman, 1969; 2nd ed., 1976.)

Craik and Lockhart (1972) propose an alternative to this common multistore model of information processing. They propose that it is the manner of encoding and not the variety of stores on which we should focus our attention. The processing of information (including linguistic information) proceeds at different *levels*. The *depth* to which one can drive the process of encoding depends on the type of stimulus input, the nature of the task, the available time, etc. The central theme of Craik and Lockhart's model of memory is that the deeper the level of encoding, the more stable will be the memory trace, and the better will be the retention. This model of information processing has consequences for a psycholinguistic theory of understanding.

Mistler-Lachmann (1972) presented her subjects with three different tasks. In the first of these, the subject had to determine whether or not a sentence made sense; in the second, he was to say whether it fit with the context; in the third, the subject was required to formulate a sentence of his own to follow the one that was presented to him. It was found that the first task appeared to be more "shallow" than the others. Subjects not only responded more rapidly, they also retained the sentences more poorly.

Let us be clear that this approach also implies that understanding must be differentially conceptualized. In the first task, the sentences are understood as well, but at a more superficial level, than in task two and three. The first task (determining whether a sentence is meaningful) requires a less profound semantic analysis than the second task (determining *what* meaning the sentence has) and less still than the third task (requiring the production of a sentence to follow meaningfully the sentence which has been presented).

Bock (1976) presented data that showed that it is in fact the encoding process (and not some factor intervening in the retention interval) that determines the depth and thereby the efficacy of retention. He presented his subjects with lists of 15 bird names and 15 names of tools. In one condition they were instructed to check off "everything living" (or "not living") and in another condition "all birds" (or "all tools"). Without the subjects' prior knowledge this was followed by a test for retention. As expected, the more general task results in less retention. Such findings prevail even if, between the checking-off and the test, the subject is told, "You probably noticed that all living things were birds," or "all not living things were tools." It is the listener's set to process at a particular level during acquisition that plays the decisive role. The coding that took place during this phase cannot be moved later to a "lower" depth.

A study by Jörg (1976) goes one step further. Whereas Mistler-Lachmann had varied the depth of linguistic coding and examined the effect of this variation on the retention of verbal utterances, Jörg presented her subjects with pictures and verbal labels. The level of verbal description was varied and the effect of this variation on retention of the pictures was examined. Each sheet, presented separately, showed four pictures. Two of these were related by means of the verbal description, "The butterfly is sitting next to the flower." What is varied is the level of generality of the concepts comprising the description. A more specific level of the above example would be, "The monarch is sitting next to the tulip." After presentation of the sentence/picture combination, the subject was shown five modifications of each original picture showing increasingly more deviation from the original. The task was to identify the picture originally seen.

The results of this study show that it is the level of generality of the verbal concepts that is responsible for determining the point of maximal differentiation between the pictures. If the sentence contains specific concepts, the pictures that are most similar to the original are well discriminated, but this is not the case for the dissimilar ones. In contrast, if the verbal labels contain general concepts, slight deviations from the original are hardly noticed; however, there is differentiation among the more strongly deviant versions.

We should also mention a second important finding of this study. In a test of recognition for those pictures not referred to by the caption (in each case, only two of the four pictures on a page were labeled), the level of discriminability corresponds to the captioned pictures on that page. Apparently, setting the level of description tunes the subject's "processing mechanism" to a particular level of differentiation that also determines the processing or coding of those pictures that are not labeled verbally.

Now we can see how the speech form and the speech level used by the individual in his interaction with reality influence the nature of his comprehension and the storage of this reality in memory. This brings us to a major topic in the study of language. Beginning with Herder and Humboldt, via Sapir and Whorf to Bernstein, the question that always resurfaces is whether and to what extent a person's thoughts and world view are influenced by the forms of expression provided by the language that he employs. This is the problem to which we now turn.

Looked at naively, language is the means whereby one can represent the reality one perceives independent of language. When, for example, in Bühler's model (see pp. 21 ff.), language is characterized by the remark of "one person talking to another about things," then the things about which the one person talks to the other have an existence and form of appearance which is quite independent of whether and in what way they are talked about.

The question of the influence of language upon the way a speaker sees his world and thinks about it originated, as was seen in the last chapter, in the developmental characteristics of categorical behavior. If the question is to be discussed in the present chapter as a problem in its own right, it takes us back to the philosophical thought reported in Chapter 7. These reflections form the wider horizon against which to view these questions.

In Chapter 7 we discussed in detail the philosophical argument which caused the independence of thing and language (or of *res* and *intellectus*) to be called into question. We noted at that point how the world-creating rather than the world-representing function of language, which appears with particular clarity in Wittgenstein's "language-game," had been developed—in the work of Peirce and Morris—as a result of taking into account pragmatic elements in the complex of *meaning*.

The problem of the influence of language upon man's view of the world has a respectable philosophical ancestry. Kant postulated that space and time are modes of perception of the human mind, which, therefore, to put it crudely, the human mind adds to objective reality. Objective reality can only be recognized with the help of the spectacles of these modes of perception (which may actually distort reality).

The chief criticism that Herder made of Kant's *Critique of Pure Reason* was that Kant completely neglected the problem of language. Is it not possible that analogously language can influence the process of perception?

When Humboldt said, "Language is the thought-forming organ" (1949 edition, p. 52), he made the decisive move away from the copying function of language, implied in Herder's criticism. Or, to quote Humboldt again, "It is the subjective activity of thinking which creates an object. For there is no single kind of idea which can be regarded as a purely receptive contemplation of an object previously given. The activity of the senses must be combined into a synthesis with the inner activity of the mind . . . To do this language is essential" (p. 55). Humboldt further wrote in the *Academy Treatise on Comparative Philology*,[1] "The mutual interdependence of

---

[1] *Translator's note:* The German title of this treatise is: *Akademie-Abhandlung über das vergleichende Sprachstudium.*

thought and word makes it evident that languages are not really means of representing already known truth, they are means of discovering hitherto unknown truth'' (1905a, p. 27).

There is no doubt that this thesis has far-reaching implications. If it is right to say that world or truth is not something to be known prior to language or independently of it (merely to be put into words), but that it can only be perceived and thought about with the help of speech, it may lead to the assumption that a particular language is a codeterminant of the world-view of the members of a speech community; the particular language would further determine the world view differently from the way another language would determine the world view of another speech community.

Humboldt saw this consequence of his thesis with complete clarity: ''The mental characteristics and the development of language of a nation are so intimately bound up with each other that if the one were known the other could be completely deduced from it. For intellect and language permit and develop only forms which are mutually compatible. Language can be said to be the outward manifestation of the mind of nations. Their language is their mind, and their mind their language. One must imagine them as completely identical'' (p. 41).

It follows that the image which man receives through cognition (Kant) or language (Humboldt) does not depend alone on the nature of the perceived object, but always includes an active contribution of the cognizing individual or speaker. It is, as Cassirer put it, not imitation (*Abbild*) but creation (*Urbild*).

The characteristic way in which every language organizes its content, the world view of the language, is called by Humboldt the *inner form of the language*.

Humboldt's idea has been developed further in several directions and by several disciplines. To name a few of such developments: Cassirer in philosophy, Sapir and Whorf in ethnology, Weisgerber in linguistics, Korzybski and Hayakawa in General Semantics. As early as 1931, Weisgerber formulated the fundamental principle of all such developments in the following terms: ''It must be recognized to what extent the individual by virtue of his membership of a language community incorporates its characteristic mentality and is shaped by it in such a way that his mental activity is more strongly determined by the world-view of his native tongue than by his individual personality'' (*Report of the Twelfth Congress of the German Psychological Association, 1931* [1932, p. 197]).

In a certain way one can refer to this, quite realistically, as word magic; for—in Aldous Huxley's terms—the word forms the mind of him who uses it. ''Conduct and character are largely determined by the nature of the words we currently use to discuss ourselves and the world around us'' (1940, p. 9).

In the same year as Weisgerber (1931), Sapir, in an American investigation on the conceptual categories in primitive language, wrote, certainly completely independently of Weisgerber, "The relation between language and experience is often misunderstood. Language is not merely a more or less systematic inventory of the various items of experience which seem relevant to the individual . . . but is also a self-contained creative symbolic organization, which not only refers to experience largely acquired without its help but actually defines experience for us by reason of its formal completeness and because of our unconscious projection of its implicit expectations into the field of experience" (1931, p. 578).

Thus, language is included among the factors that modern psychology recognizes as codeterminants in the development and quality of the processes of perceiving, learning and thinking. Gestalt psychology (in particular the Berlin School) laid emphasis upon the sensory determination of units in the field of perception and therefore looked for structuring factors in the interaction between stimulus intensity and sense organ. The "new look" of social perception stressed the contribution of motivational and experiential factors in the organization of perception and learning. Among these autonomous factors of perception or cognition, speech occupies a special position: it is less powerful than the biological and physiological factors which apply virtually to the entire species, but its influence is more powerful than that of all other sociological, situational, or personality determinants. It is not so much that an individual's direct experience and his personal motives contribute to his world view, rather it is that language—comparable to the sense organs of our physical equipment—puts at his disposal the tools necessary for gathering experience; and these are tools which the individual cannot help using. "To find words for what we have before our eyes can be most arduous. But once they have appeared, they work upon reality as if they were little hammers used by a craftsman to hammer an image out of a copperplate" (Benjamin, 1963, p. 44).

In attempting to solve the problem that we have just raised, one may be tempted to juxtapose and compare the categories of thought and the categories of language (Seiler, 1960). However, just the *attempt* is unrealistic because it already assumes that categories of thought or concepts can be understood without reference to language.

There is simply no patent recipe to solve "finally" or "decisively" the problem of the influence of language upon the world view of man. What we may reasonably expect and what we are going to attempt to do is, by approaching the problem from various angles, to delineate the presuppositions and variables which are implicit in the study of this problem.

In the preceding paragraphs a great deal of importance was attributed to the process of categorization or formation of classes. It is, therefore, natural to ask whether this process is not the basic mechanism that accounts for the variations in world-views determined by language. Even in the work of Weisgerber, whose frame of reference is entirely unpsychological, thoughts leading in this direction occur: "I can call the shape I hold in my hand a 'rose', because I recognize and identify it as a rose" (1962a, I, p. 55). The process of identification is without doubt the same as the process of classification; the exemplar in question is classified as a rose because its properties are identified sufficiently in agreement with the criterial attributes of this class. What is happening is more than mere recognition; there is also a component of a subjective judgment: "The attributes I recognize are sufficient to identify the exemplar as a rose."

What Weisgerber is describing here as a fully conscious act of recognition is surely not paradigmatic for the processes taking place in the child who is learning his language. These are the processes that are of interest to us now, because as we saw earlier (e.g., in Nelson's model p. 258), there is an interweaving of biologically predetermined conceptual roles ("agent," "object," "instrument" . . .) with the verbal labels that the environment contributes. We have encountered the strategies according to which the child first assigns the role of agent to the first unit of the adult's verbal utterance; the role of action to the second and that of object to the third. The formal and the subjective aspects of the evolving categorization are not yet differentiated. The practical consequence of this could be that the child ascribes to a word functioning as a noun properties of substance, and to words functioning as verbs the characteristics of action.

Brown spent a month recording utterances which he heard in pre-school sessions. A comparison of the words he noted with words which appeared in the language of adults produced the following results. While 16 percent of the nouns used by adults refer to objects with a visual contour, in the case of children this applies to 67 percent of the nouns used. This finding could be formulated equally as follows: children use more concrete nouns than adults. As for the verbs used by adults, only one third of the adults' verbs but two thirds of the children's verbs refer to movement.

The semantic implications which a noun has as "the name of a thing" and a verb as "referring to action" is more consistent in children's speech than in the speech of adults. At the later stages the notional or semantic uniformity of the formclasses declines. The same rules which are applied to "car," "block," "ball," and "auntie" are applied to the nonconcrete words that belong to the formclass of nouns.

What function does this initially high correlation between formclass and semantic content fulfill? It has a dual function: in the first phase it facilitates learning; at a later stage it acts as a "lure to cognition"—and this is what this final chapter is about.

Suppose an adult shows a glass of water to a child and says "water," the child is not yet able to say what this unknown word refers to: vessel, color, content, drinking, or the like. The child does not yet know what feature is to be picked out by the new word as an invariant category. He can gain this knowledge only by observing that in other situations only one feature is constant: water; everything else changes: form of vessel, location, and color. The constant feature among all the variations is then associated with the constant term.

This process is extremely lengthy and its result is uncertain. The child is helped in picking out the relevant aspects from the total situation by the adult guiding his learning. The new word is not isolated; it is presented in a sentence; in this way the child is informed about the part of speech to which the word belongs. We don't say "dog," but "Look at the little dog running along the road" and thus mark the word "dog" as something that can walk, but as a substantive as well. This embedding of the word in a verbal context limits the possible meanings of "dog," but it also provides the language learner with a hint about the formclass to which *a word of this type* belongs.

> In this sense Leisi (1961) speaks of linguistic hypostatizing. Every word category hypostatizes something specific: the noun represents the referent as an object, the adjective represents it as a property and the verb as an activity. Weisgerber (II, 1962b, p. 301) calls these three representations of the word "not only copies of reality but guides to reality."

The formclass of a word is, in Brown's view, therefore an attention-directing device. Brown has tested this assumption empirically by presenting to children artificial words which clearly belong to a certain formclass and then questioning the children about their meaning. He made use of three formclasses: verb, mass noun, and count noun.

> As is known, English treats certain nouns such as "snow," "milk," "rice," or "dirt" differently from others such as "house" or "dog"; we say "some milk," but "a dog." When we use a count noun, e.g., "dog," and say "some dogs," "dog" is plural, whereas in the case of a mass noun, e.g., "milk," it always remains in the singular; hence, "some milk."

After Brown had noticed that the children use words such as "milk," "orange juice" or "dirt" correctly, i.e., only in the singular, he undertook the experiment proper: first, they are shown a picture of a pair of hands kneading a mass of confetti-like material in a striped container. The movement would be described by a verb, the confetti-like mass by a mass noun, and the container by a count noun. It was justifiable to assume that the children had no words for any of these.

If we now investigate whether a child has an idea of the common notional significance of verbs (action or movement), the child is asked the following question: "Do you know what it means to sib? In this picture you can see sibbing. Now show me another picture of sibbing," and he is immediately presented with three further pictures which show either only the movement (applied to a different kind of material) or only the material (with different movements) or only the container (with another material).

> If one wished to study whether the child has an idea of the common notional significance of all count nouns, the question is: "Do you know what a sib is? In this picture you can see a sib. Now show me another picture of a sib."

Table 19. Picture selections for words belonging to various parts of speech.

Depicted category	Verbs	Count nouns	Mass nouns
Actions	10	1	0
Objects	4	11	3
Substances	1	2	12
No response	1	2	1

Based on Brown, 1957, p. 4.

The results of this investigation are presented in Table 19.

The result can be interpreted to mean that classification of an unknown word under a particular formclass offers the learner a hint as to the kind of substantive meaning of this particular word.

It appears that the acquisition of the system of formclasses of a language is generalizable to a high degree and intervenes as a steering device in the acquisition of semantic relationships.

On the other hand, the inherent suggestion to classify a word as belonging to the formclass of nouns ("This is probably a thing or a substance"), which helps the child in the acquisition of language, can also mislead, or misdirect the child's (or the adult's) thoughts or expectations. "When the word *justice* comes into one's vocabulary it comes as a noun and may, as a consequence, be endowed with thing-like attributes borrowed from blocks and trucks. It would then be quite natural to make statues and paintings of justice" (Brown, 1958a, p. 247).

This taxonomy of formclasses may already be a primary determining factor for the acquisition and use of language. A second factor for possible differentiation of linguistic and linguistically determined nonverbal behavior could be the "level" of categorization. Jörg's experiment, described above, showed the influence of these factors on the individual's ability for recognition. Whereas Jörg's subjects were presented with particular conceptual levels (which they had mastered, of course), we are now concerned with the availability of various levels of categorization. An example will illustrate this point: A brown shadowy movement is seen outside. We say this must be:

"an animate being"
"a quadruped"
"a dog"
"a boxer"
"the landlord's dog, named Prince"

If we say "a dog" we have decided upon a particular level. We might equally have chosen the level of "quadruped," because for the use of this category or this level a smaller number of criterial attributes is sufficient.

The question arises here, How large is the area of freedom within which we can move in a given case and what factors determine the decision? We can here immediately recognize the overwhelming influence of language: in practice we can only choose a level for which our language offers us a term. We can only classify according to categories available in the particular language. Whorf's great merit has been to draw attention to the differences between these possibilities in different languages.

Before we consider his contribution in more detail, a question which has already been mentioned here must be discussed: Which factors influence the decision to select from two or more categories available in *one* language a particular one and no other?

This is, first of all, a factor determined by age and stage of development, because the attributes which are regarded as critical for a given category change and are revised in the course of individual growth. The study of these changes is closely associated with Piaget's name. Thus, the child has, for example, a category "weight" for which the attribute of conservation or constancy is not yet critical. And, vice versa, whereas form is still a critical attribute of mass for the child, this is not so for the adult; thus, a child might say that a plasticine cube becomes "smaller" when it is flattened.

The degree of flexibility and adequacy of the categories available for labeling is determined by the level of development; it should be emphasized that this has an effect on the degree of differentiation within the intentional dynamics of the communicative situation discussed by Olson (see p. 266). Herrmann (1974, 1976) has shown that "the context specific, appropriate word choice used in labeling constant objects must be explained not only in terms of the situational context parameters (Olson) but also in terms of interindividual differences in the idiosyncratic labeling flexibility of the language user" (1974, p. 172).

In addition to these developmentally determined limitations in the flexibility of naming, are there also sociologically determined limitations? Since the early works of Bernstein (1958, 1962), this question has generated considerable controversy, undoubtedly because it led to the formation of a new branch of sociolinguistics that shows strong emancipatory tendencies. At that time, Bernstein assumed that members of the lower class used a more "restricted" verbal code, providing them with less potential for expression (and therefore fewer chances for advancement) than the more "elaborate" verbal code used by members of the middle class. According to this view, man is a prisoner of the linguistic potential forced upon him by his social class. Without it being particularly noticed, Bernstein's formulation reintroduces notions first proposed by the Marxist theoretician, N. Marr. According to the latter, language is a function of society or, more specifically, social class, and therefore reflects corresponding differences (which lead to problems in communication). But this view violates the fundamental Marxist doctrine that the human mind can grasp the unmediated reality of the world. Furthermore, this notion of linguistic relativity is apt to raise questions about the validity of verbally formulated ideologies. Therefore, it is understandable that Stalin (1950) himself confronted Marr's deviation with the view that language is universally binding for all members of society.

Meanwhile, Bernstein himself has revised his original notion in favor of a more differentiated sociolinguistic formulation that is beyond the scope of our present discussion. We should simply note that the structure of the social situation exercises a restrictive and selective function on the production and reception of verbal utterances. It codetermines which code (i.e., dialect or literary language) is to be used, and presumably it also determines the length of the utterance, the degree of politeness (Schönbach 1974), etc.

Let us now return from this rather sociolinguistically oriented problem of the use of various codes to the psycholinguistic search for the determining factors of the code, how one encodes within a particular coding system, and, conversely, how the level of coding affects nonverbal behavior, thinking, and perception. Certainly a further factor which determines the level of categorization is its usefulness or importance. Thus, when talking about an automobile one may well refer to it as a "Volkswagen" or "Ford" or "Cadillac," but in the case of coins we are hardly likely to speak of a 1960 dime or a 1962 dime. Brown, who has discussed this question in a valuable investigation, "How Shall a Thing be Called?" (1958b), comments that we make distinctions where it matters. Among coins we have to distinguish nickels, dimes, and quarters, but for anyone who is not a coin collector it is of no importance whether a dime carries the 1960 or the 1962 imprint.

At this point we can pursue two lines of thought; one leads us back to a group of problems discussed previously and the other takes us further in the discussion of the theme of the present chapter.

We can think, first, of the number of words to be subsumed under one concept (e.g., under the concept "vehicle": "Ford," "convertible," "Mercedes," "truck," etc.), and, second, of the degree of completeness or appropriateness of comprehension. If a given group of persons are in agreement as to which words to classify under a certain concept (e.g., words suggested by the term "vehicle"), this leads to safer and better communication (see Johnson, 1962).

Let us now briefly sketch the second line of thought (we distinguish among cars but not among dimes). In general we operate at the level of categorization which is common to the majority of language users. At this level the most usual term is applied; and this level also provides a norm of constancy. It serves as a reference level. Dogs are generally called 'dogs' because this term delimits a category which for society is functionally defined. It makes little sense to say that one was disturbed in one's sleep by the barking of a mammal; but it is equally pointless to indicate the color or breed of the barking mammal. As Brown expressed it, "Our naming practices for people and coins correspond to our nonlinguistic practices" (1958b, p. 16). It is immaterial with which coin we pay, but it is not immaterial with which person we go out for the evening.

As a child learns the common terms, he learns to make those distinctions which his parents make and fails to make distinctions which, following the model of his parents and other language users, are unnecessary in the particular cultural context.

It can be predicted that such distinctions correlating with language occur particularly wherever "reality" does not in an obvious way provide classifications and gradations. We shall see later how restricted in fact the area is which is determined by "reality." In Chapter 7 we had already seen how altogether difficult it is to operate in a philosophically adequate manner with the notion of "reality."

One area in which language can presumably exercise a determining influence upon perception and thinking is the sphere of religion. Here words are particularly powerful because religion is concerned with things which are "difficult to put into words." It is a major issue to what extent thought on Christianity is affected by linguistic relativity. What changes in the "deeper substance" of the Christian faith are produced by translations into Greek, Latin, German, or Swahili? Is it still the same message in all the languages? Modern theological work very largely consists in a search for the undistorted below layers of distortions.

In the social field the classifications implicit in *kinship terms* offer an excellent illustration for the fact that relationships which appear to be completely determined by "reality" can be viewed linguistically in the most varying ways. The lexical units of kinship terminology, following Lounsbury (1963), can differ in two aspects: the "personnel-designating" aspect and the "role-symbolizing" aspect. The meanings of the "father" terms in two languages can in one case be distinguished as to who may be named "father," and, second, what it means to be a "father" in that linguistic community. In the European languages an individual employs the word "father" only to refer to the male parent (apart from the exception of "stepfather," "father-in-law," or the priest addressed as "Father"). In all those societies having what anthropologists call "Iroquois-type" kinship systems, it is not only the father in the European sense who is called "father" but also the brothers of the father and male cousins. In societies having "Crow-type" kinship systems (the Crows—like the Iroquois—are North American Indian tribes), the term "father" applies to the father, the father's brothers, the father's sister's sons, the sons of the father's sister's daughters, and at times also to the brothers of the father's mother.

Let us consider the following tabulation (cf. Lounsbury, 1963, p. 571):

1. Brother, sister
2. Father's brother's son, father's brother's daughter

3. Mother's sister's son, mother's sister's daughter
4. Father's sister's son, father's sister's daughter
5. Mother's brother's son, mother's brother's daughter

In our kinship usage, types 2 to 5 are classed as cousins. In the Iroquois-type usages, the 1, 2, and 3 types are all brothers and sisters; only 4 and 5 are classed as cousins. In the Crow-type usages 1, 2, and 3 are classed as brothers and sisters, 4 as father and aunt whereas the relationships under 5 are designated as son and daughter by a man while a woman refers to them as nephew and niece.

Corresponding to this linguistic division, our society attributes greatest importance to degree of collaterality, whereas it is only of secondary importance to which generation a person belongs. In the Iroquois system, generation and bifurcation are the principal dimensions, while in the Crow system a peculiar, skewed generation membership is of particular importance (i.e., females rank a social generation higher than their male siblings). The undifferentiated use of the term "cousin," as it is customary in our society, would be experienced as either ridiculous or immoral in some other communities (cf. Shlien, 1962, p. 161).

Here, then, the linguistic term is closely linked with the social structure which is perceived as the norm (an extreme adherent of the Whorf thesis of linguistic relativity might say: the linguistic designation determines the social structure perceived as norm). In the same way, the availability of a term describing a social relationship can legitimize this relationship which, if it were not for this term, might not be sanctioned by the moral system of the society. Thus, the invention in Germany of the term "Onkelehe," "uncle marriage," was a factor in the development of postwar German society, the importance of which should not be underrated.[2]

> From this angle it is possible to approach Korzybski's, Hayakawa's, and Johnson's General Semantics. But we will leave this until later, so that for the present we may complete the discussion of kinship terms.

Kinship terminology not only reflects the sociological structure of a society or linguistic community, but beyond that implicitly suggests psychological relations which are both the basis and result of this sociological structure. Kroeber has emphatically declared that kinship terminology is a subject of social *psychology*. In a similar manner, Gifford considers that kinship terms are primarily *linguistic* phenomena, whereas the social phenomena are secondary; they reveal the modes of thought in a given society's language. Kinship terms have a high degree of stability and they

---

[2] *Translator's note.* The term "Onkelehe" refers to a man and a woman living together as husband and wife, without being legally married, in order to evade higher income tax or loss of social security benefits.

can only partially or occasionally be influenced by social structure (Shlien, 1962).

Whether or not one is inclined to regard the linguistic aspect so unreservedly as primary, it is incontestable that an established kinship terminology exercises a structuring and structure-preserving influence.

The subject of kinship terminology was on the border between psycholinguistics and sociolinguistics. The next topic, forms of address, takes us plainly back into the field of psycholinguistics. Each time someone is addressed a renewed act of decision occurs between forms which the language puts at the speaker's disposal (e.g., "Mr. Smith"—"John," or in German the formal "Sie" versus the familiar "du"). Here psychological factors of more restricted scope can manifest themselves whereas kinship terms represent a supraindividual deposit preserved in the repertoire of the language available to all speakers alike. In kinship terminology the issue was how we speak *about* a person; here we consider how we speak *to* him. We therefore inquire into differences in behavior which are related to differences in linguistic forms.

"Forms of address are relational forms—the selection is not governed by properties of the speaker alone or of the addressee alone but by the properties of the dyad", i.e., the sociopsychological structure of the dyadic group (Brown, 1962, p. 664). Titles, first names, family names and pronouns of address are forms which can connect all members of a society with each other.

Brown—partly in collaboration with Gilman—has investigated the dual forms of address in 30 different languages (1960). To begin with he distinguishes two types: a reciprocal or symmetrical pattern and a nonreciprocal, asymmetrical pattern. In the case of the reciprocal type, both members of the dyad use the same form. Thus both parties can address each other with a first name or both use "Mr. + family name" or, in German, both use the familiar "du" or the formal "Sie."

> Brown describes pronouns of the type "du" (German), "tu" (Italian and French) comprehensively as belonging to the T class, which he contrasts with the V class pronouns: "vous," "vos," "lei," "Sie."

The difference between reciprocal patterns is one of degree of intimacy, friendship or familiarity or, as Brown puts it, of solidarity, based on shared interests and values.

In the nonreciprocal pattern, one of the parties, for example, uses the Christian name, "Jim," whereas the other says, "Mr. Jackson." One partner in German might use the formal "Sie" and the other the informal "du." In medieval Europe the knight spoke to the commoner in the T form and the commoner to the knight in the V form. Even today the nonreciprocal form of address expresses a status distinction, an unequal possession of attributes valued by the society. This status distinction is chiefly manifested in different degrees of social power.

It appears to be a linguistic universal (i.e., a phenomenon common to all languages) that forms of address code the two dimensions of solidarity and status. These two dimensions can have common *formal* definitions for all languages; solidarity is based on equality, and status on inequality with regard to valued characteristics. From the point of view of *content,* there are marked differences between different languages with regard to what creates equality or solidarity and inequality or differential status: age, vocation, lineage, wealth, religion, education and so forth.

But not only is it common to all languages to code solidarity and status in the form of the address, a second phenomenon is also universal: the form of address (e.g., the T form) used reciprocally between intimates is used equally in the nonreciprocal pattern downward from the higher to the lower status, whereas the form of address normally used reciprocally between distant acquaintances is, in the nonreciprocal pattern, used upwards. The intimate address form is, therefore, always also the condescending form, whereas the more formal address is, at the same time, always also the deferential mode of address.

There is no logical reason why the relationship could not equally well be reversed. But since this does not appear to happen, it is natural to ask whether this finding can be explained on psychological grounds. Brown puts forward the following hypothesis: although in Europe inequality of status is generally no longer expressed in a nonreciprocal form of address (the European "boss" addresses his subordinates in the V form), such inequality has an important part to play in the shift from one form of address to the other. Two people nowadays are likely to use a mutual V form of address to begin with. There may well be a move to a reciprocal use of the T form. The transition has, however, a nonreciprocal aspect. The person of higher status must initiate the change. This element of nonreciprocity becomes particularly evident in languages such as German where this transition almost amounts to a rite, *Brüderschaft.*[3] The speed of transition from status difference to solidarity is always determined by the person of higher status, although the person of inferior status is more highly motivated towards such a transition because solidarity enhances his status.[4]

Up to this point we have considered the two areas of religion and society to find out how far the forms implicit in the structure of language determine the thinking which takes place in the language. But in other areas, too, in which no abstract concepts are involved, but which deal with concrete

---

[3] *Translator's note.* The transition from the V form to the T form (*Brüderschaft*) is marked by the rite of both parties drinking each other's health with arms linked.

[4] The fusion of intimacy and condescension which was common in 19th century Europe is still shown in Yiddish today (Slobin, 1963).

objects, the formative force of language can be seen. If, however, language determines how the members of the speech community view the world and think about it, the differences among various languages lead necessarily to the conclusion that members of different language communities see and think of the world in different ways or, in other words, that each language implies a particular world view.

The foregoing sentence summarizes Whorf's interpretation of the arguments of his "predecessors" (from Humboldt to Sapir). The first proposition contained in it ("Language determines thought") is frequently referred to as the *principle of linguistic determinism,* the second ("Every language embodies a definite world view") is known as the *principle of linguistic relativity.* The first is of primary importance because, if it is valid, the second is a necessary consequence.

In the last two decades, the Whorf hypothesis has been received by scholars with much interest and sympathy. What is its position within the whole field of psycholinguistics? The Whorf hypothesis is concerned with the relationship between linguistic data (e.g., the structural organization of word classes) on the one hand and nonlinguistic data (e.g., processes of perception or thinking) on the other. But this relationship has been the major theme of psycholinguistics since its beginnings. To give only one illustration from this book, the investigation by Miller and Selfridge, discussed on pp. 104 f., also had as its subject the relationship between a linguistic set of data (i.e., approximation levels of verbal material to normal text) and a nonlinguistic set of data (i.e., speed of learning of such verbal material).

Therefore, in short, the Whorf hypothesis represents a special case of what in general terms is the subject of psycholinguistics as a whole. What accounts for the fact that this particular case has aroused such widespread interest in so many different disciplines leading to an overall intensification of psycholinguistic research? It is certain that there are several reasons.

Our age no doubt provides the right climate for it. International tensions and misunderstandings are brought close to us through press and radio. We know that such tensions and misunderstandings can threaten our existence directly. Thanks to good communications and a change-oriented structure of society, we are informed of strange ways of life which are most clearly manifested in a foreign language. And, finally, the ideological debates whose din reverberates around us let us feel bitterly the relativity of words ("Christian," "democratic," "freedom," and "socialism"). Thus, Whorf, by considering the linguistic aspect of the relationship, postulates interlinguistic rather than intralinguistic distinctions, and by attempting to match them with differences in ideologies, has found a cause which we experience as our own. It can, in fact, be argued that this special position of the Whorf thesis is not justified. For even within one idiom, as Plessner once expressed it, language may think for us or against us, in any case beyond us. In a later discussion, we will see that General Semantics represents a movement which aims at the elucidation of relativity and determinism within a single language.

Another reason for the receptivity to Whorf's hypothesis lies in the fact that Whorf had the great skill of presenting his thesis in an exceedingly vivid and convincing way by comparing heterogeneous languages. He confronts American Indian languages and Eskimo with what he calls "Standard Average European" (SAE), interpreted by him as the undifferentiated communality of English, French, German, Italian, and so on. The structure of Indian languages is so radically different from SAE that culture-bound or language-bound differences between the corresponding speech communities can be particularly clearly and persuasively demonstrated. Such comparisons will now be illustrated, first by a lexical example, and then by some grammatical items.

In SAE there is a uniform category called "snow." That is to say that a single word ("snow" in English) is used to refer to falling snow, snow on the ground, packed snow, slushy snow, etc. To an Eskimo, to whom snow matters more than to an average European, this would seem extraordinary. He sees different things—and designates them by different words—in these varying modes of appearance of a substance which is always the same to us. To use the terminology of the previous paragraphs, the Eskimo categorizes on a different level. By contrast, Aztecs, for whom snow is probably less important, treat this aspect in an even more undifferentiated manner: "cold," "ice," and "snow" are all represented by the same root with different endings.

In this case, an intercultural comparison lends support to the view discussed above, i.e., that one cannot acquire the language of a community without at the same time adopting the perceptual distinctions which are normally—and perhaps inevitably—made in that society.

In order to be able to employ correctly the English word "snow" (or its equivalents in other European languages), one must learn to distinguish, on the one hand, snow from grass, earth, rain, etc., but, on the other hand, one must also learn to treat as equivalent slushy snow, powdery snow, dirty snow, icy snow, falling snow and snow on the ground. And since in English there is the uniform category "snow," it can be argued on the basis of the thesis of linguistic determinism that the user of English learns to regard snow as something unified. At this point we again encounter the process of categorization in the act of recognition which was discussed on p. 271.

Even more impressive than such differences in the vocabulary of a language are the examples of structural differences gathered by Whorf. In SAE we divide most of our words into nouns and verbs. "Our language thus gives us a bipolar division of nature. But nature herself is not thus polarized. If it be said that "strike, turn, run," are verbs because they denote temporary or short-lasting events, i.e., actions, why then is "fist" a noun? It also is a temporary event. Why are "lightning, spark, wave, eddy, pulsation, flame, storm, phase, cycle, spasm, noise, emotion" nouns? They are temporary events. If "man" and "house" are nouns because they are long-lasting and stable events, i.e., things, what then are "keep, adhere, extend, project, continue, persist, grow, dwell," and so on doing among the verbs? If it be objected that "possess, adhere" are verbs because they are stable relationships rather than stable percepts, why then should "equilibrium, pressure, current, peace, group, nation, society, tribe, sister," or any kinship term be among the nouns? It will be found that an "event" to us means "what our language classes as a verb" or something analogized therefrom. And it will be found that it is not possible to define "event, thing, object, relationship," and so on, from nature, but that to define them always involves a circuitious return to the grammatical categories of the definer's language" (Whorf, 1956, p. 215).[5]

In Hopi, one of the North American Indian languages, events are indeed defined according to duration. "Lightning, wave, flame, meteor, puff of smoke or pulsation" are necessarily verbs here, while "cloud" and "storm" are approximately at the lower limit of duration for nouns. In Hopi there is therefore a closer correlation between formal and semantic pecularities of word classes (at least in this example) so that there is less danger in Hopi than in SAE of thought being misled by the formal attributes of words.

In the following example taken from Whorf a structural distinction between SAE and Hopi has been pursued because of its nonlinguistic implications for world view: "In our language, that is SAE, plurality and cardinal numbers are applied in two ways: to real plurals and imaginary plurals . . . We say 'ten men' and also 'ten days'. Ten men either are or could be objectively perceived as ten, ten in one group perception—ten men on a street corner, for instance. But 'ten days' cannot be objectively experienced. We experience only one day, today; the other nine (or even all ten) are something conjured up from memory or imagination. If 'ten days' be regarded as a group it must be as an 'imaginary', mentally constructed group. Whence comes this mental pattern?" It originates ". . . from the fact that our language confuses the two different situations, has but one pattern for both. When we speak of 'ten steps forward, ten strokes on a bell', or any similarly described cyclic sequence, 'times' of any sort, we are doing the same thing as with 'days'. Cyclicity brings the response of imaginary plurals. But a likeness of cyclicity to aggregates is not unmistakably given by experience prior to language, or it would be found in all languages . . ." (p. 139); i.e., they would be what Carroll calls "conceptual invariants." "In Hopi there is a different linguistic situation. Plurals and cardinals are used only for entities that form or can form an objective group. There are no imaginary plurals, but instead ordinals used with singulars. An expression such as 'ten days' is not used. The equivalent statement is an operational one that

---

[5] The studies and experiments by Brown started out from this line of argument.

reaches one day by a suitable count. 'They stayed ten days' becomes 'they stayed until the eleventh day' . . . Our 'length of time' is not regarded as a length but as a relation between two events in lateness. Instead of our linguistically promoted objectification of . . . 'time', the Hopi language has not laid down any pattern that would cloak the subjective 'becoming later' that is the essence of time'' (Whorf, p. 140).

Whorf characterizes the thought habits, corresponding to and related to these different linguistic structures, thus: "The Hopi microcosm seems to have analyzed reality largely in terms of events (or better 'eventing') . . ." (p. 147). "A characteristic of Hopi behavior is the emphasis on preparation. This includes announcing and getting ready for events well beforehand . . ." (p. 148). They do not have a number of separate time elements but one continuum. Prayer, song, the preparation of special food, running, racing, dancing, all these are preparatory acts which are frequently repeated. And since time for the Hopi is not a motion but a ''getting later'' of all previous events, repetition is not wasted but accumulated.

In contrast to this, SAE, corresponding to our quantified and spatial conception of time, expresses our interest in exact chronological localization, bookkeeping, time wages (equal portions of time have equal value), also our interest in speed and economy of time.

Whorf is not the only one to have demonstrated by means of such intercultural comparisons (i.e., by comparing two speech communities) parallels between linguistic and nonlinguistic facts. For example, Hoijer (1951, 1953, 1954) has pointed out the fact that in Navaho, another North American Indian language, two kinds of verbs perform an important function. Neuter verbs appear to designate "eventings solidified" into states of being, by virtue of the withdrawal of movement. Active verbs, on the other hand, represent "eventings in motion." The nature, direction and status of a movement can be described in this language in a most precise way.

Corresponding to these linguistic facts there are certain parallels in cognition, culture and ideology. The Navahos are nomads. Their gods, too, wander from place to place seeking to maintain by their motion the dynamic flux which, in the Navaho conception, characterizes the universe.

Whereas in SAE sentences frequently present an action and its agent, a person in Navaho is not cause or originator of an action but only associated with it. This is in keeping with what Kluckhohn and Leighton (1946) have said about the Navahos and their ideology: they do not strive to master nature but to influence her with songs and rituals.

These examples must suffice. Although they impress, they leave a certain uneasiness. The impression is gained that Whorf, Hoijer, and other workers in this area with enormous skill and subtlety have searched out and discovered parallels between intangible sociocultural phenomena and linguistic structures.

It is, however, possible to question the parallelism between them. Whorf's principle of linguistic relativity and linguistic determinism does not say anything about the manner in which the two are related, nor does it predict where such parallelism is to be expected. However impressive the data are, as scientific evidence they are far too anecdotal and do not lead to precise and testable hypotheses. Nevertheless, these data have enormous value in providing suggestive leads.

> Equally suggestive are also the acute observations of poets and writers who have spoken of language as guides to thought. Simone de Beauvoir (1958) recounts how her early experiences remained shapeless without words and how the simple vocabulary of her parents, which she adopted, modelled and distorted her experiences without her being able to prevent it, although she was aware of the distortions. The German dramatist Kleist (1806) spoke of the word as the flywheel on the axle of thought (in Mueller, 1946).

The critique of Whorf's views—which, by the way, was less directed against Whorf himself than against some of his over-eager adherents —can be summarized as follows: cases that fit and have a certain plausibility are reported; but no question is raised whether there are not also other cases which do not fit. Since it is impossible to estimate the number of possible kinds of relationships between linguistic and nonlinguistic data, it is not possible to say how much importance can be attributed to the individual case in which the relationship has been proved.

The method which has been employed in this area has been made clear by Lenneberg and Roberts (1956) in a fictitious but by no means absurd illustration. Let us assume the claim that there is a relationship between language (C) and national character (K); accordingly, the matched pairs in Table 20 are produced.

Such matchings are entertaining, perhaps even impressive, but they have no scientific value. The vigor of the Whorfian thought is indicated by the fact that psychologists and anthropologists have felt impelled to take up these ideas and during the past decades have tried to support the Whorf thesis by empirical inquiries.

Table 20

Language conditions (C's)	National character traits (K's)
Japanese: harsh sounds	purported to correspond to: harsh discipline
German: complicated sentence structure	purported to correspond to: complicated philosophical thoughts
English: preponderance of monosyllabic words	purported to correspond to: conciseness; thriftiness

The basic design of such investigations has been outlined by Lenneberg in a fundamental article (1956). Variations of linguistic conditions are matched with variations of nonlinguistic behavior in the following manner:

C_1 corresponds to K_i
C_2 corresponds to K_{ii}
C_3 corresponds to K_{iii}
. . . .
C_n corresponds to K_N

The first criterion which must be met in such an investigation consists in defining what varies under C and what varies under K. In the fictitious example quoted above, it is clear that neither in C nor in K are the variations in the same dimensions. Lenneberg speaks of the *criterion of variation*.

He, secondly, introduces the *criterion of universality*. The feature investigated must be present in all cultures under investigation. For example, the question of whether the Germans have developed their philosophy because of their language or whether the Bororo Indians—equally on account of their language—lack any formal epistemology is in principle unanswerable.

The third of Lenneberg's criteria is that of *simplicity*. Commensurability presupposes the construction of descriptive parameters. Thus it is possible to compare measurements of weight because they vary along a single dimension. But if we want to describe the social actions which can be designated by the term "justice," we need a large number of parameters. The system of coordinates required would be so incredibly complex that it would be impossible to describe exactly the difference between the actions to which the term "justice" applies in the two different cultures.

Lenneberg now singles out one area which satisfies all three criteria and which is excellently suited to test the Whorf hypothesis: the language of sensory perception, i.e., the words and structures used to designate the sensations of temperature, humidity, light or color. Thus, we reach the major testing ground of the Whorf hypothesis: color coding.

> Even in this specialized field there are historically interesting predecessors of modern thought. Homer's translators had great difficulties in translating the Greek color terms so that for a time it was thought the Greeks were color blind. We note here again the tendency to explain a behavioral feature found in many people in terms of a universal physiological characteristic instead of attempting to find an exogenous (sociological or linguistic) determinant of the common feature. In quite a similar way, it has long been customary to account for the phenomena of adolescence in terms of biological changes until anthropologists reported the absence of these phenomena in other cultures where the biological changes of puberty are the same as in our own culture.

The earlier examples of the use of the word "snow" illustrated how a certain sector of nature is coded uniformly in SAE, i.e., is conceived as a single word, while in another language, Eskimo, instead of being coded uniformly, it is subdivided. The two languages dispose of different numbers of words for a certain sector of physical reality. Lenneberg and Brown have spoken of the varying degrees of "codability" of this sector in different languages.

> The concept of codability is not confined in its application to lexical items and physical reality; it can equally be applied to grammatical operations (e.g., the differences in arrangement of word classes discussed and to non-physical realities (e.g., kinship structures).

Prima facie, therefore, this presents only a coding phenomenon or differentiation of linguistic organization. This observation becomes an argument in favor of Whorf only through the claim that nonlinguistic distinctions correspond to the linguistic differentiation.

How does this apply now to color perception? The human organism can distinguish approximately 7,500,000 hues. English has nearly 4,000 color terms, but only eight of these are used frequently. Broadly expressed, it can be said that in order to encode 7,500,000 possibilities, 4000 terms (and eight common words) are available. In this area too—as always in most natural languages—coding involves a marked reduction of multiplicity.

Different languages use different color categories. In the Iakuti language there is only one term for what is named by two in SAE: blue and green. In SAE, therefore, one region or dimension of experience is differentiated which is undifferentiated in the Iakuti language.

Now all color dimensions are continuous: red is linked to orange through gradual transition; orange merges gradually into yellow and then into green, and so on.

> One objection may be expected at this point; what about the "primary colors"? Where do they come in? Why is there a tendency to regard red, blue and yellow as primary colors, or why is it sometimes claimed that red, blue, yellow and green are primary colors? There are no arguments on physical grounds for the assumption of certain colors as primary. All that the so-called color-mixing rules claim is that one has to operate with three colors if one wants to produce all the shades of the color circle. Even certain findings made by Granit, which may establish probable physiological connections with the primary color problem do not affect the conclusion that the question, What are the primary colors? should be treated mainly as a semantic problem (cf. Weisgerber, 1962b).

Where language draws sharp boundaries there are no corresponding physical boundaries. There is no physical criterion to determine up to what point one has to use the term "red" and from which point onwards one has to say "yellow."

Let us assume a speaker of SAE is asked to name a point × on the spectral continuum (Fig. 60). He will probably hesitate whether to call it green, blue, or blue-green, etc. The Iakuti speaker, on the other hand, will use the term

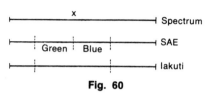

Fig. 60

applicable to the whole area without hesitation. The hue × is more difficult to code in SAE than in Iakuti.

From this observation, we are led to the fundamental question of psycholinguistic interest, Does the difference in codability affect the nonverbal behavior? A positive reply to this question would broadly lend support to the validity of the Whorf thesis at least in its general form.

This question has been studied experimentally by Brown and Lenneberg (1954). Their experiment, which is particularly noteworthy because it stands in contrast to the prevailing tendency to speculate about this question, deserves to be examined in detail.

As a first step, the concept of codability had to be defined operationally. This was done by asking five judges to pick out the "best" red, orange, yellow, green, blue, purple, pink and brown from 240 chips showing all the hues of the color circle. This indicated a very high degree of agreement among the judges. A further 16 hues were added to those eight so that the choices ranged as evenly as possible over the whole color circle.

In the first experiment carried out with the material which had thus been prepared, 24 subjects had the task of naming as rapidly as possible each color chip as it was presented. Among the measures calculated were the following:

1. the number of syllables which on the average were used to name a particular color;

The authors thus follow a suggestion made by Doob (1952), i.e., to relate the Whorf thesis to the results of Zipf's investigations. According to Zipf, the more frequently a term is used in a language, the shorter it is likely to be. From this, one can in turn infer that the number of syllables (or phenomes) offers a clue to the currency of a term in a particular language. Brown defines this conclusion as follows: the existence of a monosyllabic term in preference to a polysyllabic one suggests a high degree of cognitive availability of the particular principle of categorization.

2. average reaction time from the moment of presentation of the color to the utterance of the color term as another measure of the relationship between codability and availability;
3. the degree of agreement in the terms used by the subjects for a particular color.

These (and some other) measures were correlated. Table 21 presents the results.

Table 21.   Correlation matrix for five indices of codability.

Measure	1	2	3	4	5
Number of syllables					
Number of words	.425*				
Reaction-time	.387	.368			
Interpersonal agreement	.630*	.486*	.864*		
Intrapersonal agreement	.355	.537*	.649*	.773*	
k from second factoring	.589	.587	.787	.976	.795
Communality from first factoring	.403	.378	.671	.873	.653

*p ≤ .05
Based on Brown and Lenneberg, 1954, p. 459.

If one factor is extracted from this matrix, only a few correlations are left. This means that a single factor is sufficient to account mathematically for these coefficients of correlation. Brown and Lenneberg have named this factor "codability."

In this way, it was, first of all, possible to define operationally the factor of codability as the exact composite value of the above measures; and only after that was done was the attempt made to correlate it with nonlinguistic behavior.

The nonlinguistic behavior selected by the authors was color recognition. A set of four colors was presented to each subject simultaneously. After an interval the subjects were asked to pick out the same colors from a color chart consisting of 120 different colors.

The question to be studied was whether codability had an influence upon retention and recognition. The answer to this question lies in the correlation coefficient between codability and recognition score: 0.415. The more easily a color is coded, the better it is remembered. The conclusions of the Brown-Lenneberg study can be formulated as follows. Differences in codability are related to differences in availability. And if instead of this restricted formulation one prefers a more generalized one, it may be said that a connection between verbal and nonverbal behavior—as postulated by the Whorf hypothesis—is probably established.[6]

This investigation was made within one culture; that is to say, it investigated distinctions, matched by verbal differences, within one culture or speech community. The fundamental relevance of such studies for the discussion and evaluation of the Whorf hypothesis has already been explained above (p. 283). Nevertheless, complementary cross-cultural comparisons

---

[6] Later, in the context of Lenneberg's investigations, we shall return to Lantz and Steffire's (1964) study. There we will see that the question about the validity of Whorf's theory must encompass the communicative intention of speaker and listener.

are also of great interest; such a study was carried out by Lenneberg and Roberts (1953, cited in Brown and Lenneberg, 1954, p. 461).

In Zuni there is only one term for yellow and orange. If the above experiment is repeated with Zuni Indians, it appears that yellow and orange are confused much more frequently by Zuni Indians than by English-speaking Americans. It is interesting to note that the performance of those Zunis who also speak English falls between that of monolingual Zunis and monolingual English-speaking Americans.

Confirmation of the evidence provided in these investigations for the validity (or, perhaps better, the fruitfulness) of the Whorf hypothesis, can be found in numerous studies quite unconnected with psycholinguistics, which have demonstrated the positive influence of verbal coding on learning and retention. Anything which can be named or can be given a verbal label is learned more easily and less easily forgotten. The concept of "schema," which has been profitably employed by investigators, ranging from Head via Bartlett to Piaget, in the study of memory and cognitive psychology, generally refers to a verbally encoded schema.

In a way we have now returned to the starting point of our deliberations. After examining language-determined intra- and intercultural differences, we have now returned to the problem of how the code form which we apply to what we hear determines the corresponding "depth" of our understanding, and how, in speech production, the encoding potentials, provided by our language, define our conceptualization of reality and thereby determine the success of the cummunicative act. The psychology of information processing—with its multi-store models as well as Craik and Lockhart's "coding depth" approach—implies that all verbal and many nonverbal stimuli undergo a translation or verbal encoding phase on their way to becoming apperceptions. If this notion is valid, then it is reasonable to assume that such apperceptions—our view of the external world and our thinking about it—are partly determined by the verbal containers and structures which are at the disposal of the receiving individual for this intermediate phase. It is now possible to understand that not only those items which are available in verbal concepts (which belong to what Weisgerber would call "the linguistic intermediate sphere") are subject to linguistic relativity; even the things of direct reality are passed through a grid of verbal structures and distorted. Whether certain plants are "weeds" in a country depends on the language of the inhabitants of this country. Likewise, whether the snow falling from the sky melts in spring is a problem of semantics. If Aristotle had spoken a different language, say Chinese or Hopi, instead of Greek, we would operate today with a different kind of logic.

The thesis of language as a determiner of thought and perception and especially the thesis of psycholinguistic relativity of the thought in a given language have both been very influential in recent years. Nevertheless, criticisms have been voiced and objections have been raised which have somehow reduced the claim of absolute validity with which the Whorf hypothesis (less by Whorf himself than by his disciples) has been put forward.

The criticism of Whorf's method of inquiry has already been reported. In the following paragraphs the objections to be outlined are those that have been made from the psycholinguistic and philosophical point of view.

Among these are certain findings in developmental psychology which need mentioning first of all. The absence of parallelism in linguistic and cognitive growth in childhood has been stressed repeatedly—to name only a few—by Köhler, Vigotsky, and Piaget, who have demonstrated, in different ways, intelligent and cognitive operations in nonverbal behavior.

If, for a moment, we assume the validity of the Whorf thesis, it would mean that it would be impossible for intercultural differences in nonverbal areas (e.g., of concepts) to be greater than the differences in verbal fields. It is certain that Whorf has given a picture of the differences between languages which is too one-sided. Besides the differences to which Whorf has drawn attention, there are also communalities which we are inclined to accept as a matter of course. Greenberg, Osgood, Miller and others have opposed the concept of language universals to the Whorf notion of linguistic relativity.

We have already encountered such language universals in our earlier discussions of those primitive concepts, agent, patient, object, instrument. Presumably they have universal characteristics because the "mental apperception mechanism" (Bierwisch) of humans who use language is the same or at least similar everywhere. But in addition and beyond that there are universals at different levels. Thus, for example, all languages can be analyzed into sequences of relatively few, different phonemes.

Approximately a dozen phonological features are sufficient to signal the required distinctions. In all languages a restricted number of syntactic classes can be found. In all languages the admissible word sequences (sentences) are produced with the help of a finite number of grammatical rules. All languages have subject-predicate constructions.

All languages know the principal verbal operators ("and," "not," "or"); all languages tackle in some way the notions of space and time. "I," "you," and "he" occur in all languages. Everywhere, questions and answers follow an alternating pattern.[7]

These language universals are so much a matter of course that they are noticed less than the more striking interlinguistic differences which constitute the basis of the thesis of linguistic relativity.

Osgood (1962a), for example, recognizes the evidence reported above for the reality of linguistic relativity. He calls it "denotative relativity"; but on

---

[7] This does not mean to say that both partners cannot talk simultaneously. The masking capacity of the human voice is not sufficiently great to exclude this possibility.

the basis of his own inquiries he is able to oppose it with the existence of "connotative universality." In different languages, ratings on the semantic differential of a particular word and its translation into other languages produce congruent results.

Such observations suggest that it depends on the subject of investigation whether we will find relativity or universality. Investigations on denotative relations produce evidence for the thesis of relativity; inquiries on connotative relations yield results supporting the thesis of universality.

At any rate, the existence of such language universals draws attention once more to the biologic basis of language, hence to features which apply to the whole species. The arbitrariness of the decision to play a certain language-game, as suggested by Wittgenstein, is kept within bounds by what is biologically given (Lenneberg, 1960).

The Whorf thesis assumes the unidirectional determination of language giving form to thought. If linguistic universals are taken into account, the view reached will be that of Miller, who writes, "If it is true, as Whorf and Sapir believed, that our language shapes our psychology, then it is at least equally true that our psychology shapes our language" (1963, p. 418).

The relationship between codability and availability, which has been adduced as evidence for the validity of the case for relativity, has been critically examined by French (1963), among others. In the Brown-Lenneberg type of investigation, codability has generally been interpreted either as uniformity of designation attributed to an object by different speakers or as brevity of designation. But there are, of course, also unusual "original" terms which, in spite of their novelty, may be understood by the listener immediately. If a speaker calls a particular color "Swiss-cheese colored," he employs an unusual term of considerable phonemic length which nevertheless conveys a uniform meaning to speakers of English.

Here an impression is encoded in an unusual form; but a nonlinguistic uniformity within the linguistic community, i.e., everybody knows Swiss cheese, guarantees the consistency of the listener's reaction to this unusual creation: a member of the speech community will, for example, easily remember the color so described.

This leads us to one of the principal objections to Whorf's procedures. They are linguistically too atomistic. He takes isolated words from different languages ("snow") and, comparing these, notes that the category which this word designates in one language has not the same coverage as the category designated by the translation "equivalent" (which is not an equivalent). As the grids in the two languages do not coincide, he is led to the conclusions which are embodied in the theory of linguistic relativity.

In the analysis of structural peculiarities, too, Whorf proceeds in the same atomistic manner: for example, he notes that the verb in one language functions differently from the verb in another language. However, the work and function of a language do not result from the sequential arrangement of separate words, nor from the stringing together of single word classes or other grammatical structures. If the word A in language Alpha is not matched by a similarly defined word A′ in language Beta, who can say that in Beta one cannot express with the words A′ + F′ + N′ what in language Alpha has been expressed with A? Even if—in contrast to Navaho—we have no special class of verbs to express "eventings solidified" by class membership, we may still be capable, by means of corresponding adjectives and adverbs, to express the state which the Indian speaker wants to express and no doubt expresses more succinctly.

The Whorf view is based entirely on the notion of an independent study of semantics. But in an earlier part of this book we have already explained in detail why the meaning of a word cannot be reduced to an unambiguous and simple word-thing relationship. The inclusion of the language-user and of the situation leads beyond the simple reference function of language which Whorf had in mind. (Whorf, so to speak, "blames" language for imperfections in the word-thing relationship.) Longacre (1956), in a subtle criticism of the Whorf thesis in which he contrasts the views of Whorf and Urban, emphatically stresses that language is less a grid than a calculus.

This is also demonstrated by a study that conceptualizes Lenneberg's notion of codability somewhat differently. Lantz and Steffire (1964) defined codability not as interindividual agreement on the label but as "communicative precision," i.e., the precision with which a listener identifies a particular color chip after it has been verbally designated. This communicative precision represents a dimension that correlates more highly with retention, which was also one of Lenneberg's dependent variables, than with the interindividual agreement on the label. This study also indicates that in designating a color the formulation chosen by the subject is dependent on the context. We are reminded here of Olson, who strongly emphasized that it is not so much the speaker's vocabulary but his intention which determines the assigned label. It is not the (more or less appropriate, available) words that determine what will be said and possibly retained, but it is the words (and much else) that the speaker uses as instruments to express meaning.[8]

Whorf is so concerned with the process of classification—a process which is undoubtedly present in language—that his thesis is basically more a thesis of the relativity of lexical and grammatical features than of the relativity of language in general. In spite of difficulties, translation *is* possible, and the distinction between "amour" in French and "love" in English is no greater than the distinction between the meanings of Jack's "love" and of Jill's "love."

Whorf emphasizes the differences between languages. He denies the justification of speaking of language in general: " 'It may even be in the cards that there is no such thing as "Language" (with a capital L) at all' " (from

---

[8] Cf. Hörmann (1976).

Longacre 1956, p. 300). Opposed to this we find Bühler's view that the whole enterprise of language theory (and we might add of psycholinguistics) is based on the presupposition of the existence of "human language in the singular" (1934, p. 141).

Gipper (1972) presents one of the most thoughtfully expressed positions on the Sapir-Whorf hypothesis. After extensive studies of American Indians and their languages he comes to the following conclusion: "Man's thought is 'relative' with respect to the possibilities of expression afforded by the available language systems and their semantic structures insofar as it can only take on form by complying with these given conditions. But if human thought becomes objectified in relation to the available language it does not mean that it is also mentally determined in this manner. Relativity does not imply determinism. The human spirit has the freedom to put to infinite use the finite means of the available language. However, whatever he may be able to express verbally he will never be able to achieve total independence and absoluteness. Only in this restricted sense can one speak of a linguistic relativity principle" (p. 248).

The view that different languages reflect reality in different ways and therefore necessarily introduce an element of distortion (because reality can only be reached by means of language) has been attacked from two sides: by St. Augustine and Wittgenstein. St. Augustine says, "If no one asks me, I know; but if I want to explain to someone who asks me, I do not know." This refers to a form of knowing preceding verbal formulation and at the same time resisting such formulation. If this kind of knowledge is possible, language is a prison which man enters by speaking.

On the other hand, Wittgenstein adopts an extreme Whorfian view by making such statements as, "Grammar tells what kind of object anything is" (1958, § 373). Wittgenstein goes so far as to make the question of the relationship between language and reality meaningless—a question which is central to Whorf—because, according to Wittgenstein, reality is only constituted in language and by means of language. There is no fixed reference point by means of which the internally completely consistent language-game could be made relative to something else. Whereas in St. Augustine's view man enters the prison of language only by speaking, in Wittgenstein's view there is no question of imprisonment because there is nothing outside it.

The attempt to establish a philosophical formulation of Whorf's metalinguistics leads to no conclusion, except to the skeptical questioning whether language is always an instrument in the hands of human thought or whether thought is drawn along avenues prepared by familiar language.

From this skeptical position two trends of thought have developed: one, in a somewhat naive way, aims at language improvement in the expectation of making language more effective, and the other, more profoundly, tries to change our attitude to language and therefore to reduce human conflicts. The first can be found here and there in different places, while the second has been formalized under the name of General Semantics.

The attempt to improve the effectiveness of language—which inevitably leads to the question of the criterion by which to measure such improvement—can be illustrated for example by Steger's argument:[9] the standard language must always be a tool which is appropriate to the thought of a given age. The boldest discoveries of our time are expressed in the special languages of chemistry, mathematics and physics; for example, in our everyday standard language, the sun still "rises" and "sets" in spite of the fact that it has been known for 500 years that the sun does not do anything of the sort. Our language can make the poetry of the 18th and 19th centuries ring in our ears, yet it is quite incapable of expressing the newer discoveries about the universe. "An improved, i.e., more consistent use of language than the common standard language would be able to express thoughts in a more profound and more comprehensive way" (1962, p. 196).

This view—like, incidentally, also that of the General Semanticists—expresses an enviable belief in progress. Yet a thoughtful observer will ask whether the sun does not "rise" and "set" after all: in other words, whether the world of the physicist or of the scientist in general must necessarily form the basis of everyday language. Is everyday language most effective when it is determined by the sciences? In Steger's view everyday language should be guided by the current state of knowledge—but is it not equally possible that the current thought of an age is guided by everyday language? It would be a rewarding task for diachronic psycholinguistics to analyze the *Zeitgeist* ("mind of an age") from this point of view.

A further attempt to improve the effectiveness of language is a partial task of what is commonly known as "cybernetics." The application of a terminology, originally developed in technology, to such areas as biology, psychology, sociology, and even educational science has undoubtedly enormously enriched these disciplines. Formulations have been found for new relationships, and new connections have been made visible, thus confirming in a most eloquent way the interdependence between language and thought. Equally, however, this kind of development reveals the other side of the coin: the terminology developed round the original cybernetic model exercises a directing influence upon the biologist, psychologist, or any other scientist who operates with it. It is quite possible that those who make use of these concepts do not even know to what extent their thinking follows avenues determined by the language they employ.

General Semantics is less concerned with the improvement of the effectiveness of language than with the improvement of human relationships. This discipline is, in a way, an "applied" science. It aims at creating an

---

[9] *Translator's note.* Hugo Steger is a distinguished contemporary Germanist.

awareness of linguistic relativity and linguistic determinism in order to prevent language from taking over thought.

As a school of thought, General Semantics was established by Korzybski, a Pole who came to live in the United States. His principal work significantly carries the title of *Science and Sanity*. His views largely coincide with those expressed by Whorf, although both developed their ideas independently of each other. One difference, however, is that Korzybski and, following him, Hayakawa, Johnson, Rapaport, and others have drawn pedagogical consequences from the interdependence of language and thought. In Whorf's work the relationship between language and *thought* is central, while in General Semantics the central relationship is between language and *thinker* (or more precisely the relationship between language and the inadequate thinker). The individual who is the primary concern of General Semantics is the person who identifies the structure of language with the structure of reality. The chief principle of General Semantics is that language and reality are related in the same way as a map is to the terrain to which it refers (i.e., the principle of *nonidentity*). Language, therefore, is not an image of *reality*: at best it is an image of the *structure* of reality.

From this follow a number of interesting implications. In Whorf's view—inasmuch as he comments on this at all—reality is unstructured. It is given structure by the language in which it is conceived. For Korzybski, however, reality *is* structured: the map, therefore, can be more or less accurate. The structural concordance between map and terrain, which is of interest to General Semantics, is akin to the principle of isomorphism of Gestalt psychology where, equally, similarity of structure, for example, links different levels: stimulus, retina, cortex, etc., in an act of perception (cf. Köhler, 1924).

The second principle of General Semantics is *incompleteness*. The representations in language are always less than what is represented. The map inevitably ignores details of the terrain.

Finally, the third principle of General Semantics is that of *self-reflexiveness*. We use language to speak about language; we make judgments about judgments; we evaluate values.

All these principles can be considered to be features of the process of abstraction which is fundamental to all language. This process of abstraction can be removed to varying degrees from the level of the concrete event. If, for example, we speak of "a statement about a statement," the word "statement" is used on two different levels of abstraction. Such terms are described in General Semantics as multiordinal; "yes," "no," "true," "false," "agreement," "nonagreement," "relationship," "number," "structure," "love," "hate"—all these and many other words are multi-ordinal. It is characteristic of these multiordinal words that they have different meanings on different levels of abstraction; the first "statement" in our example is on a higher level of abstraction than the second.

The multiordinality of many words enriches our vocabulary in an extraordinary way, but it is also a source of misunderstandings and conflicts if one is not aware of them.

In this connection the reader will recall the discussion in chapter 7 of Bertrand Russell's theory of types. The example of the lying Cretan showed that, if a judgment is made about all judgments of a given class, this judgment does not itself fall into the same class. General Semantics would in this instance point out the multiordinality of the word 'judgment' and recommend as a measure of precaution the distinguishing subscripts judgment$_1$ and judgment$_2$.

There is a certain Socratic note about General Semantics which rests upon the conviction that making oneself aware of the traps of language is sufficient to circumvent them.

Once we know that a verbal statement is not reality, that past is not present, that Communism$_{1950}$ is not Communism$_{1965}$, that intelligent$_{John}$ is not intelligent$_{Jack}$, we will no longer regard the linguistic event as the signal for a ready-made, prejudiced reaction ("He is an American, no wonder . . ."). Instead, we will conceive the verbal event as such, i.e., as a symbol; therefore we will not react to the verbal event but to the nonverbal reality symbolized by the verbal event.

General Semantics sees as its aim an education for "extensional orientation," i.e., an orientation towards the reality of the world. This stands in contrast to "intensional orientation," orientation towards words or verbal labels. Man's behavior must not be directed by "semantic" or "signal" reactions, i.e., reactions evoked by the sound of what is heard or thought, therefore reactions which are prefabricated and hence prejudiced. In order to react it is not sufficient to identify the stimulus in a rough and ready manner (e.g., as the term "police") and then to make the stereotyped response (e.g., to police-in-general). It is important to control behavior in such a way that pauses may be interposed between the verbal stimulus and the response, so as to identify the symbol as a symbol, to advance from the symbol to the object symbolized and to grasp it with its differentiations (which are always simplified by the symbol). In this way the delayed symbol reaction will not be guided by a word but by reality.

This shows that General Semantics for 40 years pursued pedagogical and therapeutic goals that communications therapy now claims to have discovered.

The thesis of linguistic determinism leads to this realization: language is not simply an instrument we control; it controls us. The same language which adds a dimension of freedom to our existence appears to us at the end of this book as a power in its own right and, indeed, as overpowering. To a certain extent language seems to travel past what we proudly feel to be our "real" capacities. Through language many bygone generations help to shape our thoughts. As we speak we "educate" future generations as yet unborn.

We can look at language in another way, somewhat less pessimistically. Man is not always and not only the victim of his language. Whoever creates language, which in its purest form will be poetic creation—but in effect such creations can occur anywhere—shares in the creation of our world. Whoever forms new sentences about a sunset enriches the nation whose language he speaks. The psychology of language ends where poetry begins. Somewhere between the gain and loss of freedom which the possession of language implies is the true center of human existence. The self is surrounded by the mirrors of language.

Bibliography

Ach, N.: Zur psychologischen Grundlegung der sprachlichen Verständigung. Ber. 12. Kongr. Dtsch. Ges. Psychol. (Hamburg 1931), Jena: Fischer 1932, 122–133.

Adelson, M., F. A. Muckler, and A. C. Williams: Verbal learning and message variables related to amount of information. In: Quastler, H. (Ed.): Information theory in psychology. Glencoe, Ill.: Free Press 1955, 291–299.

Aebli, H.: Über die geistige Entwicklung des Kindes. Stuttgart: Klett 1963.

Ajdukiewicz, K.: Sprache und Sinn. Erkenntnis 4 (1934) 100–138.

Ajdukiewicz, K.: Die wissenschaftliche Weltperspektive. Erkenntnis 5 (1935), 22–30 and 165–168.

Ajuriaguerra, J. de, F. Bresson, P. Fraisse, B. Inhelder, P. Oleron and J. Piaget (Eds.): Problemes de psycholinguistique. Paris: Presses Universitaires de France 1963.

Albrecht, E.: Beiträge zur Erkenntnistheorie und das Verhältnis von Sprache und Denken. Halle (Saale): Niemeyer 1959.

Allesch, J. v.: Über das Verhältnis der Ästhetik zur Psychologie. Z. Psychol. 54 (1909), 401–536.

Allesch, J. v.: Zur nichteuklidischen Struktur des phänomenalen Raumes. Jena: Fischer 1931.

Allesch, J. v.: Über das Verhältnis des Allgemeinen zum realen Einzelnen. Arch. ges. Psychol. 111 (1942), 23–38.

Ammer, K.: Sprache, Mensch und Gessellschaft. Halle (Saale): Niemeyer 1961.

Apel, K.-O.: Sprache und Wahrheit in der gegenwärtigen Situation der Philosophie. Philos. Rdsch. 7 (1959a), 161–184.

Apel, K.-O.: Der philosophische Wahrheitsbegriff einer inhaltlich orientierten Sprachwissenschaft. In: Sprache—Schlüssel zur Welt. Festschrift fur L. Weisgerber, Düsseldorf: Päd. Verlag Schwann 1959b. 11–38.

Apel, K.-O.: Sprache and Ordnung. In: Kuhn, H. und F. Wiedmann (Eds.): Das Problem der Ordnung. 6. Dtsch. Kongr. Philos. (München, 1960). Meisenheim a. Glan: A. Hain 1962, 200–225.

Apel, K.-O.: Die Idee der Sprache in der Tradition des Humanismus von Dante bis Vico. Arch. Begriffsgesch. 8 (1963).

Apel, K.-O.: Sprachanalyse als Metaphysikkritik. Paper presented at Freie Universität Berlin, 22.2. 1965.

Arnheim, R.: Perceptual abstraction and art. Psychol. Rev., 54 (1947), 66–82.

Attneave, F.: Applications of information theory to psychology: A summary of basic concepts, methods, and results. New York: Holt, Rinehart and Winston 1959.

Austin, J. L.: How to do things with words. Oxford: Oxford University Press 1962.

Barclay, J. R., J. D. Bransford, J. J. Franks, N. S. McCarrell, and K. Nitsch: Comprehension and semantic flexibility. J. Verb. Learn. Verb. Behav. **13** (1974), 471–481.

Bartlett, F. C.: Remembering. Cambridge: Cambridge University Press 1950 (1st Ed., 1932).

Beauvoir, S. de: Memoires d'une jeune fille rangée. Paris: Gaillimard 1958.

Becker, K. F.: Organismus der Sprache. Frankfurt (Main): G. F. Kettenbeil 1841.

Begg, J. and A. Paivio: Concreteness and imagery in sentence meaning. J. Verb. Learn. Verb. Behav. **8** (1969), 821–827.

Bellugi, U. and R. W. Brown (Eds.): The acquisition of language. Monogr. Soc. Res. Child Develpm. **29** (1964), 1 (Serial No. 92).

Benjamin, W.: San Gimignano. In: Benjamin, W., Städtebilder, Frankfurt (Main): Suhrkamp 1963.

Bentley, M. and E. Varon: An accessory study of phonetic symbolism. Amer. J. Psychol. **45** (1933), 76–86.

Bergson, H.: L'Evolution créatrice. Paris: Félix Alcan 1907. English Edition: Creative Evolution. Translated by Mitchell, A. London: Macmillan 1954.

Berko, J.: The child's learning of English morphology. Word **14** (1958), 150–177.

Berko, J. and R. W. Brown: Psycholinguistic research methods. In: Mussen, P. H. (Ed.), Handbook of research methods in child development. New York: Wiley 1960, 517–557.

Berlyne, D. E.: Novelty and curiosity as determinants of exploratory behavior. Brit. J. Psychol. **41** (1950), 68–80.

Berlyne, D. E.: Knowledge and stimulus-response psychology. Psychol. Rev. **61** (1954a), 245–254.

Berlyne, D. E.: A theory of human curiosity. An experimental study of human curiosity. Brit. J. Psychol. **45** (1954b), 180–191.

Bernstein, B.: Some sociological determinants of perception. An inquiry into subcultural differences. Brit. J. Sociol. **9** (1958), 159–174.

Bernstein, B.: Linguistic codes, hesitation phenomena, and intelligence. Language and Speech **5** (1962), 31–46.

Bernstein, B.: Elaborated and restricted codes: Their social origins and some consequences. In: Gumperz, J. J. and D. Hymes (Eds.): The ethnography of communication. American Anthropologist **66**, 6 (1964), 55–69.

Bever, T. G.: The cognitive basis for linguistic structures. In: Hayes, J. R. (Ed.): Cognition and the development of language. New York: Wiley 1970, 279–352.

Bierwisch, M.: Aufgaben und Form der Grammatik. In: Zeichen und System der Sprache, Vol. III. Berlin: VEB-Verlag 1966, 28–69.

Bierwisch, M.: Some semantic universals of German adjectivals. Found. Lang. **3** (1967), 1–36.

Bierwisch, M.: On certain problems of semantic representations. Found. Lang. **5** (1969), 153–184.

Bierwisch, M.: Review of Hörmann, H.: Psycholinguistics, 1971. In: Z. Psychol. **180/181** (1972/73), 92–96.

Bixler, R. H. and H. C. Yeager: It may have begun with "Mama". Psychol. Rep. **4** (1958), 471–475.

Bloch, E.: Tübinger Einleitung in die Philosophie, I. Frankfurt (Main): Suhrkamp 1963.

Bloomfield, L.: A set of postulates for the science of language. Language 2, 153–164
(1926). Reprinted in Saporta, S. (Ed.): Psycholinguistics. New York: Holt,
Rinehart and Winston 1961, 26–33.

Bloomfield, L.: Language. New York: Henry Holt 1933.

Blumenthal, A. L.: Prompted recall of sentences. J. Verb. Learn. Verb. Behav. 6
(1967), 203–206.

Blumenthal, A. L.: Language and psychology: Historical aspects of psycholinguistics. New York: Wiley 1970.

Bock, M.: The influence of instructions on feature selection in semantic memory. J.
Verb. Learn. Verb. Behav. 15 (1976), 183–191.

Bond, Z. S. and J. Gray: Subjective phrase structure: An empirical investigation. J.
Psycholing. Res. 2 (1973), 259–266.

Bousfield, W. A.: The occurrence of clustering in the recall of randomly arranged
associates. J. Gen. Psychol. 49 (1953), 229–240.

Bousfield, W. A.: The problem of meaning in verbal learning. In: Cofer, C. N. (Ed.):
Verbal learning and verbal behavior. New York: McGraw-Hill 1961, 81–91.

Bousfield, W. A., G. A. Whitmarsh, and H. Berkowitz: Partial response identities in
associative clustering. J. Gen. Psychol. 63 (1960), 233–238.

Brackbill, Y. and K. B. Little: Factors determining the guessing of meanings of
foreign words. J. Abnorm. Soc. Psychol. 54 (1957), 312–318.

Braine, M. D. S.: On learning the grammatical order of words. Psychol. Rev. 70
(1963a), 323–348.

Braine, M. D. S.: The ontogeny of English phrase structure: The first phrase.
Language 39 (1963b), 1–13.

Bransford, J. D., J. R. Barclay, and J. J. Franks: Sentence memory: A constructive
versus interpretive approach. Cognitive Psychology 3 (1972), 193–209.

Bridgman, P. W.: The nature of physical theory. Princeton: Princeton University
Press, 1936.

Bridgman, P. W.: The operational aspect of meaning. Synthese 8 (1950/51), 251–259.

Bridgman, P. W.: The way things are. Cambridge, Mass.: Harvard University Press
1959.

Broadbent, D. E.: Perception and communication. London: Pergamon Press 1958.

Broadbent, D. E.: Behaviour. New York: Basic Books 1961.

Broadbent, D. E.: Perceptual and response factors in the organization of speech. In:
Reuck, A. V. S. De and M. O'Connor (Eds.): Disorders of language. London: J.
and A. Churchill 1964, 79–92.

Brown, R. W.: Language and categories. In: Bruner, J. S., J. J. Goodnow, and G. A.
Austin (Eds.): A study of thinking. New York: Science Editions 1956, Appendix,
247–312.

Brown, R. W.: Linguistic determinism and the part of speech. J. Abnorm. Soc.
Psychol. 55 (1957), 1–5.

Brown, R. W.: Words and things. Glencoe. Ill.: Free Press 1958a.

Brown, R. W.: How shall a thing be called? Psychol. Rev. 65 (1958b), 14–21.

Brown, R. W.: The language of social relationship. Proc. 16th Int. Congr. Psychol.,
Bonn, 1960. Amsterdam: North-Holland 1961, 663–667.

Brown, R. W.: A first language. Cambridge, Mass.: Harvard University Press 1973.

Brown, R. W. and U. Bellugi: Three processes in the child's acquisition of syntax.
Harv. Educ. Rev. 34 (1964), 133–151.

Brown, R. W. and J. Berko: Word association and the acquisition of grammar. Child Develpm. **31** (1960), 1–14.

Brown, R. W., A. Black, and A. Horowitz: Phonetic symbolism in natural languages. J. Abnorm. Soc. Psychol. **50** (1955), 388–393.

Brown, R. W. and D. E. Dulaney: A stimulus-response analysis of language and meaning. In: Henle, P. (Ed.): Language, thought, and culture. Ann Arbor, Mich.: University of Michigan Press 1965, 49–95.

Brown, R. W. and M. Ford: Address in American English. J. Abnorm. Soc. Psychol. **62** (1961), 375–385.

Brown, R. W. and C. Fraser: The acquisition of syntax. In: Cofer, C. N. and B. S. Musgrave (Eds.), Verbal behavior and learning. New York: McGraw-Hill 1963, 158–197.

Brown, R. W. and A. Gilman: The pronouns of power and solidarity. In: Sebeok, T. A. (Ed.): Style in language. New York: Wiley 1960, 253–276.

Brown, R. W. and R. J. Herrnstein: Psychology. Boston: Little, Brown & Co. 1975.

Brown, R. W. and E. H. Lenneberg: A study in language and cognition. J. Abnorm. Soc. Psychol. **49** (1954), 454–462.

Brown, R. W. and D. McNeill: The "tip of the tongue" phenomenon. J. Verb. Learn. Verb. Behav. **5** (1966), 325–337.

Brown, R. W. and R. Nuttall: Method in phonetic symbolism experiments. J. Abnorm. Soc. Psychol. **59** (1959), 441–445.

Bruner, J. S.: Going beyond the information given. In: Bruner, J. S., et al.: Contemporary approaches to cognition. Cambridge, Mass.: Harvard University Press 1957a, 41–69.

Bruner, J. S.: On perceptual readiness. Psychol. Rev. **64** (1957b), 123–152.

Bruner, J. S.: Nature and uses of immaturity. Amer. Psychol. **27** (1972), 1–22.

Bruner, J. S.: From communication to language: A psychological perspective. Cognition **3** (1974/75), 255–287.

Bruner, J. S., E. Brunswick, L. Festinger, F. Heider, K. F. Muenzinger, C. E. Osgood, and D. Rapaport: Contemporary approaches to cognition. Cambridge, Mass.: Harvard University Press, 1957.

Bruner, J. S., J. J. Goodnow, and G. A. Austin: A study of thinking. New York: Science Editions, 1956.

Brutyan, G. A.: A marxist evaluation of the Whorf hypothesis. ETC. **19** (1962), 199–220.

Bühler, K.: Das Ganze der Sprachtheorie, ihr Aufbau and ihre Teile. Ber. 12. Kongr. Dtsch. Ges. Psychol. (Hamburg 1931), Jena: Fischer 1932, 95–122.

Bühler, K.: Sprachtheorie. Jena: Fischer 1934.

Carmichael, L. (Ed.): Manual of child psychology. New York: Wiley 1954.

Carmichael, L. (Ed.): The early growth of language capacity in the individual. In: Lenneberg, E. H. (Ed.): New directions in the study of language. Cambridge, Mass.: M.I.T. Press 1964, 1–22.

Carnap, R.. Philosophy and logical syntax. London: K. Paul, Trench, Trubner 1935.

Carnap, R.: The logical syntax of language. London: Routledge and K. Paul 1937.

Carnap, R.: Introduction to semantics. Cambridge, Mass.: Harvard University Press 1948.

Carnap, R.: Empiricism, semantics, and ontology. Rev. Int. de Philos. **4** (1950), 20–40.

Carroll, J. B.: Diversity of vocabulary and the harmonic series law of word-frequency distribution. Psychol. Rec. **2** (1938), 379–386.

Carroll, J. B.: The study of language. Cambridge, Mass.: Harvard University Press 1955.

Carroll, J. B.: Review of Osgood, C. E., et al.: The measurement of meaning. In: Language **35** (1959), 58–77.

Carroll, J. B.: Language and thought. Englewood Cliffs, N. J.: Prentice-Hall 1964a.

Carroll, J. B.: Words, meanings, and concepts. Harv. Educ. Rev. **34** (1964b), 178–202.

Carroll, J. B., P. M. Kjeldergaard, and A. S. Carton: Number of opposites versus number of primaries as a response measure in free-association tests. J. Verb. Learn. Verb. Behav. **1** (1962/63), 22–30.

Carterette, E. C. and A. Moller: The perception of real and synthetic vowels after very sharp filtering. Proc. Speech Communication Seminar (1962) II, Stockholm: Speech Transmission Laboratory, Royal Institute of Technology 1963.

Cassirer, E.: Die Sprache und der Aufbau der Gegenstandswelt. Ber. 12 Kongr. Dtsch. Ges. Psychol. (Hamburg 1931). Jena: Fischer 1932, 134–145.

Cassirer, E.: An essay on man. An introduction to a philosophy of human culture. New Haven: Yale University Press 1944.

Cassirer, E.: Philosophie der symbolischen Formen. I: Die Sprache. Darmstadt: Wissenschaftliche Buchgesellschaft 1964. English Ed.: The philosophy of symbolic forms. I: Language. Translated by Manheim, R. New Haven: Yale University Press 1953.

Cattell, J. McK.: Über die Zeit der Erkennung und Benennung von Schriftzeichen, Bildern und Farben. Philos. Stud. **2** (1885), 635–650.

Cattell, J. McK.: Psychometrische Untersuchungen. Philos. Stud. **3** (1886), 452–492.

Chafe, W. L.: Meaning and the structure of language. Chicago: University of Chicago Press 1970.

Chafe, W. L.: Linguistics and human knowledge. Georgetown University Monograph Series on Languages and Linguistics **25** (1971), 57–69.

Cherry, C.: On human communication. A review, a survey, and a criticism. New York: Wiley 1957.

Chomsky, N.: Syntactic structures. Gravenhage: Mouton 1957.

Chomsky, N.: Review of Skinner, B. F.: Verbal behavior, 1957. In: Language **35** (1959), 26–58.

Chomsky, N.: Some methodological remarks on generative grammar. Word **17** (1961), 219–239.

Chomsky, N.: Aspects of the theory of syntax. Cambridge, Mass.: M. I. T. Press 1965.

Chomsky, N.: Cartesean linguistics. New York: Harper and Row 1966.

Chomsky, N.: The formal nature of language. In: Lenneberg, E. H. (Ed.): Biological Foundations of Language. New York: Wiley 1967, 483–539.

Chomsky, N.: Deep structure, surface structure, and semantic interpretation. In: Steinberg, D. and L. A. Jakobovits (Eds.): Semantics. Cambridge: Cambridge University Press 1971, 183–216.

Church, J.: Language and the discovery of reality. New York: Random House 1961.

Clark, E. V.: What's in a word? On the child's acquisition of semantics in his first language. In: Moore, T. E. (Ed.): Cognitive development and the acquisition of language. New York: Academic Press 1973, 65–110.

Clark, H. H.: Word association and linguistic theory. In: Lyons, J. (Ed.): New horizons in linguistics. Baltimore: Penguin Books 1970, 271–286.

Clark, H. H.: Semantics and comprehension. In: Sebeok, T. A. (Ed.): Current trends in linguistics. Vol. 12. The Hague: Mouton 1973, 1291–1498.

Cofer, C. N. (Ed.): Verbal learning and verbal behaviour. New York: McGraw-Hill 1961.

Cofer, C. N. and B. S. Musgrave (Eds.): Verbal behavior and learning: Problems and processes. New York: McGraw-Hill 1963.

Cohen, B. H.: Role of awareness in meaning established by classical conditioning. J. Exp. Psychol. **67** (1964), 373–378.

Coleman, E. B.: Sequential interferences demonstrated by serial reconstructions. J. Exp. Psychol. **64** (1962), 46–51.

Coleman, E. B.: Approximation to English: Some comments on the method. Amer. J. Psychol. **76** (1963), 239–247.

Collins, A. M., and M. R. Quillian: Retrieval time from semantic memory. J. Verb. Learn. Verb. Behav. **8** (1969), 241–248.

Collins, A. M., and M. R. Quillian: Experiments on semantic memory and language comprehension. In: Gregg, L. W. (Ed.), Cognition in Learning and Memory. New York: Wiley 1972, 117–148.

Craik, F. I. M., and R. S. Lockhart: Levels of processing: A framework for memory research. J. Verb. Learn. Verb. Behav. **11** (1972), 671–684.

Curtius, G.: Grundzüge der griechischen Etymologie. Leipzig: Teubner 1858. English Ed.: Principles of Greek etymology. Translated by Wilkins, A. S. and E. B. England. London: Murray 1886.

Davis, E. A.: The development of linguistic skill in twins, singletons and only children from age five to ten years. Minneapolis: University of Minnesota Press 1937.

Davis, R.: The fitness of names to drawings: A cross-cultural study in Tanganyika. Brit. J. Psychol. **52** (1961), 259–268.

Day, E. J.: The development of language in twins. Child Develpm. **3** (1932), 179–199.

Deese, J.: Serial organization in the recall of disconnected items. Psychol. Rep. **3** (1957), 577–582.

Deese, J.: Influence of inter-item associative strength upon immediate free recall. Psychol. Rep. **5** (1959a), 305–312.

Deese, J.: On the prediction of occurrence of particular verbal intrusions in immediate recall. J. Exp. Psychol. **58** (1959b), 17–22.

Deese, J.: From the isolated verbal unit to connected discourse. In: Cofer, C. N. (Ed.): Verbal learning and verbal behavior. New York: McGraw-Hill 1961a, 11–41.

Deese, J.: Associative structure and serial reproduction experiment. J. Abnorm. Soc. Psychol. **63** (1961b), 95–100.

Deese, J.: On the structure of associative meaning. Psychol. Rev. **69** (1962), 161–175.

Deese, J.: Form class and the determinants of association. J. Verb. Learn. Verb. Behav. **1** (1962/63), 79–84.

Deese, J.: Meaning and change of meaning. Amer. Psychologist **22** (1967), 641–651.

Deese, J.: Associate and memory. In: Dixon, T. R. and D. L. Horton (Eds.): Verbal behavior and general behavior theory. Englewood Cliffs, N.J.: Prentice-Hall 1968, 97–108.

Deese, J.: Behavior and fact. Amer. Psychologist **24** (1969), 515–522.

Deutsch, J. A. and Deutsch, D.: Attention: some theoretical considerations. Psychol. Rev. **70** (1963), 80–90.

Doob, L. W.: Social psychology: an analysis of human behavior. New York: Holt 1952.

Durkheim, E.: Les règles de la méthode sociologique. Paris: F. Alcan, 1918. English Ed.: The rules of sociological method. Translated by Solovay, S. A. and J. H. Mueller. New York: Free Press of Glencoe 1938.

Engelkamp, J.: Semantische Struktur und die Verarbeitung von Sätzen. Bern: Huber 1973.

Engelkamp, J.: Psycholinguistik. München: W. Fink 1974.

Engelkamp, J. and H. Hörmann: Semantische Faktoren beim Behalten der Verneinung von Sätzen. Psychol. Forsch. **35** (1972), 93–116.

Engelkamp, J. and H. Hörmann: The effect of non-verbal information on the recall of negation. Quart. J. Exp. Psychol. **26** (1974), 98–105.

Entwisle, D. R., D. F. Forsyth, and R. Muus: The syntactic-paradigmatic shift in children's word associations. J. Verb. Learn. Verb. Behav. **3** (1964), 19–29.

Epstein, W.: The influence of syntactical structure on learning. Amer. J. Psychol. **74** (1961), 80–85.

Epstein, W.: A further study of the influence of syntactical structure on learning. Amer. J. Psychol. **75** (1962), 121–126.

Erdmann, B. and R. Dodge: Psychologische Untersuchungen über das Lesen auf experimenteller Grundlage. Halle (Saale): Voss 1898.

Erdmann, K. O.: Die Bedeutung des Wortes. Leipzig: Avenarius 1925.

Ertel, S.: Die emotionale Natur des ''semantischen'' Raumes. Psychol. Forsch. **28** (1964), 1–32.

Ertel, S.: Weitere Untersuchungen zur Standardisierung eines Eindrucksdifferentials. Z. exp. angew. Psychol. **12** (1965), 177–208.

Ertel, S.: Allgemeinqualität und Relation. Arch. Psychol. **119** (1967), 26–56.

Ertel, S.: Psychophonetik. Göttingen: 1969.

Ertel, S. and W. D. Bloemer: Affirmation and negation as constructive action. Psychol. Res. **37** (1975), 335–342.

Ertel, S. und R. Dorst: Expressive Lautsymbolik. Z. exp. angew. Psychol. **12** (1965), 557–569.

Ervin, S. M.: Changes with age in the verbal determinants of word-association. Amer. J. Psychol. **74** (1961a), 361–372.

Ervin, S. M.: Learning and recall in bilinguals. Amer. J. Psychol. **74** (1961b), 446–451.

Ervin, S. M.: The connotations of gender. Word **18** (1962), 249–261.

Ervin, S. M.: Correlates of associative frequency. J. Verb. Learn. Verb. Behav. **1** (1962/63), 422–431.

Ervin, S. M. and G. Foster: The development of meaning in children's descriptive terms. J. Abnorm. Soc. Psychol. **61** (1960), 271–275.

Ervin, S. M. and C. E. Osgood: Second language learning and bilingualism. In: Osgood, C. E. and T. A. Sebeok (Eds.): Psycholinguistics. J. Abnorm. Soc. Psychol. **49**, Suppl., Baltimore 1954, 139–146.

Esch, H.: Über die Schallerzeugung beim Werbetanz der Honigbiene. Z. vergl. Physiol. **45** (1961), 1–11.

Figge, U. L.: Strukturale Linguistik. In: Koch, W. A. (Ed.): Perspektiven der Linguistik, Vol. 1. Stuttgart: Kröner 1973.

Fillenbaum, S.: Semantic generalization in verbal satiation. Psychol. Rep. 13 (1963), 158.

Fillenbaum, S.: Semantic association and decision latency. J. Exp. Psychol. 68 (1964), 240–244.

Fillenbaum, S.: Memory for gist: Some relevant variables. Lang. Speech 9 (1966), 217–227.

Fillenbaum, S. and A. Rapaport: Structures in the subjective lexicon. New York: Academic Press 1971.

Fillmore, C. J.: The case for case. In: Bach, E. and R. Harms (Eds.): Universals in linguistic theory. New York: Holt, Rinehart and Winston 1968a, 1–90.

Fillmore, C. J.: Lexicals entries for verbs. Found. Lang. 4 (1968b), 373–393.

Fischer, H.: Die Allgemeine Semantik. Eine nichtaristotelische Wertungslehre A. Korzybskis. Stud. Gen. 6 (1953), 361–388.

Fishman, J. A.: A systematization of the Whorfian hypothesis. Behav. Sci. 5 (1960), 323–339.

Fishman, J. A.: Who speaks what language to whom and when. La Linguistique 2 (1965), 67–88.

Flanagan, J. L.: Speech analysis. Synthesis and perception. Berlin: Springer 1965.

Flavell, J. H.: A test of the Whorfian theory. Psychol. Rep. 4 (1958), 455–462.

Flesch, R.: The art of plain talk. New York: Harper 1946.

Flesch, R.: Measuring the level of abstraction. J. Appl. Psychol. 34 (1950), 384–390.

Flores d'Arcais, G. B.: Cognitive principles in language processing. Leiden: University of Leiden Press 1973.

Fodor, J. A. and T. G. Bever: The psychological reality of linguistic elements. J. Verb. Learn. Verb. Behav. 4 (1965), 414–420.

Forschhammer, E.: Über einige Fälle von eigentümlichen Sprachbildungen bei Kindern. Arch. ges. Psychol. 104 (1939), 395–438.

Freeman, R. B.: Zerebrale Asymmetrie der Sprachwahrnehmung bei Neugeborenen. 15. Tagung exp. arb. Psychologen. Erlangen 1973.

French, D.: The relationship of anthropology to studies in perception and cognition. In: Koch, S. (Ed.): Psychology. A study of a science. Vol. VI. New York: McGraw-Hill 1963, 388–428.

French, N. R. and J. C. Steinberg: Factors governing the intelligibility of speech sounds. J. Acoust. Soc. Amer. 19 (1947), 90–119.

Freytag-Loeringhoff, B.: Diskussionsbemerkung. In: Kuhn, H. and F. Wiedmann (Eds.). Das Problem der Ordnung. 6. Dtsch. Kongr. Philos. (München 1960), Meisenheim a. Glan: A. Hain 1962, 240.

Frisch, K. v.: Über die "Sprache" der Bienen. Eine tierpsychologische Untersuchung. Jena: Fischer 1923.

Frisch, K. v.: Erinnerungen eines Biologen. Berlin/Göttingen/Heidelberg: Springer 1962a. English Ed.: A biologist remembers. Translated by Gombrich, L. Oxford: Pergamon Press 1967.

Frisch, K. v.: Dialects in the language of the bees. Sci. Amer. 207 (1962b), H. 2, 79–87, 1965.

Frisch, K. v.: Tanzsprache und Orientierung der Bienen. Berlin: Springer 1965.

Gabelentz, G. v. d.: Die Sprachwissenschaft, ihre Aufgaben, Methoden und bisherigen Ergebnisse, Leipzig: Tauchnitz 1901.

Gadamer, H.-G.: Die Natur der Sache und die Sprache der Dinge. In: Kuhn, H. und F. Weidmann (Eds.): Das Problem der Ordnung. 6. Dtsch. Kongr. Philos. (München 1960). Meisenheim a. Glan: A. Hain 1962, 26–36.

Galton, F.: Psychometric experiments. Brain 2 (1880), 149–162.

Gardner, R. A., and B. T. Gardner: Teaching sign language to a chimpanzee. Science 165 (1969), 664–672.

Garfinkel, H.: Remarks on ethnomethodology. In: Gumperz, J. J., and D. Hymes (Eds.): Directions in sociolinguistics. New York: Holt, Rinehart and Winston 1972.

Garrett, M., T. G. Bever and J. A. Fodor: The active use of grammar in speech perception. Perc. Psychophys. 1 (1965), 30–32.

Gehlen, A.: Der Mensch, seine Natur und seine Stellung in der Welt. Bonn: Athenäum-Verlag 1950.

Gifford, W. W.: A problem in kinship terminology. Amer. Anthrop. 42 (1940), 193–194.

Gipper, H. Sessel oder Stuhl. In: Festschrift Weisgerber. Düsseldorf: Päd. Verlag Schwann 1959.

Gipper, H.: Gibt es ein sprachliches Relativitätsprinzip? Frankfurt: 1972.

Glanzer, M.: Toward a psychology of language structure. J. Speech Hear. Res. 5 (1962), 303–314.

Glanzer, M.: Grammatical category: A rote learning and word association analysis. J. Verb. Learn. Verb. Behav. 1 (1962/63), 31–41.

Glanzer, M. and W. H. Clark: Accuracy of perceptual recall: An analysis of organization. J. Verb. Learn. Verb. Behav. 1 (1962/63), 289–299.

Glanzer, M. and W. H. Clark: The verbal loop hypothesis: Binary numbers. J. Verb. Learn. Verb. Behav. 2 (1963), 301–309.

Glanzer, M. and W. H. Clark: The verbal-loop hypothesis: Conventional figures. Amer. J. Psychol. 77 (1964), 621–626.

Glinz, H.: Die Leistung der Sprache für zwei Menschen. In: Sprache–Schlüssel zur Welt. Festschrift für L. Weisgerber. Düsseldorf: Päd, Verlag Schwann 1959, 87–105.

Glinz, H.: Grammatik und Sprache. In: Moser, H. (Ed.): Das Ringen um eine neue deutsche Grammatik. 1962, 42–60.

Glinz, H.: Ziele und Arbeitsweisen der modernen Sprachwissenschaft. Archiv für neue Sprachen 200 (1964), 161–181.

Goldman-Eisler, F.: Psycholinguistics: Experiments in spontaneous speech. London: Academic Press 1968.

Goldman-Eisler, F.: Hesitation, information and levels of speech production. In: Reuck, A. V. S. De and M. O'Connor (Eds.): Disorders of language. London: J. and A. Churchill 1964, 96–111.

Goldman-Eisler, F.: Pauses, clauses, sentences. Lang. and Speech 15 (1972) 103–113.

Goldstein, K.: Die pathologischen Tatsachen in ihrer Bedeutung für das Problem der Sprache. Ber. 12. Kongr. Dtsch. Ges. Psychol. (Hamburg 1931), Jena: Fischer 1932, 145–164.

Goldstein, K.: Language and language disturbance. New York: Grune and Stratton 1948.

Goodall, J.: My life among wild chimpanzees. Natl. Geogr. Mag. **124** (1963), 272–308.

Goss, A. E.: Early behaviorism and verbal mediating responses. Amer. Psychologist **16** (1961), 285–298.

Goss, A. E.: Verbal mediation. Psychol. Rec. **14** (1964), 363–382.

Granit, R.: Sensory mechanisms of the retina. New York: Hafner 1963.

Greenberg, J. H.: Concerning inferences from linguistic to nonlinguistic data. In: Hoijer, H. (Ed.): Language in culture. Chicago: University of Chicago Press 1954, 3–19.

Greenberg, J. H.: Essays in linguistics. New York: Wenner-Gren Foundation for Anthropological Research 1957.

Greenberg, J. H.: Review of Hockett, C. F., A course in modern linguistics. In: Amer. Anthropologist **63** (1961), 1140–1145.

Greenberg, J. H. (Ed.): Universals of language. Cambridge, Mass.: M.I.T. Press 1963.

Greenfield, P. M., K. Nelson and E. Saltzman: The development of rulebound strategies for manipulating seriated cups: A parallel between action and grammar. Cognitive Psychology 3 (1972), 291–310.

Groeben, N.: Literaturpsychologie. Stuttgart: Kohlhammer 1972.

Groeben, N.: Verstehen, Behalten, Interesse. Unterrichtswissenschaft **2** (1976), 128–142.

Gumperz, J. J. and D. Hymes (Eds.): The ethnography of communication. Special issue of Amer. Anthropologist, 1964, 66.

Habermas, J.: Vorbereitende Bemerkungen zu einer Theorie der kommunikativen Kompetenz. In: Habermas, J. and N. Luhmann (Eds.): Theorie der Gesellschaft oder Sozialtechnologie. Frankfurt: Suhrkamp 1971, 101–141.

Halle, M. and K. N. Stevens: Analysis by synthesis. In: Wathen-Dunn (Ed.), Models of vision and speech. Proceedings of the seminar on speech compression and processing. Cambridge, Mass.: M.I.T. Press 1959.

Halle, M. and K. N. Stevens: Speech recognition: A model and a program for research. IRE Transactions on Information Theory IT-8 (1962), 155–159.

Hare, R. D.: Cognitive factors in transfer of meaning. Psychol. Rep. **15** (1964), 199–206.

Harlow, H. F.: Mice, monkeys, men, and motives. Psychol. Rev. **60** (1953), 23–32.

Harlow, H. F. and C. N. Wollsey (Eds.): Biological and biochemical bases of behavior. Madison, Wis.: University of Wisconsin Press 1958.

Hayakawa, S. I.: Language in thought and action. New York: Harcourt, Brace and World 1949.

Hayakawa, S. I.: The aims and tasks of general semantics, implications of time-binding theory. ETC-8 (1951), No. 4, 243–253.

Hebb, D. O.: The organization of behavior. New York: Wiley 1949.

Heidegger, M.: Was heißt Denken? Tübingen: M. Niemeyer, 1954. English Edition: What is called thinking? Translated by Wieck, F. D. and J. G. Gray. New York: Harper and Row 1968.

Heider, F.: Trends in cognitive theory. In: Bruner, J. S. et al. (Eds.): Contemporary approaches to cognition. Cambridge, Mass.: Harvard University Press 1957, 201–210.

Henley, N. M.: A psychological study of the semantics of animal terms. J. Verb. Learn. Verb. Behav. **8** (1969), 176–184.

Henle, P. (Ed.): Language, thought, and culture. Ann Arbor, Mich.: University of Michigan Press 1965.

Herdan, G.: Language as choice and chance. Groningen: Noordhoff 1956.

Herdan, G.: Type-token mathematics. Den Haag: Mouton 1960.

Herder, J. G.: Abhandlung über den Ursprung der Sprache. Berlin: C. F. Voss 1772.

Herrmann, T.: Syntaktische Untersuchungen zum unmittelbaren Behalten von Wortketten. Z. exp. angew. Psychol. **9** (1962), 397–416.

Herrmann, T.: Über Benennungsflexibilität. Bericht 29. Kongr. Deutsche Ges. Psychol. 1974, 168–173.

Herrmann, T. and W. Deutsch: Psychologie der Objektbenennung. Bern: Huber 1976.

Hobbes, T.: Leviathan. London: A. Crooke 1651.

Hockett, C. F.: Review of "The mathematical theory of communication" by Shannon, C. E., and W. Weaver. In: Saporta, S. (Ed.): Psycholinguistics. New York: Holt, Rinehart and Winston 1961, 44–67.

Höpp, G.: Evolution der Sprache und Vernunft. Berlin: Springer 1970.

Hörmann, H.: Aussagemöglichkeiten psychologischer Diagnostik. Göttingen: Verlag für Psychologie 1964.

Hörmann, H.: Semantic factors in negation. Psych. Forsch. **35** (1971), 1–16.

Hörmann, H.: Semantic factors in psycholinguistic processes. 20th Int. Congr. Psychology, Tokyo 1972.

Hörmann, H.: Semantische Anomalie. Metapher und Witz. Folia Ling. **5** (1972/73), 310–330.

Hörmann, H.: Psycholinguistik. In: Koch, W. A. (Ed.): Perspektiven der Linguistik, II. Stuttgart: Kröner 1974, 138–156.

Hörmann, H.: Meinen und Verstehen. Frankfurt: Suhrkamp 1976.

Hörmann, H., G. Lazarus and H. Lazarus: The role of the predicate in sentence perception. Bochum 1975, Unpubl. paper.

Hörmann, H. and G. Terbuyken: Situational factors in meaning. Psych. Forsch. **36** (1974), 297–310.

Hofstätter, P. R.: Farbsymbolik und Ambivalenz. Psychol. Beitr. **2** (1955), 526–540.

Hofstätter, P. R.: Über sprachliche Bestimmungsleistungen: das Problem des grammatischen Geschlechts von Sonne und Mond. Z. exp. angew. Psychol. **10** (1963), 91–108.

Hoijer, H.: Cultural implications of some Navaho linguistic categories. Language **27** (1951), 111–120.

Hoijer, H.: The relation of language to culture. In: Kroeber, A. L. (Ed.): Anthropology today. Chicago: University of Chicago Press 1953, 554–573.

Hoijer, H.: (Ed.): Language in culture. Chicago: University of Chicago Press 1954.

Holenstein, E.: Linguistik, Semiotik, Hermeneutik. Frankfurt:Suhrkamp 1976.

Holland, M. K. and M. Wertheimer: Some physiognomic aspects of naming, or, maluma and takete revisited. Percept. Mot. Skills **19** (1964), 111–117.

Holyoak, K. J.: The role of imagery in the evaluation of sentences. J. Verb. Learn. Verb. Behav. **13** (1974), 163–166.

Howes, D. H.: On the interpretation of word frequency as a variable affecting speed of recognition. J. Exp. Psychol. **48** (1954), 106–112.

Howes, D. H.: On the relation between the probability of a word as an association and in general linguistic usage. J. Abnorm. Soc. Psychol. **54** (1957), 75–85.

Howes, D. H.: Application of the word-frequency concept to aphasia. In: Reuck, A. V. S. de and M. O'Connor (Eds.): Disorders of language. London: J. and A. Churchill 1964, 47–75.

Howes, D. H. and C. E. Osgood: On the combination of associative probabilities in linguistic contexts. Amer. J. Psychol. **67** (1954), 241–258.

Hull, C. L.: Knowledge and purpose as habit mechanisms. Psychol. Rev. **37** (1930), 511–525.

Humboldt, W. v.: Über das vergleichende Sprachstudium in Beziehung auf die verschiedenen Epochen der Sprachentwicklung. Gesammelte Schriften, Vol. 4. Berlin: Königlich-Preußische Akademie der Wissenschaften, 1905a (1st published as Abhandlungen hist.-philol. Kl. Königl. Preuß. Akad. Wiss. 1820–1821. 1822, 239–260).

Humboldt, W. v.: Über den Nationalcharakter der Sprachen. Gesammelte Schriften, Vol. 4. Berlin: Königlich-Preußische Akademie der Wissenschaften, 1905b (1st published in Z. Völkerpsychol. u. Sprachwiss. **13**, 1882, 211–232).

Humboldt, W. v.: Über die Verschiedenheit des menschlichen Sprachbaues und ihren Einfluß auf die geistige Entwicklung des Menschengeschlechts. Gesammelte Schriften, Vol. VII, Part 1. Berlin: Königlich-Preußische Akademie der Wissenschaften, 1907 (also introduction to Über die Kawi-Sprache auf der Insel Java. Darmstadt 1949. 1st published in Berlin, 1836.)

Humphrey, G.: There is no problem of meaning. Brit. J. Psychol. **42** (1951), 238–245.

Husserl, E.: Logische Untersuchungen. Halle (Saale): Niemeyer 1913.

Husserl, E.: Formale und transzendentale Logik. Halle (Saale): Niemeyer 1929.

Huttenlocher, J., K. Eisenberg and S. Straus: Comprehension: Relation between perceived actor and logical subject. J. Verb. Learn. Verb. Behav. **7** (1968), 527–530.

Huxley, A.: Words and their meanings. Los Angeles: Ward Ritchie Press 1940.

Hymes, D.: Towards communicative competence. Philadelphia: University of Pennsylvania Press 1972.

Ipsen, G.: Der alte Orient und die Indogermanen. In: Stand und Aufgaben der Sprachwissenschaft. Festschrift für W. Streitberg. Heidelberg: C. Winter 1924, 200–237.

Ipsen, G.: Der neue Sprachbegriff. Z. Deutschk. **46** (1932), 1–18.

Irwin, R. J.: Can animals talk? Percept. Mot. Skills **18** (1964), 369–374.

Jakobovits, L. A. and W. E. Lambert: Semantic satiation among bilinguals. J. Exp. Psychol. **62** (1961), 576–582.

Jakobovits, L. A. and W. E. Lambert: Mediated satiation in verbal transfer. J. Exp. Psychol. **64** (1962a), 346–351.

Jakobovits, L. A. and W. E. Lambert: Semantic satiation in an addition task. Canad. J. Psychol. **16** (1962b), 112–119.

Jakobovits, L. A. and W. E. Lambert: Stimulus-characteristics as determinants of semantic changes with repeated presentation. Amer. J. Psychol. **77** (1964), 84–92.

Jakobson, R.: Kindersprache, Aphasie und allgemeine Lautgesetze. Universitets Arsskrift (Uppsala) **9** (1942), 1–83.

Jakobson, R.: Aphasia as a linguistic problem: In: Werner, H. (Ed.): On expressive language. Worcester, Mass.: Clark University Press 1955, 69–81.

Jakobson, R.: Why 'Mama' and 'Papa'? In: Kaplan, B. and S. Wapner (Eds.): Perspectives in psychological theory. Essays in honor of Heinz Werner. New York: International Universities Press 1960, 124–134.

Jakobson, R.: Toward a linguistic typology of aphasic impairments. In: Reuck, A. V. S. de and M. O'Connor (Eds.): Disorders of language. London: J. and A. Churchill 1964, 21–40.

Jakobson, R.: Main trends in the science of language. New York: Harper & Row 1973.

Jakobson, R. and M. Halle: Fundamentals of language. Gravenhage: Mouton 1956.

Jakobson, R. and M. Halle: Phonology and phonetics. In: Jakobson, R. and M. Halle (Eds.): Fundamentals of language's Gravenhage: Mouton 1956, 1–51.

Jenkins, J. J. (Ed.): Associative processes in verbal behavior. Minnesota Conference 1955.

Jenkins, J. J.: Cited in Howes, D. H.: On the relation between the probability of a word as an association and in general linguistic usage. J. Abnorm. Soc. Psychol. 54 (1957), 75–85.

Jenkins, J. J. (Ed.): The change in some American word association norms in the twentieth century. Proc. 15th Int. Congr. Psychol. (Brüssel 1957). Amsterdam: North-Holland 1959, 583–584.

Jenkins, J. J. (Ed.): Communality of association as an indicator of more general patterns of verbal behavior. In: Sebeok, T. A. (Ed.): Style in language. New York: Wiley 1960, 307–329.

Jenkins, J. J. (Ed.): Mediated association: Paradigms and situations. In: Cofer, C. N. and B. S. Musgrave (Eds.), Verbal behavior and learning. New York: McGraw-Hill 1963, 210–245.

Jenkins, J. J. (Ed.): Mediation theory and grammatical behavior. In: Rosenberg, S. (Ed.): Directions in psycholinguistics. New York: Macmillan 1965, 66–96.

Jenkins, J. J. and D. S. Palermo: Mediation processes and the acquisition of linguistic structure. In: Bellugi, U. and R. Brown (Eds.): The acquisition of language. Monogr. Soc. Res. Child Developm. 29 (1964), 1 (Serial No. 92).

Jenkins, J. J. and W. A. Russell: Associative clustering during recall. J. Abnorm. Soc. Psychol. 47 (1952), 818–821.

Jenkins, P. M. and C. N. Cofer: An exploratory study of discrete free association to compound verbal stimuli. Psychol. Rep. 3 (1957), 599–602.

Jespersen, O.: Language, its nature, development, and origin. New York: W. W. Norton 1964.

Johnson, N. F.: Linguistic models and functional units of language behavior. In: Rosenberg, S. (Ed.): Directions in psycholinguistics. New York: Macmillan 1965, 29–65.

Johnson, R. C.: Linguistic structure as related to concept formation and to concept content. Psychol. Bull. 59 (1962), 468–476.

Johnson, W.: Studies in language behavior. I. A program of research. Psychol. Monogr. 56 (1944), No. 2.

Jörg, S.: Der Einfluß sprachlicher Bezeichnungen auf das Wiedererkennen von Bildern. Phil. Diss. Ruhr-Universität Bochum 1976.

Jorgensen, C. C. and W. Kintsch: The role of imagery in the evaluation of sentences. Cognit. Psychol. 4 (1973), 110–116.

Jung, C. G.: Diagnostische Assoziationsstudien. Leipzig, Vol. I, 1906; Vol. II, 1910.

English Ed.: Studies in word-association. Translated by Eder, M. D. London: W. Heinemann 1918.

Kaeding, F. W.: Häufigkeitswörterbuch der deutschen Sprache. Berlin: Selbstverlag des Herausgebers, Mittler Sohn 1897.

Kainz, F.: Psychologie der Sprache. Vol. II: Vergleichend-genetische Sprachpsychologie. Stuttgart: Enke 1943.

Kainz, F.: Die Sprache der Tiere, Tatsachen—Problemschau—Theorie. Stuttgart: Enke 1961.

Kaminski, G.: Ordnungsstrukturen und Ordnungsprozesse. In: Bergius, R. (Ed.): Handbuch der Psychologie, Vol. 1. Allgemeine Psychologie, Part 2. Lernen und Denken. Göttingen: Verlag für Psychologie 1964, 373–492.

Kanungo, R. and W. E. Lambert: Semantic satiation and meaningfulness. Amer. J. Psychol. 76 (1963), 421–428.

Kasschau, R. A.: Semantic satiation as a function of duration of repetition. J. Verb. Learn. Verb. Behav. 8 (1969), 36–42.

Katz, J. J. and J. Fodor: The structure of a semantic theory. Lang. 39 (1963), 170–260.

Katz, J. J. and P. Postal: An integrated theory of linguistic descriptions. Cambridge, Mass.: M.I.T. Press 1964.

Kelchner, M.: Kummer und Trost jugendlicher Arbeiterinnen. In: Forschungen zur Völkerpsychologie und Soziologie, Vol. VI. Leipzig: C. L. Hirschfeld 1929.

Keller, H.: The story of my life. New York: Grosset and Dunlop, 1905.

Kendall, M. G. and W. R. Buckland: A dictionary of statistical terms. Edinburgh: Oliver and Boyd for the International Statistical Institute 1960.

Kent, H. G. and A. J. Rosanoff: A study of association in insanity. Amer. J. Insanity 67 (1910), 37–96, 317–390.

Kintsch, W.: Learning, memory, and conceptual processes. New York: Wiley 1970a.

Kintsch, W.: Recognition memory in bilinguals. J. Verb. Learn. Verb. Behav. 9 (1970b), 405–409.

Kintsch, W.: The representation of meaning in memory. Hillsdale, N. J.: Lawrence Erlbaum Associates 1974.

Kirchhoff, R.: (Ed.): Handbuch der Psychologie, Vol. 5: Ausdruckspsychologie. Götttingen: Verlag für Psychologie 1965.

Kleist, H. v.: Über die allmähliche Verfertigung der Gedanken beim Reden (1806). In: Mueller, A. H. (Ed.), Vom Gespräch. Hamburg: Hauswedell 1946, 24–32.

Kluckhohn, C. and D. Leighton: The Navaho. Cambridge, Mass.: Harvard University Press 1946.

Koch, S. (Ed.): Psychology, a study of a science. Vol. I-VI. New York: McGraw-Hill 1959–1963.

Köhler, W.: Die physischen Gestalten in Ruhe und im stationären Zustand. Erlangen: Philosophische Akademie 1924.

Köhler, W.: Gestalt Psychology. New York: Liveright 1947.

Köhler, W.: Intelligenzprüfungen an Menschenaffen. Berlin: Abhandlungen d. Preuß. Akademie d. Wissenschaften 1917. Later Ed.: Berlin: Springer. English Ed.: The mentality of apes. Translated by Winter, E. London: Routledge and K. Paul 1956.

Korzybski, A.: Time-binding: The general theory. Lakeville, Conn.: Institute of General Semantics 1949.

Korzybski, A.: Science and sanity. An introduction to Non-Aristotelian systems and General Semantics. Lakeville, Conn.: International Non-Aristotelian Library 1950.

Kroeber, A. L.: Classificatory systems of relationship. J. Royal Anthropological Institute 39 (1909), 77–84.

Küpfmüller, K.: Die Entropie der deutschen Sprache. Fernmeldetechn. Z. 7 (1954), H. 6, 265–272.

Ladefoged, P.: The perception of speech. Proc. Symposium on Mechanization of Thought Processes (Teddington 1958), London: Her Majesty's Stationery Office 1959, Vol. I, 399–409.

Ladefoged, P. and D. E. Broadbent: Information conveyed by vowels. J. Acoust. Soc. Amer. 29 (1957), 98–104.

Laffal, J.: Psycholinguistics and the psychology of language. Amer. Psychologist 19 (1964). 813–815.

Laguna, G. A. de: Speech: Its function and development. Bloomington, Ind.: Indiana University Press 1963.

Lambert, W. E. and L. A. Jakobovits: Verbal satiation and cnanges in the intensity of meaning. J. Exp. Psychol. 60 (1960), 376–383.

Lambert, W. E., J. Havelka, and C. Crosby: The influence of language-acquisition contexts on bilingualism. J. Abnorm. Soc. Psychol. 56, 239–244 (1958). Reprinted in: Saporta, S. (Ed.): Psycholinguistics. New York: Holt, Rinehart and Winston 1961, 407–414.

Lane, H.: Psychophysical parameters of vowel perception. Psychol. Monogr. 76 (1962), H. 44.

Lane, H.: The motor theory of speech perception: A critical review. Psychol. Rev. 72 (1965), 275–309.

Langer, J. and F. Schulz von Thun: Messung komplexer Merkmale in Psychologie und Pädagogik. München, Basel: Reinhardt 1974.

Langer, S. K.: Philosophy in a new key. Cambridge, Mass.: Harvard University Press 1963.

Lantz, D. L. and V. Stefflere: Language and cognition revisited. J. Abnorm. Soc. Psychol. 69 (1964), 472–481.

Lashley, K. S.: Studies of cerebral function in learning. IV: Vicarious function after destruction of the visual areas. Amer. J. Physiol. 59 (1922), 44–71.

Lashley, K. S.: Learning. I: Nervous mechanisms in learning. In: Murchison, C. (Ed.): The foundations of experimental psychology. Worcester, Mass.: Clark University Press 1929, 524–563.

Lashley, K. S.: Basic neural mechanisms in behavior. Psychol. Rev. 37 (1930), 1–24.

Lashley, K. S.: The problem of serial order in behavior. In: Jeffress, L. A. (Ed.): Cerebral mechanisms in behavior. The Hixon Symposium. New York: Hafner 1951, 112–136.

Lashley, K. S.: In search of the engram. In: Beach, F. A. et al. (Eds.): The neuropsychology of Lashley. Selected papers of K. S. Lashley. New York: McGraw-Hill 1960, 478–505.

Leibniz, G. E.: Unvorgreifliche Gedanken betreffend die Ausübung und Verbesserung der teutschen Sprache. Beiträge zur deutschen Sprachkunde, vorgelesen in der Akademie der Wissenschaften zu Berlin, I, 1794.

Leisi, E.: Der Wortinhalt. Seine Struktur im Deutschen und Englischen, Heidelberg: Quelle Meyer 1961.

Lenneberg, E. H.: Cognition in ethnolinguistics. Language **29** (1953), 463–471.

Lenneberg, E. H.: A note on Cassirer's philosophy of language. Phil. Phenomenol. Res. **15** (1955), 512–522.

Lenneberg, E. H.: Language, evolution, and purposive behavior. In: Diamond, S. (Ed.): Culture in history: Essays in honor of Paul Radin. New York: Columbia University Press 1960.

Lenneberg, E. H.: Understanding language without ability to speak: A case report. J. Abnorm. Soc. Psychol. **65** (1962), 419–425.

Lenneberg, E. H. (Ed.): New directions in the study of language. Cambridge, Mass.: M.I.T. Press 1964a.

Lenneberg, E. H.: A biological perspective of language. In: Lenneberg, E. H. (Ed.): New directions in the study of language. Cambridge, Mass.: M.I.T. Press 1964b, 65–88.

Lenneberg, E. H. and J. M. Roberts: The denotata of color terms. Paper read at the Linguistic Society of America, Bloomington, Ind., August, 1953. Cited in Brown, R. W. and E. H. Lenneberg: A study in language and cognition. (p. 461). J. Abnorm. Soc. Psychol. **49**, No. 3, 454–462 (1954).

Lenneberg, E. H. and J. M. Roberts: The language of experience. In: Saporta, S. (Ed.): Psycholinguistics. New York: Holt, Rinehart and Winston 1961, 493–502.

Leontiev, A. N.: Learning as a problem in psychology. In: O'Connor, N. (Ed.): Recent Soviet psychology. Oxford: Pergamon Press 1961, 227–246.

Leontiev, A. N.: Soviet psycholinguistics–New trends. 20th Intern. Congr. Psychology, Tokyo 1972.

Levelt, W. J. M.: Some psychological aspects of linguistic data. Linguistische Berichte **17** (1972), 18–30.

Levelt, W. J. M.: Formal grammars in linguistics and psycholinguistics, Vol. **I–III**. The Hague: Mouton 1974.

Levelt, W. J. M.: What became of LAD? Lisse: Peter de Ridder Press 1975.

Lewandowski, T.: Linguistisches Wörterbuch. Heidelberg: Quelle und Meyer 1973.

Lewis, M. M.: Infant speech: A study of the beginnings of language. New York: Humanities Press 1951.

Lewis, M. M.: Language, thought, and personality in infancy and childhood. London: George G. Harrap 1963.

Liberman, A. M.: Some results of research on speech perception. J. Acoust. Soc. Amer. **29** (1957), 117–123; Reprinted in: Saporta, S. (Ed.): Psycholinguistics. New York: Holt, Rinehart and Winston 1961, 142–153.

Liberman, A. M., F. S. Cooper, K. S. Harris, and P. F. MacNeilage: A motor theory of speech perception. Proc. Speech Communication Seminar (1962) II. Stockholm: Speech Transmission Laboratory, Royal Institute of Technology 1963.

Liberman, A. M., P. C. Delattre, and F. S. Cooper: The role of selected stimulus-variables in the perception of the unvoiced stop consonants. Amer. J. Psychol. **65** (1952), 497–516.

Liberman, A. M., P. C. Delattre, F. S. Cooper, and L. J. Gerstman: The role of consonant-vowel transitions in the perception of the stop and nasal consonants. Psychol. Monogr. **68** (1954), No. 8.

Liberman, A. M., P. C. Delattre, F. S. Cooper, and L. J. Gerstman: Tempo of frequency change as a cue for distinguishing classes of speech sounds. J. Exp. Psychol. **52** (1956), 127–137.

Liberman, A. M., K. S. Harris, H. S. Hoffman, and B. C. Griffith: The descrimination of speech sounds within and across phoneme boundaries. J. Exp. Psychol. **54** (1957), 358–368.

Licklider, J. C. R.: Effects of amplitude distortion upon the intelligibility of speech. J. Acoust. Soc. Amer. **18** (1946), 429–434.

Licklider, J. C. R. and G. A. Miller: The perception of speech. In: Stevens, S. S. (Ed.): Handbook of experimental psychology. New York: Wiley 1951, 1040–1074.

Lindauer, M.: Communication among social bees. Cambridge, Mass.: Harvard University Press 1961.

Locke, J. L. and F. S. Fehr: Subvocal rehearsal as a form of speech. J. Verb. Learn. Verb. Behav. **9** (1970), 495–498.

Lohmann, J.: Sprache und Zeit. Stud. Gen. **8** (1955), 562–567.

Lohmann, J.: Das Ordnungsprinzip der Sprachwissenschaft. In: Kuhn, H. and F. Wiedmann (Eds.). Das Problem der Ordnung. 6. Dtsch. Kongr. Philos. (München 1960), Meisenheim a. Glan: A. Hain 1962, 225–236.

Longacre, R. E.: Review of "Language and reality" by Urban, W. M., and "Four articles on metalinguistics" by Whorf, B. L. Language **32**, No. 2 (1956), 298–308.

Lorenz, K.: Die angeborenen Formen möglicher Erfahrung. Z. Tierpsychol. **5** (1943), 235–409.

Lounsbury, F. G.: A semantic analysis of the Pawnee kinship usage. Language **32** (1956), 158–194.

Lounsbury, F. G.: Linguistics and psychology. In: Koch, S. (Ed.): Psychology, a study of a science. Vol. VI. New York: McGraw-Hill 1963, 552–582.

Lüdtke, H.: In: Zeichen und System der Sprache. Vol. I (Veröffentl. 1. Int. Symp. "Zeichen u. System der Sprache", 1959 in Erfurt). Schriften zur Phonetik, Sprachwissenschaft u. Kommunikationsforschung. Nr. 3, Berlin 1961, 249ff.

Luria, A. R.: The directive function of speech in development and dissolution. Word **15** (1959), 341–352 and 453–464.

Luria, A. R.: Human brain and psychological processes. New York: Harper and Row 1966.

Luria, A. R.: Traumatic aphasia. The Hague: Mouton 1968.

Luria, A. R. and F. I. Yudovich: Speech and development of mental processes in the child: An experimental investigation. London: Staples Press 1959.

MacKay, D. M.: Formal analysis of communication processes. In: Hinde, R. A. (Ed.): Non-verbal communication. Cambridge: Cambridge University Press 1972, 3–25.

MacNamara, J.: Cognitive basis of language learning in infants. Psychol. Rev. **79** (1972), 1–13.

MacNamara, J. and S. Kushnir: Linguistic independence of bilinguals: The input switch. J. Verb. Learn. Verb. Behav. **10** (1971), 480–487.

Malinowski, B.: The problem of meaning in primitive languages. In: Ogden, C. K. and T. A. Richards (Eds.): The meaning of meaning. London: Kegan Paul, Trench, Trubner 1936.

Malmberg, B.: Structural linguistics and human communication. Berlin: Springer 1963.

Maltzman, I., L. Morrisett, and L. O. Brooks: An investigation of phonetic symbolism. J. Abnorm. Soc. Psychol. **53** (1956), 249–251.

Marks, L. E. and G. A. Miller: The role of semantic and syntactic constraints in the memorization of English sentences. J. Verb. Learn. Verb. Behav. **3** (1964), 1–5.

Marshall, G. R. and C. N. Cofer: Associative indices as measures of word relatedness: A summary and comparison of ten methods. J. Verb. Learn. Verb. Behav. **1** (1962/63), 408–421.

Marshall, J. C.: Psychological linguistics: Psychological aspects of semantic structure. In: A. R. Meetham (Ed.): Encyclopedia of linguistics, information and control. London: Pergamon Press 1969.

Marshall, J. C.: The adequacy of grammars. Proceedings of the Joint Session of the Mind Association and the Aristotelian Society, 1970.

Martin, J. G.: Hesitations in the speaker's production and listener's reproduction of utterances. J. Verb. Learn. Verb. Behav. **6** (1967), 903–909.

Martinet, A.: A functional view of language. Oxford: Clarendon Press 1962.

Martinet, A.: Elements of General Linguistics. London: Faber and Faber 1964.

Massaro, D. W.: Preperceptual images, processing time, and perceptual units in auditory perception. Psychol. Rev. **79** (1972), 124–145.

McCarthy, D.: Language development in children. In: Carmichael, L. (Ed.): Manual of child psychology. New York: Wiley 1954, 492–630.

McKean, K., D. Slobin, and G. A. Miller: Cited in Miller, G. A.: Some psychological studies of grammar. Amer. Psychologist **17** (1962), 748–762.

McNeill, D.: The origin of associations within the same grammatical class. J. Verb. Learn. Verb. Behav. **2** (1963), 250–262.

McNeill, D.: The acquisition of language: The study of developmental psycholinguistics. New York: Harper and Row 1970.

Mehler, J.: Some effects of grammatical transformation on the recall of English sentences. J. Verbal Learn. Verb. Behav. **2** (1963), 346–351.

Mehrabian, A.: Significance of posture and position in the communication of attitude and status relationships. Psychol. Bull. **71** (1969), 359–372.

Meier, H.: Deutsche Sprachstatistik. Vols. I and II. Hildesheim: G. Olms 1964.

Menyuk, P.: Syntactic structures in the language of children. Child Develpm. **34** (1963), 407–422.

Menyuk, P.: Alternation of rules in children's grammar. J. Verb. Learn. Verb. Behav. **3** (1964), 480–488.

Merleau-Ponty, M.: Sur la phénoménologie du langage. In: Breda, H. L. van (Éd.): Problèmes actuels de la phénoménologie. Paris: Desclée de Brouwer 1952, 91–109.

Meumann, E.: Die Entstehung der ersten Worbedeutungen beim Kinde. Leipzig: W. Engelmann 1908.

Meyer-Eppler, W.: Grundlagen und Anwendungen der Informationstheorie. Berlin: Springer 1959.

Meyer-Eppler, W.: Problèmes informationnels de la communication parlée. In: Moles, A. A. and B. Vallancien (Éds.): Communications et langages. Paris: Gauthier-Villars 1963, 51–65.

Miller, G. A.: Language and communication. New York: McGraw-Hill 1951a.

Miller, G. A.: Speech and language. In: Stevens, S. S. (Ed.): Handbook of experimental psychology. New York: Wiley 1951b, 789–810.

Miller, G. A.: The magical number seven, plus or minus two: Some limits on our capacity for processing information. Psychol. Rev. **63** (1956), 81–97.

Miller, G. A.: Decision units in the perception of speech. IRE Transactions on Information Theory. IT-8 (1962a), 81–83.

Miller, G. A.: Some psychological studies of grammar. Amer. Psychologist **17** (1962b), 748–762.

Miller, G. A.: Review of Greenberg, J. H. (Ed.): Universals of language. In: Contemp. Psychol. **8** (1963), 417–418.

Miller, G. A.: Language and psychology. In: Lenneberg, E. H. (Ed.): New directions in the study of language. Cambridge, Mass.: M.I.T. Press 1964, 89–107.

Miller, G. A.: Some preliminaries to psycholinguistics. Amer. Psychologist **20** (1965), 15–20.

Miller, G. A.: Empirical methods in the study of semantics. In: Steinberg, D. D. and L. A. Jakobovits (Eds.): Semantics. Cambridge: Cambridge University Press 1971, 569–585.

Miller, G. A.: English verbs of motion: A case study in semantic and lexical memory. In: Melton, A. W. and E. Martin (Eds.): Coding processes in human memory. Washington: V. Winston 1972, 335–372.

Miller, G. A., J. S. Bruner, and L. Postman: Familiarity of letter sequences and tachistoscopic identification. J. Gen. Psychol. **50** (1954), 129–139.

Miller, G. A. and E. A. Friedman: The reconstruction of mutilated English texts. Inform. Control **1** (1957), 38–55.

Miller, G. A., E. Galanter, and K. H. Pribram: Plans and the structure of behavior. New York: Henry Holt 1960.

Miller, G. A., G. A. Heise, and W. Lichten: The intelligibility of speech as a function of the context of the test materials. J. Exp. Psychol. **41** (1951), 329–335.

Miller, G. A. and S. Isard: Some perceptual consequences of linguistic rules. J. Verb. Learn. Verb. Behav. **2** (1963), 217–228.

Miller, G. A. and J. C. R. Licklider: The intelligibility of interrupted speech. J. Acoust. Soc. Amer. **22** (1950), 167–173.

Miller, G. A. and K. McKean: A chronometric study of some relations between sentences. Quart. J. Exp. Psychol. **16** (1964), 297–308.

Miller, G. A. and P. E. Nicely. An analysis of perceptual confusions among some English consonants. J. Acoust. Soc. Amer. **27** (1955), 338–352. Reprinted in: Saporta, S. (Ed.): Psycholinguistics. New York: Holt, Rinehart and Winston 1961, 153–175.

Miller, G. A. and J. A. Selfridge: Verbal context and the recall of meaningful material. Amer. J. Psychol. **63** (1950), 176–185.

Mistler-Lachmann, J. L.: Levels of comprehension in processing of normal and ambiguous sentences. J. Verb. Learn. Verb. Behav. **11** (1972), 614–623.

Moles, A. A.: Les bases de la théorie de l'information et son application aux langages. In: Moles, A. A. and B. Vallancien (Éds.): Communications et langages. Paris: Gauthier-Villars 1963, 15–33.

Moles, A. A. and B. Vallancien (Éds.): Communications et langages. Paris: Gauthier-Villars 1963.

Morris, C. W.: Foundations of the theory of signs. International Encyclopedia of Unified Science No. 2. Chicago. University of Chicago Press 1938.

Morris, C. W.: Signs, language, and behavior. New York: G. Braziller 1955.

Morton, J.: Interaction of information in word recognition. Psychol. Rev. **76** (1969), 165–178.

Moser, H. (Ed.): Das Ringen um eine neue deutsche Grammatik. Aufsätze aus 3 Jahrzehnten. Darmstadt: Wissenschaftliche Buchgesellschaft 1965.

Mowrer, O. H.: Preparatory set (expectancy)—Some methods of measurement. Psychol. Rev. Monogr. Suppl. **52** (1940).

Mowrer, O. H.: The psychologist looks at language. Amer. Psychologist **9** (1954), 660–694.

Mowrer, O. H.: Learning theory and the symbolic processes. New York: Wiley 1960.

Müller, A. L.: Experimentelle Untersuchungen zur stimmlichen Darstellung von Gefühlen. Dissertation, Göttingen 1960.

Neisser, U.: Cognitive psychology. New York: Appleton-Century-Crofts 1967.

Nelson, K.: Concept, word, and sentence. Interrelations in acquisition and development. Psychol. Review **81** (1974), 267–285.

Neubert, A.: Semantischer Positivismus in den USA. Halle (Saale): Neimeyer 1962.

Newman, S.: Further experiments in phonetic symbolism. Amer. J. Psychol. **45** (1933), 53–75.

Norman, D. A.: Memory and attention. New York: Wiley 1976.

O'Connell, D. C.: Nonsense strings, words, and sentences: Some cross-linguistic comparisons. Psychol. Forsch. **33** (1969), 37–49.

Öhman, S.: Wortinhalt und Weltbild. Stockholm: Thesis Stockholm's Högskola 1951.

Öhman, S.: Theories of the "linguistic field". Word **9** (1953), 123–134.

Ogden, C. K. and I. A. Richards: The meaning of meaning. London: Kegan Paul, Trench, Trubner 1936.

Oldfield, R. C.: Individual vocabulary and semantic currency: A preliminary study. Brit. J. Soc. Clin. Psychol. **2** (1963), 122–130.

Oléron, P.: Reconstitution des textes français ayant subi divers taux de mutilation. Psychol. Franç. **5** (1960), 161–174.

Oléron, P.: Les habitudes verbales. In: Ajuriaguerra, J. de, et al. (Éds.): Problèmes de psycholinguistique. Paris: Presses Universitaires de France 1963, 73–103.

Olson, D. R.: Language and thought: Aspects of a cognitive theory of semantics. Psychol. Rev. **77** (1970), 257–273.

Osgood, C. E.: A behavioristic analysis of perception and language as cognitive phenomena. In: Bruner, J. S. et al. (Eds.): Contemporary approaches to cognition. Cambridge, Mass.: Harvard University Press 1957, 75–118.

Osgood, C. E.: The representational model and relevant research methods. In: Pool, I. de S. (Ed.): Trends in content analysis. Urbana, Ill.: University of Illinois Press 1959, 33–88.

Osgood, C. E.: Some effects of motivation on style of encoding. In: Sebeok, T. A. (Ed.): Style in language. New York: Wiley 1960, 293–306.

Osgood, C. E.: Comments on: Bousfield, W. A.: The problem of meaning in verbal learning. In: Cofer, C. N. (Ed.): Verbal learning and verbal behavior. New York: McGraw-Hill 1961, 91–106.

Osgood, C. E.: Psycholinguistic relativity and universality. Proc. 16th Int. Congr. Psychol. (Bonn 1960). Amsterdam, North-Holland 1962a, 673–678.

Osgood, C. E.: Studies on the generality of affective meaning systems. Amer. Psychologist **17** (1962b), 10–28.

Osgood, C. E.: Psycholinguistics. In: Koch, S. (Ed.): Psychology, a study of a science. Vol. VI. New York: McGraw-Hill 1963, 244–316.

Osgood, C. E.: Exploration in semantic space: A personal diary. J. Soc. Issues **27** (1971a), 5–64.

Osgood, C. E.: Where do sentences come from? In: D. D. Steinberg and L. A. Jakobovits (Eds.): Semantics. Cambridge: Cambridge University Press 1971b, 497–529.

Osgood, C. E. and T. A. Sebeok (Eds.): Psycholinguistics. A survey of theory and research problems. J. Abnorm. Soc. Psychol. **49** (1954), Supplement. Reprinted as: Psycholinguistics. A survey of theory and research problems. With: A survey of psycholinguistic research 1954–1964. By Diebold, A. R. Bloomington and London: Indiana University Press 1965.

Osgood, C. E., G. J. Suci, and P. H. Tannenbaum: The measurement of meaning. Urbana, Ill.: University of Illinois Press 1957.

Paivio, A.: On the functional significance of imagery. Psychol. Bull. **73** (1970), 385–392.

Palermo, D. S. and J. J. Jenkins: Sex differences in word association. J. Gen. Psychol. **72** (1965), 77–84.

Paul, H.: Prinzipien der Sprachgeschichte. Tübingen: Niemeyer 1960.

Pavlov, I. P.: Conditioned reflexes: An investigation of the physiological activity of the cerebral cortex. Translated by Anrep, A. V. New York: Dover Publications 1960.

Pavlov, I. P.: Lectures on conditioned reflexes. Translated by Gantt, W. H. New York: Internat. Publishers 1963.

Pečjak, V.: Poglavija iz psihologije, Ljubljana 1965.

Pečjak, V.: Emotional symbolism of spatial forms. Anthropos **3** (1970), 117–126.

Peirce, C. S.: Collected papers, II. Cambridge, Mass.: Belknap Press of Harvard University 1960.

Penfield, W. and L. Roberts: Speech and brain-mechanisms. Princeton, N. J.: Princeton University Press 1959.

Perfetti, C. A.: Psychosemantics. Psychol. Bull. **78** (1972), 241–259.

Piaget, J.: Le Langage et la pensée chez l'enfant. Neuchâtel et Paris: Delachaux and Niestlé 1923.

Piaget, J.: La formation du symbole chez l'enfant. Neuchâtel and Paris: Delachoux et Niestlé, 1945. English Ed.: Play, dreams and imitation in childhood. Translated by Gattegno, C., and F. M. Hodgson. London: W. Heinemann 1951.

Piaget, J.: La construction du réél chez l'enfant. Neuchâtel: Delachaux and Niestlé 1950.

Pick, A.: Die agrammatischen Sprachstörungen. Studien zur psychologischen Grundlegung der Aphasielehre. Part 1. Monographien aus dem Gesamtgebiete der Neurologie und Psychiatrie. 7. Berlin 1913.

Ploog, D.: Kommunikation in Affengesellschaften und deren Bedeutung für die Verständigungsweisen des Menschen. In: Gadamer, H.-G., and P. Vogler, P. (Eds.): Neue Anthropologie, Vol. 2, Biologische Anthropologie. Stuttgart: dtv-Thieme Verlag 1972, 98–178.

Pollack, I.: The information of elementary auditory displays. J. Acoust. Soc. Amer. **24** (1952), 745–749.

Pollack, I.: Assimilation of sequentially encoded information. Amer. J. Psychol. **66** (1953a), 421–435.

Pollack, I.: The information of elementary auditory displays. II. J. Acoust. Soc. Amer. **25** (1953b), 765–769.

Pollack, I. and L. Ficks: Information of elementary multidimensional auditory displays. J. Acoust. Soc. Amer. **26** (1954), 155–158.

Pollack, I. and J. M. Pickett: Intelligibility of excerpts from fluent speech: Auditory vs. structural context. J. Verb. Learn. Verb. Behav. **3** (1964), 79–84.

Pollio, H. R.: Composition of associative clusters. J. Exp. Psychol. **67** (1964), 199–208.

Porzig, W.: Wesenhafte Bedeutungsbeziehungen. Beiträge zur Geschichte der deutschen Sprache und Literatur **58** (1934), 70–97.

Premack, D.: Preparations for discussing behaviorism with chimpanzee. In: Smith, F. and G. A. Miller (Eds.): The genesis of language. Cambridge, Mass.: M.I.T. Press 1966, 295–335.

Premack, D.: A functional analysis of language. J. Exp. Anal. Behav. **14** (1970), 107–125.

Putnam, H.: Zu einigen Problemen der theoretischen Grundlegung der Grammatik. Sprache im technischen Zeitalter **14** (1965), 1109–1131.

Quillian, M. R.: Word concepts: A theory and simulation of some basic semantic capabilities. Behav. Sci. **12** (1967), 410–430.

Quillian, M. R.: The teachable language comprehender: A simulation program and theory of language. Communications of the ACM **12** (1969), 459–476.

Rapaport, D.: Discussion of Osgood, C. E.: A behavioristic analysis of perception and language as cognitive phenomena. In: Bruner, J. S. et al. (Eds.): Contemporary approaches to cognition. Cambridge, Mass.: Harvard University Press 1957, 120–125.

Razran, G.: Semantic and phonetographic generalizations of salivary conditioning to verbal stimuli. J. Exp. Psychol. **39** (1949), 642–652.

Razran, G.: Experimental semantics. Trans. N. Y. Acad. Sci. **13** (1950/51), 171–177.

Reese, H. W.: Imagery and contextual meaning. Psychol. Bull. **73** (1970), 404–414.

Reuck, A. V. S. de and M. O'Connor (Eds.): Disorders of language. Ciba Foundation Symposium, London: J. and A. Churchill 1964.

Révész, G.: Ursprung und Vorgeschichte der Sprache. Bern: A. Francke 1946.

Riegel, K. and M. Riegel: Changes in associative behavior during later years of life. Vita Humana **7** (1964), 1–32.

Riesman, D., R. Denney, and N. Glazer: The lonely crowd. New Haven: Yale University Press 1950.

Romney, A. K., D'Andrade, R. G.: Cognitive aspects of English kin terms. Amer. Anthropologist **66** (1964), Nr. 3, Part 2.

Rosch-Heider, E.: On the internal structure of perceptual and semantic categories. In: Moore, T. E. (Ed.): Cognitive development and the acquisition of language. New York: Academic Press 1973. 111–144.

Rosenberg, S. (Ed.): Directions in psycholinguistics. New York: Macmillan 1965.

Rosenberg, S. and N. Baker: Grammatical form class as a variable in verbal learning at three levels of linguistic structure. Cited in Rosenberg, S. and J. Koplin:

Introduction to psycholinguistics. In: Rosenberg, S. (Ed.): Directions in psycholinguistics. New York: Macmillan 1965, 3–12.

Rosenblith, W. A.: Auditory masking and fatigue. J. Acoust. Soc. Amer. 22 (1950), 792–800.

Rosenblith, W. A.: La perception catégorielle des phénomènes sonores. In: Moles, A. A. and B. Vallancien (Éds.): Communications et langages. Paris: Gauthier-Villars 1963, 67–76.

Rosenzweig, M. R.: Études sur l'association des mots. Année psychol. 57 (1957), 23–32.

Rosenzweig, M. R.: Comparisons among word-association responses in English, French, German, and Italian. Amer. J. Psychol. 74 (1961), 347–360.

Rosenzweig, M. R.: Comparisons among word-association responses in English, French, German, and Italian. Proc. 16th Int. Congr. Psychol., Bonn 1960. Amsterdam: North-Holland 1962, 704–705.

Rosenzweig, M. R.: Word associations of French workmen: Comparisons with associations of French students and American workmen and students. J. Verb. Learn. Verb. Behav. 3 (1964), 57–69.

Rosenzweig, M. R. and W. A. Rosenblith: Some electrophysiological correlates of the perception of successive clicks. J. Acoust. Soc. Amer. 22 (1950), 878–880.

Rubenstein, H. and M. Aborn: Immediate recall as a function of degree of organization and length of study period. J. Exp. Psychol. 48 (1954), 146–152.

Rubenstein, H. and M. Aborn: Psycholinguistics. Annu. Rev. Psychol. 11 (1960), 291–322.

Russell, W. A.: Bi-directional effects in word association. In: Jenkins, J. J. (Ed.): Associative processes in verbal behavior. Minnesota Conference 1955, 1–12.

Russell, W. A. and O. R. Meseck: Der Einfluß der Assoziation auf das Erinnern von Worten in der deutschen, französischen und englischen Sprache. Z. exp. angew. Psychol. 6 (1959), 191–211.

Russell, W. A. and L. H. Storms: Implicit verbal chaining in paired associate learning. J. Exp. Psychol. 49 (1955), 287–293.

Sachs, J.: Recognition memory for syntactic and semantic aspects of connected discourse. Perception and Psychophysics 2 (1967), 437–442.

Sachs, J.: Memory in reading and listening to discourse: Memory and Cognition 2 (1974), 95–100.

Salzinger, K., S. Portnoy, and R. S. Feldman: The effect of order of approximation to the statistical structure of English on the emission of verbal responses. J. Exp. Psychol. 64 (1962), 52–57.

Sapir, E.: A study in phonetic symbolism. J. Exp. Psychol. 12 (1929), 225–239.

Sapir, E.: Conceptual categories in primitive language. Science 74 (1931).

Sapir, E.: Language. Encyclopedia of the social sciences 9 (1933), 155–168.

Sapir, E.: Selected writings. Ed. Mandelbaum, D. G., Berkeley, Cal.: University of California Press 1949.

Sapir, E.: Language. In: E. Seligman, (Ed.): Encyclopedia of the social sciences. Vol. IX & X. New York: Macmillan 1963.

Saporta, S.: Frequency of consonant clusters. Language 31 (1955a), 25–30.

Saporta, S.: Linguistic structure as a factor and as a measure in word association. In: Jenkins, J. J. (Ed.): Associative processes in verbal behavior. Minnesota Conference 1955b, 210–214.

Saporta, S.: (Ed.): Psycholinguistics. A book of readings. New York: Holt, Rinehart and Winston 1961.

Saussure, F. de: Cours de linguistique générale. Paris: Payot 1916. English Ed.: Course in general linguistics. Translated by Baskin, W. New York: Philosophical Library 1959.

Schank, R. C.: Conceptual dependency: A theory of natural language understanding. Cognitive Psychol. 3 (1972), 552–631.

Schlesinger, I. M.: A note on the relationship between psychological and linguistic theories. Found. Lang. 3 (1967), 397–402.

Schlesinger, I. M.: Learning of grammar: From pivot to realization rule. In: Huxley, R. and E. Ingram (Eds.): Language acquisition: Models and methods. London: Science Series 1971a, 79–93.

Schlesinger, I. M.: Production of utterance and language acquisition. In Slobin, D. (Ed.): The ontogenesis of grammar. New York: Academic Press 1971b, 63–101.

Schmeiterer, L.: Sprache und Informationstheorie. In: Sprache und Wissenschaft. Vorträge der Tagung der Jungius-Gesellschaft in Hamburg 1959. Göttingen: Vandenhoeck Ruprecht 1960, 155–168.

Schmitt, A.: Helen Keller und die Sprache. Münster-Köln: Böhlau 1954.

Schnelle, H.: Zur Entwicklung der theoretischen Linguistik. Studium Generale 23 (1970), 1–29.

Schönbach, P.: Soziolinguistik. In: Koch, W. A. (Ed.): Perspektiven der Linguistik, II. Stuttgart: Kröner 1974, 156–177.

Searle, J. R.: Speech acts. Cambridge: Cambridge University Press 1969.

Sebeok, T. A. (Ed.): Style in language. New York: Wiley 1960.

Sebeok, T. A.: Review of "Communication among social bees" by Lindauer, M.; "Porpoises and Sonar" by Kellogg, W. N.; "Man and dolphin" by Lilly, J. C. Language 39, No. 3, 448–466 (1963).

Segerstedt, T. T.: Die Macht des Wortes, Zürich: Panverlag 1947.

Seiler, H.: Sprachsysteme und systematische Sprachbetrachtung. In: Sprache und Wissenschaft. Vorträge der Tagung der Jungius-Gesselschaft in Hamburg 1959. Göttingen: Vandenhoeck & Ruprecht 1960, 43–50.

Shannon, C. E.: Prediction and entropy of printed English. Bell System Techn. J. 30 (1951), 50–64.

Shannon, C. E. and W. Weaver: The mathematical theory of communication. Urbana, Ill.: University of Illinois Press 1949.

Shipinowa, Y. and M. Surina: Cited in Lewis, M. M.: Language, thought, and personality in infancy and childhood. London: G. G. Harrap 1963, p. 36; also in Simon, B. (Ed.): Psychology in the Soviet Union. London: Routledge and Paul 1957, 198.

Shipley, W. C.: Indirect conditioning. J. Gen. Psychol. 12 (1935), 337–357.

Shlien, J.: Mother-in-law: A problem in kinship terminology. ETC. 19 (1962), 161–171.

Skinner, B. F.: The distribution of associated words. Psychol. Rec. 1 (1937), 71–76.

Skinner, B. F.: Verbal behavior. New York: Appleton-Century-Crofts 1957.

Slobin, D.: Some aspects of the use of pronouns of address in Yiddish. Word 19 (1963), 193–202.

Slobin, D.: (Ed.): The ontogenesis of grammar. New York: Academic Press 1971.

Smirnov, A. A.: Sprachbewegungen und Retention. Proc. 16th Int. Congr. Psychol., Bonn, 1960. Amsterdam: North-Holland 1961, 678–683.

Sokolov, A. N.: Speech-motor afferentiation and the problem of brain mechanism of thought. Voprosy psikhologii 13 (1967), (3), 41–54.

Sokolov, A. N.: Internal speech and thought. Internat. J. Psychol./Journal International de Psychologie 6 (1971), 79–92.

Sommerfelt, A.: Diachronic and synchronic aspects of language. Selected articles. Gravenhage: Mouton 1962a.

Sommerfelt, A.: La linguistique: Science sociologique. In: Sommerfelt, A.: Diachronic and synchronic aspects of language. Gravenhage: Mouton 1962b, 36–51.

Staats, A. W.: Verbal habit-families, concepts, and the operant conditioning of word classes. Psychol. Rev. 68 (1961), 190–204.

Staats, A. W. and C. K. Staats: Attitudes established by classical conditioning. J. Abnorm. Soc. Psychol. 57 (1958), 37–40.

Staats, A. W., C. K. Staats, and D. A. Biggs: Meaning of verbal stimuli changed by conditioning. Amer. J. Psychol. 71 (1958), 429–431.

Staats, A. W., C. K. Staats, and W. G. Heard: Denotative meaning established by classical conditioning. J. Exp. Psychol. 61 (1961), 300–303.

Staats, C. K. and A. W. Staats: Meaning established by classical conditioning. J. Exp. Psychol. 54 (1957), 74–80.

Steger, H.: Sprachnorm, Grammatik und technische Welt. Sprache im technischen Zeitalter 3 (1962), 183–198.

Steinberg, D. D. and L. A. Jakobovits: Semantics. Cambridge: Cambridge University Press 1971.

Steinbuch, K.: Automat und Mensch. Berlin: Springer 1965.

Steinthal, H.: Einleitung in die Psychologie und Sprachwissenschaft. Berlin: F. Dümmler's Verlagsbuchhandlung 1871.

Stenzel, J.. Sinn, Bedeutung, Begriff, Definition. Jb. Philologie 1 (1925), 160–201.

Stenzel, J.: Philosophie der Sprache. Munich: Oldenbourg 1934.

Stern, C. and W. Stern: Die Kindersprache. Eine psychologische und sprachtheoretische Untersuchung. Leipzig: Barth 1907.

Stern, W.: Psychologie der frühen Kindheit. Leipzig: Quelle and Meyer 1930.

Stevens, S. S. (Ed.): Handbook of experimental psychology. New York: Wiley 1951.

Stevens, S. S. and H. Davis: Hearing. New York: Wiley 1938.

Stevenson, C. L.: Ethics and language. New Haven: Yale University Press 1944.

Studdert-Kennedy, M., A. M. Liberman, K. S. Harris, and F. S. Cooper: Motor theory of speech-perception: A reply to Lane's critical review. Psychol. Rev. 77 (1970), 234–249.

Stumpf, C.: Die Sprachlaute, Berlin: J. Springer 1926.

Sumby, W. H. and I. Pollack: Visual contribution to speech intelligibility in noise. J. Acoust. Soc. Amer. 26 (1954), 212–215.

Szalay, L. B., and J. A. Bryson: Measurement of Psychocultural Distance: a comparison of American Blacks and Whites. J. Pers. Social Psychology 26 (1973), 166–177.

Szalay, L. B., and R. G. D'Andrade: Scaling versus content analysis: Interpreting word association data from Americans and Koreans. Southw. J. Anthropology 28 (1972), 50–68.

Szalay, L. B. and B. C. Maday: Verbal associations in the analysis of subjective culture. Current Anthropology **14** (1973), 33–42.

Szalay, L. B., C. Windle, and D. A. Lysne: Attitude measurement by free verbal associations. J. Soc. Psychol. **82** (1970), 53–55.

Taylor, I. K.: Phonetic symbolism re-examined. Psychol. Bull. **60** (1963), 200–209.

Taylor, W. L.: Cloze procedure, a new tool for measuring readability. Journalism Quart. **30** (1953), 415–433.

Teuber, H. L.: Discussion. In: Reuck, A. V. S. de and M. O'Connor (Eds.): Disorders of language. London: J. and A. Churchill 1964, 255.

Thorndike, E. L.: Educational psychology. New York: Lemcke and Buechner 1903.

Thorndike, E. L.: Man and his works. Cambridge, Mass.: Harvard University Press 1943.

Thorndike, E. L. and I. Lorge: The teacher's word book of 30,000 words. New York: Bureau of Publications, Teacher's College, Columbia University 1944.

Thumb, A. und K. Marbe: Experimentelle Untersuchungen über die psychologischen Grundlagen der sprachlichen Analogiebildung. Leipzig: Engelmann 1901.

Tichomirow, O. K.: Review of Skinner, B. F.: Verbal Behavior, 1957. In: Word **15** (1959), 362–367.

Tinbergen, N.: The study of instinct. Oxford: Clarendon Press 1951.

Titchener, E. B.: A text-book of psychology. Part II. New York: Macmillan 1910.

Tolman, E. C.: Cognitive maps in rats and men. Psychol. Rev. **55** (1948), 189–208.

Tolman, E. C.: Principles of purposive behavior. In: Koch, S. (Ed.): Psychology, a study of a science. Vol. II. New York: McGraw-Hill 1959, 92–157.

Toulmin, St.: Brain and language: A commentary. Synthese **23** (1971), 369–395.

Trautscholdt, M.: Experimentelle Untersuchungen über die Association der Vorstellungen. Philos. Stud. (Ed. W. Wundt) **1** (1883), 213–250.

Treisman, A. M.: Contextual cues in selective listening. Quart. J. Exp. Psychol. **12** (1960), 242–248.

Treisman, A. M.: The effect of irrelevant material on the efficiency of selective listening. Amer. J. Psychol. **77** (1964), 533–546.

Treisman, A. M.: Strategies and models of selective attention. Psychol. Rev. **76** (1969), 282–299.

Trier, J.: Der deutsche Wortschatz im Sinnbezirk des Verstandes. Vol. 1. Heidelberg: C. Winter 1931.

Trier, J.: Das sprachliche Feld. Neue Jahrbücher für Wissenschaft und Jugendbildung **10** (1934), 428–449.

Trubetzkoy, N.: Zur allgemeinen Theorie der phonologischen Vokalsysteme. Prague: Travaux du Cercle linguistique de Prague. I. 1929.

Trubetzkoy, N.: Grundzüge der Phonologie. Prague: Travaux du Cercle linguistique de Prague. VII. 1939.

Tsuru, S. and H. S. Fries: A problem in meaning. J. Gen. Psychol. **8** (1933), 281–284.

Uexküll, J. von: Theoretische Biologie. Berlin: J. Springer 1928. English Ed.: Theoretical biology. Translated by Mackinnon, D. L. London: K. Paul, Trench, Trubner 1926.

Ullmann, S.: Semantics: An introduction to the science of meaning. New York: Barnes and Noble 1962.

Ullmann, S.: The principles of semantics. New York: Barnes and Noble 1963.

Urban, W. M.: Language and reality. London: Allen and Unwin 1939.

Van Lancker, D.: Heterogeneity in language and speech: Neurolinguistic studies. Working Papers in Phonetics 29, Los Angeles 1975.

Vigotsky, L. S.: Thought and language. Edited and translated by Hanfmann, E. and G. Vakar. Cambridge, Mass.: M.I.T. Press 1962 (Orig. Ed. Moscow 1934).

Wallach, M.: Perceptual recognition of approximations to English in relation to spelling achievement. J. Educ. Psychol. **54** (1963), 57–62.

Watson, J. B.: Psychology from the standpoint of a behaviorist. Philadelphia: Lippincott 1924.

Wegener, P.: Untersuchungen über die Grundfragen des Sprachlebens. Halle (Saale): Niemeyer 1885.

Weinreich, U.: Travels through semantic space. Word **14** (1958), 346–366.

Weir, R. H.: Language in the crib. The Hague: Mouton 1962.

Weisgerber, L.: Sprachvergleichung und Psychologie. Ber. 12. Kongr. Dtsch. Ges. Psychol: Fischer Hamburg, 1931, Jena 1932, 193–201.

Weisgerber, L.: Energetische Terminologie in der Sprachpsychologie. Z. exp. angew. Psychol. **6** (1959), 621–632.

Weisgerber, L.: Von den Kräften der deutschen Sprache. Vol. 1: Grundzüge der inhaltbezogenen Grammatik, Düsseldorf: Päd. Verlag Schwann 1962a.

Weisgerber, L.: Von den Kräften der deutschen Sprache. Vol. II: Die sprachliche Gestaltung der Welt. Düsseldorf: Päd Verlag Schwann 1962b.

Weiss, J. H.: Further study of the relation between the sound of a word and its meaning. Amer. J. Psychol. **76** (1963), 624–630.

Weiss, J. H.: Phonetic symbolism re-examined. Psychol. Bull., **61** (1964a), 454–458.

Weiss, J. H.: The role of stimulus meaningfulness in the phonetic symbolism response. J. Gen. Psychol. **70** (1964b), 255–263.

Weizsäcker, C. F. v.: Sprache als Information. In: Die Sprache. Vortragsreihe der Bayrischen Akademie der Schönen Künste. Darmstadt: Wissenschaftliche Buchgesellschaft 1959, 33–53.

Weizsäcker, C. F. v.: Die Sprache der Physik. In: Sprache und Wissenschaft. Vorträge der Tagung der Jungius-Gesellschaft in Hamburg 1959. Göttingen: Vandenhoeck Ruprecht 1960, 137–153.

Werner, H.: Grundlagen der Sprachphysiognomik. Leipzig: Barth 1932.

Werner, H.: (Ed.): On expressive language. Worcester, Mass.: Clark University Press 1955.

Werner, H.: Einführung in die Entwicklungspsychologie. Munich: Barth, 1953. English Ed.: Comparative psychology of mental development. Translated by Garside, E. B. New York: International Universities Press 1957.

Werner, H. and B. Kaplan: Symbol formation. New York: Wiley 1963.

Werner, H. and E. Kaplan: The acquisition of word meanings: A developmental study. Monogr. Soc. Res. Child Develpm. **15** (1952), 190–200.

Wertheimer, M.: The relation between the sound of a word and its meaning. Amer. J. Psychol. **71** (1958), 412–415.

Wettler, M.: Über die Struktur des semantischen Langzeitgedächtnisses. Istituto per gli Studi Semantici e Cognitivi, Castagnola, Switzerland 1974.

Whitehurst, G. J. and R. Vasta: Is language acquired through imitation? J. Psycholing. Res. **4** (1975), 37–60.

Whorf, B. L.: Language, thought, and reality. Edited by Carroll, J. B. Cambridge, Mass.: M.I.T. Press 1956.

Wiener, M., S. Devoe, S. Rubionow and J. Geller: Nonverbal behavior and nonverbal communication. Psychol. Rev. **79** (1972), 185–214.

Wilde, K.: Naive und künstlerische Formen des graphischen Ausdrucks. Ber. 21. Kongr. Dtsch. Ges. Psychol., Bonn, 1957, Göttingen: Verlag für Psychologie 1958, 157–159.

Wissemann, H.: Untersuchungen zur Onomatopoiie. Part 1: Die sprachpsychologischen Versuche, Heidelberg: Winter 1954.

Wittgenstein, L.: Schriften: Tractatus logico-philosophicus. Tagebücher 1914–1916. Philosophische Untersuchungen. Frankfurt (Main): Suhrkamp 1963. English Eds.: Philosophical Investigations. Translated by Anscombe, G. E. M. Oxford: Basil Blackwell 1958; and Tractatus Logico-Philosophicus. Translated by Pears, D. F. and B. F. McGuinness. London: Routledge and Kegan Paul 1966.

Woodrow, H. and F. Lowell: Children's association frequency tables. Psychol. Monogr. **22** (1916), (Whole No. 97).

Woodworth, R. S., and H. Schlosberg: Experimental psychology. New York: Holt, Rinehart and Winston 1954.

Wreschner, A.: Die Reproduktion und Assoziation von Vorstellungen, Z. Psychol. Physiol. Sinnesorg., 1907, Supplement 3, 1–599.

Wundt, W.: Grundzüge der physiologischen Psychologie. 4th ed. Vols. I and II. Leipzig: W. Engelmann 1893; 6th rev. ed. Vol. I 1908, Vol. II 1910, Vol. III 1911.

Yavuz, H. S. and W. A. Bousfield: Recall of connotative meaning. Psychol. Rep. **5** (1959), 319–320.

Yelen, D. R. and R. W. Schulz: Verbal satiation? J. Verb. Learn. Verb. Behav. **1** (1962–63), 372–377.

Zazzo, R.: Les jumeaux, le couple et la personne. Paris: Presses Universitaires de France 1960.

Zemanek, H.: Elementare Informationstheorie. Munich: Oldenbourg 1959.

Zipf, G. K.: The psycho-biology of language. Boston: Houghton Mifflin 1935.

Zipf, G. K.: The meaning-frequency relationship of words. J. Gen. Psychol. **33** (1945), 251–256.

Zipf, G. K.: Human behavior and the principle of least effort. Cambridge, Mass.: Addison-Wesley 1949.

Author Index

Aborn, M., 105, *323*
Ach, N., *301*
Adelson, M., 105, *301*
Aebli, H., *301*
Ajdukiewicz, K., 141, *301*
Ajuriaguerra, J. de, *301*
Albrecht, E., 10, *301*
Allesch, J. v., 24, *301*
Ammer, K., 141, *301*
Apel, K.-O., 13, 137, 139, 141, 142, 149, *301*
Arnheim, R., 75, 267, *301*
Attneave, F., 65, *301*
Austin, G. A., 259, *303*
Austin, J. L., *301*

Barclay, J. R., 267, *302, 303*
Bartlett, F. C., 267, *302*
Beauvoir, S. de, 287, *302*
Becker, K. F., 13, *302*
Begg, J., 229, *302*
Bellugi, U., 240, 241, 242, 243, *302, 303*
Benjamin, W., 273, *302*
Bentley, M., 194, *302*
Bergson, H., *302*
Berko, J., 39, 244, *302, 304*
Berkowitz, H., 166, *303*
Berlyne, D. E., *302*
Bernstein, B., 93, 277, *302*
Bever, T. G., 214, 262, *302, 308*
Bierwisch, M., 38, 228, *302*
Bixler, R. H., *302*
Black, A., 195, *304*
Bloch, E., 253, *302*
Bloemer, W. D., 200, *307*
Bloomfield, L., 162, 171, *303*
Blumenthal, A. L., 215, *303*
Bock, M., 269, *303*
Bond, Z. S., 231, *303*
Bousfield, W. A., 129, 166, *303*
Brackbill, Y., 196, *303*
Braine, M. D. S., 239, *303*
Bransford, J. D., 267, *302, 303*
Bresson, F., *301*
Bridgeman, P. W., 143, *303*
Broadbent, D. E., 108, *303*
Brooks, L. O., 195, *318*

Brown, R. W., 29, 39, 92, 145, 146, 161, 188,
  195, 196, 198, 225, 234, 235, 240, 241, 242,
  243, 259, 260, 263, 276, 281, 290, 291, 292,
  302, 303, 304
Bruner, J. S., 68, 95, 169, 259, *303, 304*
Brutyan, G. A., *304*
Bryson, J. A., 121, *325*
Buckland, W. R., 99, *314*
Bühler, K., 21, 22, 23, 190, 296, *304*

Carmichael, L., 28, 237, *304*
Carnap, R., 142, *304*
Carroll, J. B., 17, 40, 45, 92, 179, 180, 257, *305*
Carterette, E. C., 76, *305*
Carton, A. S., *305*
Cassirer, E., 3, 7, 30, 188, 189, 258, *305*
Cattell, J. McK., 106, 114, *305*
Chafe, W. L., 108, *305*
Cherry, C., 82, 90, *305*
Chomsky, N., 48, 49, 51, 157, 159, 204, *305*
Church, J., 248, *305*
Clark, E. V., *305*
Clark, H. H., 126, *306*
Clark, W. H., *309*
Cofer, C. N., 166, *306*
Cohen, B. H., 176, *306*
Coleman, E. B., 202, 203, *306*
Collins, A. M., 226, *306*
Cooper, F. S., 36, 69, *316*
Craik, F. I. M., 269, 306
Crosby, C., 178, *315*
Curtius, G., 186, *306*

D'Andrade, R. G., 135, *322*
Davis, E. A., 251, *306*
Davis, H., *325*
Davis, R., 190, *306*
Day, E. J., *306*
Deese, J., 130, 132, 133, 134, 161, 202, *306,
  307*
Delattre, P. C., *316*
Denney, R., 322
Deutsch, D., 107, 307
Deutsch, J. A., 107, *307*
Devoe, S., 30, 200, 265, *328*
Dodge, R., *307*

Doob, L.W., 290, *307*
Dorst, R., 197, *307*
Dulaney, D. E., 235, *304*
Durkheim, E., *307*

Eisenberg, K., *312*
Engelkamp, J., 128, 220, 224, 230, *307*
Entwisle, D. R., 122, *307*
Epstein, W., 204, 205, *307*
Erdmann, B., *307*
Erdmann, K. O., *307*
Ertel, S., 181, 186, 197, 199, 200, 307
Ervin, S. M., 122, 124, 125, *307*
Esch, H., 27, *307*

Fehr, F. S., 74, *317*
Feldman, R. S., *323*
Ficks, L., 67, *322*
Figge, U. L., 12, *308*
Fillenbaum, S., 135, *308*
Fillmore, C. J., 55, 230, *308*
Fischer, H., *308*
Fishman, J. A., *308*
Flanagan, J. L., 38, 69, *308*
Flavell, J. H., *308*
Flesch, R., 94, *308*
Flores d'Arcais, G. B., 268, *308*
Fodor, J. A., 214, *308*
Ford, M., *304*
Forschhammer, E., 251, *308*
Forsyth, D. F., 122, *307*
Foster, G. *307*
Fraisse, P., *301*
Franks, J. J., 267, *302, 303*
Fraser, C., *304*
Freeman, R. B., 74, 238, *308*
French, D., 294, *308*
French, N. R., 75, 76, *308*
Freytag-Loeringhoff, B., 7, *308*
Friedman, E. A., 106, *319*
Fries, H. S., 195, *326*
Frisch, K. v., 26, 27, *308*

Gabelentz, G. v.d., 189, *309*
Gademer, H. -G., 138, 159, *309*
Galanter, E., 211, *319*
Galton, F., 114, *309*
Gardner, B. T., 28, 250, *309*
Gardner, R. A., 28, 250, *309*
Garfinkel, H., 60, 141, *309*
Garrett, M., 214, *309*
Gehlen, A., 146, *309*
Geller, J., 30, 200, 265, 328
Gifford, W. W., *309*
Gilman, A., 281, *304*
Gipper, H., 228, 296, *309*
Glanzer, M., 206, *309*

Glazer, N., *322*
Glinz, H., 8, 47, *309*
Goldman-Eisler, F., 210, *309*
Goldstein, K., *309*
Goodall, J., 28, *310*
Goodnow, J. J., 259, *303*
Goss, A. E., *310*
Granit, R., *310*
Gray, J., 231, *303*
Greenberg, J. H., 28, *310*
Greenfield, P. M., 262, *310*
Groeben, N., 94, *310*
Gumperz, J. J., *310*

Habermas, J., 151, *310*
Halle, M., 39, 44, 74, 209, *310, 313*
Hare, R. D., 176, *310*
Harlow, H. F., *310*
Harris, K. S., 36, 69, *316*
Havelka, J., 178, *315*
Hayakawa, S. I., 8, *310*
Hebb, D. O., *310*
Heidegger, M., 249, *310*
Heider, F., 97, *310*
Heise, G. A., 85, 86, *319*
Henle, P., *311*
Henley, N. M., 227, *311*
Herdan, G., 14, 91, *311*
Herder, J. G., 25, *311*
Herrmann, T., 204, 277, *311*
Herrnstein, R. J., 234, *304*
Hobbes, T., *311*
Hockett, C. F., *311*
Höpp, G., 9, 24, 249, 265, *311*
Hörmann, H., 4, 19, 42, 49, 54, 55, 60, 150, 152, 162, 182, 200, 203, 231, 238, 249, 266, 295, *307, 311*
Horowitz, A., 195, *304*
Hofstätter, P. R., *311*
Hoijer, H., 286, *311*
Holenstein, E., 14, *311*
Holland, M. K., 190, *311*
Holyoak, K. J., 229, *311*
Howes, D. H., 91, *311, 312*
Hull, C.L., 164, *311*
Humboldt, W. v., 2, 12, 13, 156, 187, 193, 250, 271, 272, *312*
Humphrey, G., 154, *312*
Husserl, E., 24, 150, *312*
Huttenlocher, J., *312*
Huxley, A., 272, *312*
Hymes, D., 151, *312*

Inhelder, B., *310*
Ipsen, G., 127, *312*
Irwin, R. J., *312*
Isard, S., *319*

Jakabovits, L. A., 177, 178, *312*
Jakobson, R., 12, 14, 39, 44, *312, 313*
Jenkins, J. J., 121, 123, 129, *313*
Jenkins, P. M., *313*
Jespersen, O., *313*
Johnson, N. F., 46, 221, 222, 223, 224, *313*
Johnson, R. C., 278, *313*
Johnson W., *313*
Jörg, S., 270, *313*
Jorgensen, C. C., 229, *313*
Jung, C. G., *313*

Kaeding, F. W., 88, *314*
Kainz, F., *314*
Kaminski, G., 167, *314*
Kanungo, R., *314*
Kaplan, B., 191, 192, 193, *327*
Kaplan, E., *327*
Kasschau, R. A., 177, *314*
Katz, J. J., 52, 126, *314*
Kelchner, M., 91, *314*
Keller, H., 257, *314*
Kendall, M. G., 99, *314*
Kent, H. G., 117, *314*
Kintsch, W., 179, 229, *313, 314*
Kirchhoff, R., 25, *314*
Kjeldergaard, P. M., *305*
Kleist, H. v., 287, *314*
Kluckhohn, C., *314*
Koch, S., *314*
Köhler, W., 190, 298, *314*
Korzybski, A., *314, 315*
Kroeber, A. L., *315*
Küpfmüller, K., *315*
Kushnir, S., 179, *317*

Ladefoged, P., 98, 208, *315*
Laffal, J., *315*
Laguna, G. A. de, *315*
Lambert, W. E., 177, 178, *315*
Lane, H., 71, 72, *315*
Langer, J., 30, 94, *315*
Langer, S. K., 10, 11, 29, 30, 73, 255, *315*
Lantz, D. L., 291, 295, *315*
Lashley, K. S., 201, 212, *315*
Lazarus, G., 231, *311*
Lazarus, H., 231, *311*
Leibniz, G. E., *315*
Leighton, D., *314*
Leisi, E., 142, 145, 275, *316*
Lenneberg, E. H., 1, 73, 236, 238, 287, 288, 290, 291, 292, 294, *304, 316*
Leontier, A. N., 10, 74, *316*
Levelt, W. J. M., 233, 236, *316*
Lewandowski, T., 46, *316*
Lewis, M. M., 245, 254, 255, *316*
Liberman, A. M., 36, 69, *316, 317*

Lichten, W., 85, 86, *319*
Licklider, J. C. R., *317*
Lindauer, M., 27, *317*
Little, K. B., 196, *303*
Locke, J. L., 74, *317*
Lockhart, R. S., 269, *306*
Lohmann, J., 12, 16, *317*
Longacre, R. E., 295, 296, *317*
Lorenz, K., *317*
Lorge, I., 88, *326*
Lounsbury, F. G., 18, 279, *317*
Lowell, F., 123, *328*
Lüdtke, H., 44, 45, 46, *317*
Luria, A. R., 212, 250, 251, 252, *317*
Lysne, D. E., 121, *326*

Mackay, D. M., 30, 31, 161, *317*
MacNamara, J., 179, 248, *317*
MacNeilage, P. F., 36, 69, *316*
Maday, B. C., *326*
Malinowski, B., *317*
Malmberg, B., 14, 23, 39, 42, 43, 243, *317*
Maltzman, I., 195, *318*
Marbe, K., 114, 116, *326*
Marks, L. E., 206, *318*
Marshall, G. R., *318*
Marshall, J. C., 138, *318*
Martin, J. G., 211, *318*
Martinet, A., 13, 38, 39, *318*
Massaro, D. W., 74, *318*
McCarthy, D., *318*
McCarrell, N. S., 267, *302*
McKean, K., *318*
McNeill, D., 125, 225, 261, *318*
Mehler, J., *318*
Mehrabian, A., 265, *318*
Meier, H., 88, 89, 91, 261, *318*
Menyuk, P., *318*
Merleau-Ponty, M., 15, 24, *318*
Meseck, O. R., 118, 120, 129, 130, *313, 323*
Meumann, E., *318*
Meyer-Eppler, W., *318*
Miller, G. A., 44, 76, 77, 79, 82, 85, 86, 93, 104, 105, 106, 135, 202, 203, 206, 211, 217, 218, 219, 237, 294, *318, 319*
Mistler-Lachmann, J. L., 269, *319*
Moles, A. A., 60, 67, *319*
Möller, A., 76, *305*
Morris, C. W., 149, 161, *319, 320*
Morrisett, L., 195, *318*
Morton, J., 107, *320*
Moser, H., *320*
Mowrer, O. H., *320*
Muckler, F. A., 105, *301*
Müller, A. L., 287, *320*
Musgrave, B. S., *306*
Muus, R., 122, *307*

Neisser, U., 45, 74, *320*
Nelson, K., 258, 262, *320*
Neubert, A., 142, *320*
Newman, S., 194, *320*
Nicely, P. E., *319*
Nitsch, K., 267, *302*
Norman, D. A., 269, *320*
Nuttall, R., 196, *304*

O'Connell, D. C., *320*
O'Connor, M., *322*
Öhman, S., *320*
Ogden, C. K., 8, 148, *320*
Oldfield, R. C., *320*
Oléron, P., *301, 320*
Olson, D. R., 266, *320*
Osgood, C. E., 17, 18, 164, 170, 174, 177, 180, 181, 198, 293, *320, 321*

Paivio, A., 229, *321*
Palermo, D. S., 122, *321*
Paul, H., *321*
Pavlov, I. P., 10, *321*
Peëjak, V., 198, *321*
Peirce, C. S., 23, 321
Penfield, W., *321*
Perfetti, C. A., *321*
Piaget, J., *301, 321*
Pick, A., *321*
Pickett, J. M., *322*
Ploog, D., 29, *321*
Pollack, I., 67, 87, 106, *322, 325*
Pollio, H. R., *322*
Portnoy, S., *323*
Porzig, W., 128, *322*
Postman, L., *319*
Premack, D., 28, *322*
Pribram, K. H., 211, *319*
Putnam, H., 52, *322*

Quillian, M. R., 226, 322

Rapaport, D., 182, *322*
Razran, G., *322*
Reese, H. W., 229, *322*
Reuck, A. V. S. de, *322*
Révész, G., 7, 25, 26, *322*
Richards, I. A., 8, 148, *320*
Riegel, K., 123, *322*
Riegel, M., 123, *322*
Riesman, D., *322*
Roberts, J. M., 287, 288, 292, *316*
Romney, A. K., 135, *322*
Rosanoff, A. J., 117, *314*
Rosch-Heider, E., 228, *322*
Rosenberg, S., 207, *322*

Rosenblith, W. A., 66, 67, 68, *323*
Rosenzweig, M. R., 121, 129, *323*
Rubenstein, H., 105, *323*
Rubionow, S., 30, 200, 265, *328*
Russell, W. A., 118, 120, 129, 130, *313, 323*

Sachs, J., 268, 323
Salzinger, K., *323*
Saltzman, E., 262, *310*
Sapir, E., 29, 194, 273, *323*
Saporta, S., 72, 124, *323, 324*
Saussure, F. de, 14, 15, 16, 112, *324*
Schank, R. C., 168, *324*
Schlesinger, I. M., 203, 249, *324*
Schlosberg, H., 117, *328*
Schmetterer, L., 57, *324*
Schmitt, A., *324*
Schnelle, H., 39, *324*
Schönbach, P., 278, *324*
Schulz, R. W., *328*
Schulz von Thun, F., 30, 94, *315*
Searle, J. R., 151, *324*
Sebeok, T. A., *324*
Segerstedt, T. T., *324*
Seiler, H., 273, *324*
Selfridge, J. A., 104, 105, *319*
Shannon, C. E., 101, *324*
Shipinowa, Y., *324*
Shipley, W. C., *324*
Shlien, J., 280, 281, *324*
Skinner, B. F., 154, *324*
Slobin, D., 282, *324*
Smirnov, A. A., 74, *325*
Sokolov, A. N., 74, *325*
Sommerfelt, A., 13, *325*
Staats, A. W., *325*
Staats, C. K., *325*
Stefflre, V., 291, 295, *315*
Steger, H., 297, *325*
Steinberg, D. D., *325*
Steinberg, J. C., 75, 76, *308*
Steinbuch, K., 34, 35, 102, *325*
Steinthal, H., 9, *325*
Stenzel, J., 11, 113, 140, 144, 150, 169, 185, 193, *325*
Stern, C., *325*
Stern, W., *325*
Stevens, K. N., 74, 209, *310*
Stevens, S. S., *325*
Stevenson, C. L., *325*
Straus, S., *312*
Studdert-Kennedy, M., 73, *325*
Stumpf, C., 36, *325*
Sumby, W. H., 106, *325*
Surina, M., *324*
Szalay, L. B., 121, *325, 326*

Taylor, I. K., 198, *326*
Taylor, W. L., *326*
Terbuyken, G., 266, *311*
Teuber, H. L., 254, *326*
Thorndike, E. L., 1, 88, *326*
Thumb, A., 114, 116, *326*
Tichomirow, O. K., 155, *326*
Tinbergen, N., *326*
Titchener, E. B., 144, *326*
Tolman, E. C., *326*
Toulmin, St., 4, *326*
Trautscholdt, M., 114, *326*
Treisman, A. M., *326*
Trier, J., 127, *326*
Trubetzkoy, N., 40, *326*
Tsuru, S., 195, *326*

Uexküll, J. v., 3, *326*
Ullmann, S., *326*
Urban, W. M., *327*

Van Lancker, D., 108, 266, *327*
Varon, E., 194, *302*
Vasta, R., 233, 236, *327*
Vigotsky, L. S., 252, 253, *327*

Wallach, M., 106, *327*
Watson, J. B., 145, *327*
Weaver, W., 101, *324*
Wegener, P., *327*
Weinreich, U., 179, *327*
Weir, R. H., *327*

Weisgerber, L., 47, 144, 272, 274, 275, 289, *327*
Weiss, J. H., 197, 198, *327*
Weizsäcker, C. F. v., 57, 58, 59, 60, 143, 248, *327*
Werner, H., 191, 192, 193, *327*
Wertheimer, M., *327*
Wettler, M., 203, *327*
Whitehurst, G. J., 233, 236, *327*
Whitmarsh, G. A., 166, *303*
Whorf, B. L., 285, *328*
Wiener, M., 30, 200, 265, *328*
Wilde, K., 197, *328*
Williams, A. C., 105, *301*
Windle, C., 121, *326*
Wissemann, H., 188, *328*
Wittgenstein, L., 24, 142, 150, 288, 265, 296, *328*
Wollsey, C. N., *310*
Woodrow, H., 123, *328*
Woodworth, R. S., 117, *328*
Wreschner, A., 121, 328
Wundt, W., 12, *328*

Yavuz, H. S., *328*
Yeager, H. C., *302*
Yelen, D. R., *328*
Yudovich, F. I., 250, 251, *317*

Zazzo, R., 251, *328*
Zemanek, H., 101, *328*
Zipf, G. K., 88, *328*

Subject Index

Acoustic analysis of speech sounds, 35
Acoustic phase of speech event, 34
Acquired similarity versus acquired distinctiveness, 70–71, 74
Acquired transitional probabilities, retention of, 105
Action, grammar of, 261
Activity in Osgood's semantic differential, 173
Adequatio rei et intellectus, 139
Age differences, verbal usage and, 122–123
Allomorph, 30, 41
American Indian languages, SAE and, comparison of, 284–287
American Sign Language, Washoe the chimpanzee and, 250–251
Amplitude, discriminatory capacity for, 66–67
Analysis-by-synthesis process, speech perception as, 209
Animals, language of, 25
Anticipation, verbal usage and, 124–125
Apel, 137, 142
Aphasia
  functional disturbances in, 254
  Jakobson on, 123
  theory of, 92
Appeal as function of language, 22
Approximation, order of, *see* Order of approximation
Approximation to natural language, 101
Aristotelian concept of meaning, 138
Articulation
  dual, in language, 39–40
  of verbal and nonverbal events, 200
Articulatory phase of speech event, 34
Association
  behaviorist views of, 154
  concept of, Galton on, 113–114
  laws of, 113
  linguistic unit and, 111
  norms of, 116
  origin of, 113
Association experiments, 112–113, 114–123
  of Deese, 130–135

personality-specific speech habits and, 123–124
  S-R sequence in, 115
Association theory, Werner's theory and, 192–193
Associationist model of grammar, inadequacies of, 201–202
Associations, formation of, 153
Associative and sequential approach, distinction between, 111
Associative behavior in children, 122–123
Attention-directing device, formclass of word as, 275–276
Auditory phase of speech event, 34

Bees, language of, 26–27
Behavior
  of animals, language and, 25
  as interaction of life space and spontaneity, 5
  meaning as, 150
  norms of association and, 116–117
  perception and, 5
  purposive, signs and, 10
  symbolic, origin of language and, 29–30
  verbal, Skinner's theory of, 154–157
Behaviorism, psycholinguistics and, 145
Behaviorist view of meaning, 154
Bilingualism, 177–179
Binary opposition, principle of, 44
Biologic basis of language, 237–238
  language universals and, 294
Bipolar relationship, meaning as, 138
Bit as measuring unit for information, 61–62
Bloomfield
  definition of meaning of, 162
  diagram of speech event of, 247–248
  model of speech act of, 260
Bousfield
  on meaning response, 165–167
  model of, and Osgood's model, differences between, 170, 171

Brain wave pattern in infants, development of speech and, 74
Braine, experiments on children's grammar by, 238–240
Broadbent
   on channel capacity, 80
   on definition of logogens, 107
Brown, Roger, studies of Adam and Sarah by, 241–242
Brown and Bellugi, studies of children's grammar by, 240–241
Brown and McNeill on tip-of-the-tongue phenomena, 225–226
Brown-Lenneberg study on codability, retention, and recognition, 290–291
Bühler
   on concept of phoneme, 40, 41
   on distinction between symbol, symptom, and signal, 42
   on language of bees, 28
   organon model of, 21–24, 60, 271
      deficiencies of, 24
      sign quality and, 23–24

Carroll
   on definition of language, 17
   on semantic space, 179
Cassirer on reduplication, 189
Categories, semantic, 227–228
Channel capacity
   concept of, 75, 88
   experiments on, 80–82
   selection mechanism in, 81–82
Child psychology, Langer on, 73
Child's grammar, Braine's experiments on, 238–240
Child's speech, studies of, 240–246
Children
   associative behavior in, 122–123
   concept formation in, 257–259
Chimpanzees, communication system of, 28–29
Chomsky
   on behaviorism in psycholinguistics, 157–159
   on generative grammar, 48
   on surface and deep structures, 50
Clark on meaning as association, 126
Classical learning theory, language acquisition and, 234
Closure, discrimination of phonemes and, 96
Clustering, experiments on, 129
Codability, concept of, 290–291
Code
   as analysis of linguistic event, 18
   information transmission and, 59–60
Coding, comprehension and, 269–270

Coding systems, acquisition of, 97
Cognitive and emotional maps of meaning, 181–187
Cognitive development, influence of language on, 252
Coleman, studies of, on order of approximation, 202–204
Color coding, Whorf hypothesis and, 288–292
Color recognition, experiments on, 290–291
Communication channel, 69
Communication intentions, 30–31
Communication system of chimpanzees, 28–29
Communicative competence, 151
Competence
   communicative, 151
   grammatical, 151
   performance and, in generative grammar, 48–49
Compound bilingualism, 177, 178
Comprehension
   coding and, 269–270
   as constructive process, 267–268
   Deese on, 161–162
   levels of, 269–270
Concept, nature of, 257
Concept formation
   in children, 257–259
   mediation theories and, 167–168
Conditioning of verbal behavior, 157
Conditioning theory of meaning, 153–154, 182
   as basis for origin of sign, 146
   bilingualism and, 177–179
Connotation and denotation, distinction between, 180, 181
Consonant-vowel sequences, spectrograms of, 72
Consonants, formants in, 36
Constancies, 259
Constancy phenomenon, morphemes and phonemes and, 41
Contact-sound, speech as, 7
Content words, 206–207
Coordinate bilingualism, 177, 178

Decoding processes of sentence generation, 222; see also Encoding
Deep structure
   in Porzig field, 128
   surface structure and
      Chomsky on, 50
      psychological reality and, 215–217
Deese
   association experiments of, 130–135
   on comprehension, 161–162
   factorial structures of, 134–135
   on understanding, 183

Denotation, 168
  connotation and, distinction between, 180,
    181
Determining tendency, concept of, 212
Developmental psychology of language ac-
  quisition, 233-263
Diachronic linguistics, 15
Dialects in language of bees, 26-27
Disposition, meaning as, 160-161
Distinctive feature, definition of, 42
Dual articulation in language, 39-40
Dual-coding hypothesis of Pavio, 229-230
Duration of sound, 35
  phoneme as, 42
Durkheim on language, 13
Dyadic model of meaning, 143-144
Dyadic relationship, meaning as, 138

Egocentric speech, Piaget on, 252-253
Emotion and meaning, 168-169
Emotional and cognitive maps of meaning,
  181-187
Emotional factor in mediation model, 165, 168
Encoding
  decoding and
    concepts of, 18
    as processes of translation, 33
    as series of decisions, 19
    as transformations, 65
  levels of, 211
Energeia, language as, 13, 193
Environment, organism and, 4-5, 10
Epstein on syntactical structure's effects on
  learning and retention, 204-206
Ertel and Dorst, expressive sound symbolism
  and, 197-198
Ertel's experiments in psychophonetics,
  199-200
Evaluation as factor in Osgood's semantic dif-
  ferential, 173
Ewe language of Africa, high- and low-tone
  forms in, 189
Expression as function of language, 22
Expressive sound symbolism, Ertel and Dorst
  on, 197-198

Field of force for speech events, 7, 8
Fillmore on predicate/argument structure, 230
Formant, definition of, 35
Formants in vowels, 35-36
Formclass of word as attention-directing de-
  vice, 275-276
Forms of address, psycholinguistics and,
  281-282
Frequency
  of association, 115, 116

in sound, 35
  discriminatory capacity for, 66-67
Frequency counts of linguistic units, 88-89
Frequency indices, Thorndike and Lorge's,
  93
Frequency spectra of language
  comparison of, 91
  experiments on, 75-76
Frisch on language of bees, 26-27
Function words, 206-207

Galton on concept of association, 113-114
Gardner and Gardner on chimpanzee com-
  munication, 28-29
General Semantics, 296-299
Generative grammar, 47-48, 203
  as phrase-structure grammar with trans-
    formational component, 51
Generative linguistics
  analysis of sentence within framework of,
    51
  psychological reality and, 214
Generative semantics, 216
German language, frequencies of words in, 88
Gestalt principle of organization, 194
Gestalt psychology, psycholinguistics and,
  145
Glanzer on function and content words, 206-
  207
Glinz on grammar, 47
Goldman-Eisler study of pauses, 210
Goldstein on theory of aphasia, 92, 254
Grammar, 45
  of action, 261
  definition of, 46-47, 201
  psychological reality of, 201-232
  sentence and, 46-47
Grammar plan, 213
Grammatical competence, 151
Grammaticality, concept of, 203-204
Greenfield on nonverbal behavior in children,
  262
Group factors in verbal usage, 119-121
'Group think', 121

Halle, 43, 44
Halle-Stevens theory of analysis-by-
  synthesis process of speech
  production, 209-210
Hayakawa on sound as social contact, 8
Hierarchical structures for ordering semantic
  features, 226-227
Historical linguistics, 12-13
Hopi, plurals and cardinals in, 285-286
Hörmann on sense constancy, 152
Hull on pure stimulus acts, 164-165

Humboldt
    on fundamental nature of language, 2
    on language and world view, 270–271
    on onomatopoeia and sound symbolism,
        188
    on relationship between speech sound and
        object, 186–187
    on semantic field, 127
    versus Skinner, 156
    on transformation of world into language,
        12
    on world view and language, 13
Husserl, 13, 14

Imagery, language process and, 229–230
Imitation
    in language acquisition, 233–236
    Lewis on, 254–255
Implicit response, Watson on, 160
Information
    bit as measuring unit for, 61–62
    concept of, 57–58
    Shannon's concept of, 57
Information content, frequency and probabil-
        ity and, 85
Information loss, variables of, 87–88
Information theory
    mathematical presentation of, 63–64
    psycholinguistics and, 65
    truth-function of language and, 140
Information transmission, theory of, 59
    code and, 59–60
Information value, uncertainty and, 58–59, 61
'Inner speech', Vigotsky on, 253–254
Intensity of sound, 35
    discrimination of, 68
    phoneme as, 42
Intentions of speaker, language acquisition
        and, 249
Intonation in languages, 266

Jakobson, Roman, 42
    on aphasia, 123
    on linguistic perception, 69
Jakobson-Fant-Halle's analytic transcription
        of phonemes of English, 43
Johnson, N. F., sentence processing theory
        of, 221–224
Joint probabilities, 100–101
    of elements of sentence, 99
Jörg on levels of comprehension, 270
Jung, word association experiments of, 123–
        124

Kaeding on frequency of words used in En-
        glish, 93

Kant on language and world view, 271
Katz and Fodor, semantic theory of, 52–54
Keller, Helen, language acquisition by, 254–
        257
Kent-Rosanoff norms, 129
Kinship terminology, 279–281
Knowing, concept of, 182–183
Köhler's experiment on "maluma" and
        "takete", 190–193
Korzybski, General Semantics and, 298

LAD (Language Acquisition Device), 236–
        238
Lambert and Jakobovits on semantic satia-
        tion, 176
Langer, Suzanne
    on child psychology, 73
    on symbolic value of words, 29–30
Language
    action and, Wittgenstein on, 150
    of animals, 25
    of bees, 26–27
    Carroll on definition of, 17
    cognitive development and, 252
    as energeia, 13, 193
    Humboldt on
        fundamental nature of, 2
        inner form of, 272
        world view and, 13
    laws of nature and, 13
    Markov model of, 202
    meta-language and, 140–141
    natural, approximation to, 101
    origin of, symbolic behavior and, 29–30
    philosophy and, 137
    presence of, in man, 1–2
    probabilistic structure of, 98
    probability profile of, 88
    as product of social field, 11
    as response, 6–7
    sign as elementary unit of, 15
    social field and, 7
    as social phenomenon, Durkheim on, 13
    as specifically human possession, 1
    as stimulus-response events, 5–7
    as system of signs, 9–10
    thought and, 11
    transformation of experience into concepts
        as motive of, 11
    truth-function of, 137–140
    at word level, Markov model of, 207–208
    world view and, Humboldt on, 13
Language acquisition
    classical learning theory on, 234
    developmental psychology of, 233–263
    imitation in, 233–236
    intentions of speaker and, 249

Language acquisition (*cont'd*)
  Skinner on, 234–235
  strategies in, 262–263
  Thorndike on, 234–235
  total situation and, 250–252
Language Acquisition Device (LAD), 236–238
Language comprehension, world view and, 265–300
Language-game of Wittgenstein, 142, 150
Language process, imagery and, 229–230
Language universals, 293–294
Languages, biological component of, 237–238
Langue and *parole*, distinction between, 14–15
Lashley, reflex chain theory and, 211–212
Learning in Skinner's theory of verbal behavior, 156; *see also* Retention
Leibniz on original language of mankind, 186
Lenneberg and Roberts on Whorf's hypothesis, 287–288
Lewis on imitation, 254–255
Lexical field, Trier's concept of, 127–128
Lexically restricted spectra, stress and, 91
Lexicon
  ambiguity about nature of, 135
  dimensions of, 54
  structure of, 53–54
Liberman's motor theory of speech perception, 69, 71–74, 209
Life force and life space, relationship between, 3
Linguistic determinism, 277–278
  religion and, 279
  Whorf's principle of, 283
Linguistic event(s)
  code as analysis of, 18
  Markov process and, 99
  redundancies as, 99–100
Linguistic evolution, stages of, 7–9
Linguistic expression, structure of, human perception and, 55–56
Linguistic hypostatizing, 275
Linguistic potential, social class and, 277
Linguistic relativity
  linguistic determinism and, 277–278
  Whorf's principle of, 283
Linguistic unit(s)
  association and, 111
  concept of, 57
  frequency counts of, 88–89
Linguistics
  development of, 12–17
  psycholinguistics and, 17–19
  as science of language, 17
Listener and speaker, 7–9, 18
Listening event, description of, 34
Logarithmus dualis, 62

Logogens, definition of, 107
Logos, concept of, 137–138

MacKay on definition of information, 161
MacNamara's theory of language acquisition, 249, 262, 265
  one-word sentences and, 261
"Maluma" and "takete", experiments on, 190–193
Marbe's law, 115, 116
Markov model of language, 202
  concept of transitional probabilities in, 207
Markov process, linguistic events and, 99
Masking in experiments on speech perception, 78, 79
Meaning
  arbitrariness of, 185
  Aristotelian concept of, 138
  as association, Clark on, 126
  as behavior, 150
  behaviorist view of, 154
  as bipolar relationship, 138
  Bloomfield's definition of, 162
  concept of, psycholinguistics and, 137
  conditioning theories of, 153–154
  conditioning theory and, 182
  as context, 147–148
  as disposition, 160–161
  emotional and cognitive maps of, 181–187
  'mediating sphere' of, 144
  mediational theories of, 162–164
  Osgood's model and Bloomfield's model of, differences between, 171
  as response, 159–160
  S-R model of, 182
  situational determinants of, 266–267
  speech perception and, 6
Meaning-oriented semantic versus syntax-oriented grammar, 52
Meaningful material, retention of, 103
Meaningful response, Bousfield on, 165–167
Meaningless and meaningful utterance, difference between, 103
'Mediating sphere', 144
Mediation, mechanism of, 164
Mediation theory(ies), 162–164
  acquisition of meaning and, 167
  concept formation and, 167–168
  in psychology, 165
Meier's frequency spectra, 91
Meta-language and language, 140–141
Miller
  on concept of transformation, 217–218
  on psychological theory of retention, 219
Miller and Selfridge, 283
  on order of approximation and retention, 202

Monemes, 38
Morpheme(s), 40
   constancy phenomenon and, 41
   definition of, 38–39, 44
   phoneme and, boundary between, 186
   syllable and, 45
Morphology and syntax, 45
Morris
   on meaning as disposition, 160–161
   on scheme of 'semiotic', 148–149
Morton on model of logogens, 107–108
Mother and child, verbal interaction between,
      243
Mowrer's thesis, truth-function of language
      and, 140

Naming, developmentally and sociologically
      determined limitations to, 277
National psychology, 119
Natural language, approximation to, 101
Negation as semantic variable, 218–220
Noise
   definition of, 78
   effect of, on speech perception, 79
Nonverbal behavior in children, Greenfield's
      studies of, 262
Nonverbal communication, 265
Noun, use of, in children's and adults'
      speech, 274

Ogden and Richards, 147–148
Olson's cognitive theory of semantics, 266,
      277
One-word sentences, 260–261
Onomatopoeia
   evolution of, 188–189
   Humboldt on, 187
   sound symbolism and, evolution of speech
      and, 190
Operationalism, pragmatism and, 142–143
Order of approximation
   Coleman's studies on, 202–203
   grammaticalness and, 204
   learning and retention and, 104–105, 202
   at word level, 103
Organism
   definition of, 2–3
   environment and, 4–5, 10
Organon model, see Bühler's organon model
Organs of speech, 34
Osgood
   mediational model of, 168, 169–172
      Bousfield's model and, differences be-
         tween, 170
   semantic differential of, 172–175
   theory of

criticism of, 179–180
phonetic symbolism and, 198
universal sound symbolism and, 198

Paradigmatic associations in adults, 123
Paraphrase, 52–53
Parole and langue, distinction between,
      14–15
Pattern playback, 35
Pauses, 265
   Goldman-Eisler study of, 210
   structuring of sentence by, 215
   verbal planning and, 210–211
Pavio on imagery and language process,
      229–230
Perception
   behavior and, 5
   psychology of, 6
Perfect pitch, 68
Performance and competence in generative
      grammar, 48–49
Personality-specific speech habits, associa-
      tion tests and, 123–124
Philosophy and language, 137
Phoneme(s), 40
   Bühler's concept of, 40, 41
   closure and, 96
   constancy phenomenon and, 41
   definition of, 39, 44
   distinctive feature in, 42–44
   of English, analytic transcription of, 43
   as intensity, pitch, or duration of sound, 42
   morpheme and, boundary between, 186
Phoneme boundaries, discrimination at, 70
Phonetic symbolism, experiments on, 195–
      197
Phonetics, 40
Phonic shape, 39
Phonology, 40
Physiognomic qualities of objects, 191–192
Physiognomy, Werner's concept of, 190–193
Piaget
   on notion of egocentric speech, 252–253
   on sensori-motor period, 246
Pitch of sound, phoneme as, 42
Plan, concept of, 211–213
Plato on truth-function of language, 138, 186
Plurals and cardinals in Hopi, 285–286
Porzig, field concept of, 128–129
Potency as factor in Osgood's semantic dif-
      ferential, 173
Pragmatism, operationalism and, 142–143
Prague Circle, 40, 42
Predicate/argument structure, 230
   sentence retention and, 231
Primary colors, Whorf hypothesis and, 289
Principle of least effort, 90

Probabilistic-associationistic approach to grammar, 202–203
Probabilistic structure of language, 98
Probability in language processes, psychology of language and, 97
Probability structures in fifth-grade children, 106
Propositions, sentence retention and, 231–232
Psychoanalysis, psycholinguistics and, 145
Psycholinguistics
  behaviorism and, 145
    Chomsky on, 157–159
  concept of meaning and, 137
  concept of physiognomy in, 190–193
  concept of plan in, 211–213
  forms of address and, 281–282
  Gestalt psychology and, 145
  information theory and, 65
  linguistics and, 17–19
  morphemes versus syllables and, 45
  psychoanalysis and, 145
  psychology of learning and, 114, 115
  S-R analysis and, 5
  sequential, 111
  Shannon's information concept and, 57
  sound symbolism and, 191
  syntax versus morphology and, 46
  Whorf hypothesis and, 283–291
Psychological reality
  concept of transformation and, 217–221
  surface and deep structure and, 215–217
Psychological theory of retention, 219
Psychology
  developmental, language acquisition and, 233–263
  experimental, use of Thorndike-Lorge frequency scores in, 95
  of learning, psycholinguistics and, 114, 115
  mediational theories in, 165
  of memory, 267
  national, 119
  of perception, 6, 267
Psychophonetics, Ertel's experiments in, 199–200
Pure stimulus acts, Hull's concept of, 164–165

Rank order of frequency, 88–91
Readability of texts, 94–95
Redundancies as linguistic events, 99–100
Redundancy, effect of, on speech perception, 106
Reduplication, Cassirer on, 189
Reflex chain theory, 211–212
Reinforcement, concept of, in Skinner's theory of verbal behavior, 158
Representation as function of language, 22

Representational response, Bousfield's model of, 165–167
Response
  meaning as, 159–160
  speech as, 5
Retention, see also Learning
  Miller's psychological theory of, 219
  syntactical structure's effects on, 204–206
Révész
  on language of animals, 25, 26
  on stages of linguistic evolution, 7–9
Russell and Rosenzweig, association experiments of, 118–120

S-R analysis of speech, 5–7
S-R experiments, Deese's association experiments and, 130–135
S-R model of meaning, 182
S-R sequence in association experiments, 115
SAE (Standard Average European), 284
  American Indian languages and, comparison of, 284–287
Sapir
  on conceptual categories in primitive language, 272–273
  on symbolic value of words, 29–30
Saussure, 143
  on definition of sign, 16
  on distinction between langue and parole, 14–15
  on sign, 23
  on symbols, 111
  on syntagms, 112
Scheme, concept of, 183
Searle on speech acts, 151
Semantic abiguity, 52–53
Semantic anomaly, 52–53
Semantic categories, 227–228
Semantic description, comprehension and, 268–269
Semantic differential, 172–175
  experiments on similarity of meaning and, 175–176
Semantic features of sentence structure, 225–226
  hierarchical structures for ordering of, 226–227
Semantic field, concept of, 127–128
Semantic satiation, 176
Semantic space(s)
  Carroll on, 179
  models of, 174
Semantic structure(s)
  dynamic structures and, 229
  of Katz and Fodor, factorial structures of Deese and, 134–135
  sentence memory and, 231

Semantic theory of Katz and Fodor, 52–54
Semantics
  General, 296–299
  Olson's cognitive theory of, 266
'Semiotic', schema of, 149
Sense constancy, 55, 152
Sensory-motor stage of intelligence, 236–237
Sentence
  analysis of, within framework of generative
      linguistics, 50–51
  definition of, 201
  grammar and, 46–47
  one-word, 260–261
  transitional and joint probabilities of, 99
Sentence generation, decoding processes of,
    222
Sentence processing theory of N. F. Johnson,
    221–224
Sentence structure, semantic features of,
    225–226
Sequential psycholinguistics, 111
Sex differences, verbal usage and, 122–123
Shannon-Wiener measure of information, 64
Shannon's concept of information, 57
Shipley experiments, 162–164
Sign(s)
  Bühler's model and, 23–24
  concept of, 57
  conditioning theory as basis for, 146
  as elementary unit of language, 15
  language as system of, 9–10
  nature of, 22–23
  purposive behavior and, 10
  syntax's rules for combining of, 15
  use of, as specifically human behavior, 149
Signal-to-noise ratio, 80, 85–87
Signifiant, 23, 143
  as one definition of sign, 16
Signifié, 23, 143
  as one definition of sign, 16
Situational determinants of meaning, 266–267
Skinner, 154
  on language acquisition, 234–235
  theory of verbal behavior of, 154–157
  versus Humboldt, 156
Skinner box, 158
Slips of tongue, 212
"Snow" in SAE and Eskimo, 284
Social field as language-forming structure, 7,
    11
Social group, verbal usage and, 121–122
Social psychology, closure and, 96
Sociological structure, kinship terminology
    and, 280–281
Sound
  discrimination of, 66–67
  as social contact, Hayakawa on, 8
  threshold of detectability and, 78

Sound symbolism, 186, 197
  description of, 187–188
  Humboldt on, 187
  universality of, 195
Speaker
  intentions of, language acquisition and, 249
  listener and, 7–9, 18
Spectrograph, 35
Speech
  as contact-sound, 7
  definition of, 2
  evolution of, 190
  organs of, 34
  precondition for emergence of, 4–5
  as response, 5
  S-R analysis of, 5–6
  as stimulus, 5
Speech act
  Bloomfield's model of, 260
  Searle on, 151
Speech articulation to speech perception,
    feedback mechanism from, 71
Speech development in children, brain wave
    pattern and, 74
Speech event(s)
  attempts to define units of, 34
  Bloomfield's diagram of, 247–248
  description of, 34
  field of force for, 7, 8
  hierarchical plan as organizing principle of,
      213
  model of, 33
  processes in categorization of, 36–38
Speech patterns, synthetic, 69–70
Speech perception
  as analysis-by-synthesis process, 209
  classification in, 68, 69
  effect of noise on, 79
  effect of redundancy on, 106
  Liberman's motor theory of, 69, 71–74, 209
  masking in experiments on, 78
  meaning and, 6
  retention in, 82–83
Speech production
  temporal features of, 209–211
  Van Lancker's theory of, 108–109
Speech sounds
  acoustic analysis of, 35
  discrimination of, 67–68
  meaning content of, 186
Staats, A. and C., 175
Standard Average European, see SAE
Stenzel on emotion and meaning, 168–169
Stimulus, speech as, 5
Stimulus and response in Bühler's organon
    model, 22
Stimulus-response events, conceptualization
    of language as, 5–7; see also S-R entries

Strategies in language acquisition, 262–263
Stress, lexically restricted spectra and, 91
Structure, deep and surface, psychological
  reality and, 215–217
Substitution model, difficulties of, 159–160
Surface and deep structure
  in generative grammar, 49–50
  psychological reality and, 215–217
Syllable, morpheme and, 45
Symbol, 4, 147–148
  Saussure on, 111
Symbolic behavior, origin of language and,
  29–30
Symbolic value of words, 29–30
Synchronic linguistics, 15
  linguistic signs and, 16
Syntactical structure, effects of, on learning
  and retention, 204–206
Syntagmatic associations in children, 123
Syntagms, Saussure on, 112
Syntax
  morphology and, 45
  rules for combining of signs and, 15
Syntax-oriented grammar versus meaning-
  oriented semantic, 52

Thorndike-Lorge frequency scores, 93–95
Thorndike on language acquisition, 234–235
Thought and language, 11
Thumb and Marbe, association experiments
  of, 114–116
Tip-of-the-tongue phenomena, 225–226
Total situation, language acquisition and,
  250–252
TOTE unit (test-operate-test-exit), 213
Transformation, concept of, psychological
  reality and, 217–221
Transformational component of generative
  grammar, 49
Transitional probabilities, 100–101
  acquired, retention of, 105
  joint probabilities and, 99
  in Markov model, 207
Translation, encoding and decoding as pro-
  cesses of, 33
Trier's conception of lexical field, 127–128
Truth-function of language, 137–140
Tsuru and Fries, experiments of, using un-
  known second language, 195
TTR (type-token ratio), 92–93
Twins, language acquisition studies of, 251–
  252
Type-token ratio (TTR), 92–93

Understanding, Deese's definition of, 183

Van Lancker's theory of speech production,
  108–109
Verbal and nonverbal events, Ertel's findings
  on, 200
Verbal association in mediational theory, 165
Verbal behavior
  conditioning of, 157
  Skinner's theory of, 154–157
Verbal planning, pauses and, 210–211
Verbal satiation, 176
Verbal usage
  age and sex differences and, 122–123
  anticipation and, 124–125
  group factors in, 119–121
  social group and, 121–122
Vigotsky
  on 'inner speech', 253–254
  on language and cognitive development,
    252–253
Vocabularies, individual, Zipf's law and, 92
Vocal cords, 34
Vowels
  consonants and, categorization of, 37
  formants in, 35–36

Washoe the chimpanzee, language acquisition
  by, 28–29, 250–251
Watson, 145
  on implicit response, 160
  on reflex chain theory, 211–212
Weisgerber, 272–274
Werner's theory of symbol formation, 190–
  193
Whorf hypothesis, 283–291
  color coding and, 288–292
  Lenneberg and Roberts on, 287–288
Whorf's principle of linguistic relativity, 283
Whorf's procedures, objections to, 294–296
Wittgenstein on notion of language-game, 142,
  150, 296
Word, definition of, 45–46
Word-association experiments, 112–113
  clustering experiments and, 129
  in German, French, and English, 118–120
  of Jung, 123–124
World view
  Humboldt on, 13
  Kant on, 271
  language comprehension and, 265–300
Würzburg School's concept of determining
  tendency, 212

Zipf on human behavior, 90
Zipf's law, individual vocabularies and, 91–92
Zipf's rank order of frequency, 88–91